Forensic Approaches to Buried Remains

Forensic Approaches to Buried Remains

John Hunter

MFL (Manlove Forensics Limited),
Wantage, Oxfordshire, UK
University of Birmingham, Birmingham, UK

Barrie Simpson

MFL (Manlove Forensics Limited),
Wantage, Oxfordshire, UK

Caroline Sturdy Colls

MFL (Manlove Forensics Limited), Wantage, Oxfordshire, UK
Staffordshire University, Stoke-on-Trent, Staffordshire, UK

WILEY Blackwell

Library of Congress Cataloging-in-Publication Data

Hunter, John.
　　Forensic approaches to buried remains / John Hunter, Barrie Simpson and Caroline Sturdy Colls.
　　　　pages cm
　　Includes bibliographical references and index.
　　ISBN 978-0-470-66630-2 (cloth) – ISBN 978-0-470-66629-6 (pbk.)　　1. Forensic sciences.
2. Forensic anthropology.　3. Criminal investigation.　I. Title.
　　HV8073.H8936 2014
　　363.25–dc23
　　　　　　　　　　　　　　　　　　　　　　　　　　　　　　　　　2013015040

A catalogue record for this book is available from the British Library.

Set in 10/12pt Times by Aptara Inc., New Delhi, India
Printed and bound in Singapore by Markono Print Media Pte Ltd

1　2013

Contents

List of figures

Series foreword

Essentials of forensic science

The world of forensic science is changing at a very fast pace in terms of the provision of forensic science services, the development of technologies and knowledge and the interpretation of analytical and other data as it is applied within forensic practice. Practicing forensic scientists are constantly striving to deliver the very best for the judicial process and as such need a reliable and robust knowledge base within their diverse disciplines. It is hoped that this book series will provide a resource by which such knowledge can be underpinned for both students and practitioners of forensic science alike.

It is the objective of this book series to provide a valuable resource for forensic science practitioners, educators and others in that regard. The books developed and published within this series come from some of the leading researchers and practitioners in their fields and will provide essential and relevant information to the reader.

Professor Niamh Nic Daéid
Series Editor

Preface and acknowledgements

Forensic archaeology is no longer new and this book follows from two previous books by this co-author in that it attempts to be more evaluative than prescriptive in its content, resting on some 25 years' experience of working with police forces and other law enforcement agencies in finding and recovering buried bodies. The first two books (Hunter *et al.* 1996; Hunter and Cox 2005) were very much mission-based in a subject that was still a relatively novel area. This book, we anticipate, moves the subject a step further: it demonstrates that theory and practice are not always compatible; that it is rarely a perfect world, and that there are inevitably political, processual and contextual external forces that an objective textbook can rarely take into account. It seemed appropriate that after 25 years of experience there was much that might be set out for the benefit of future workers in the field, even if some of the comments might not be universally popular. Forensic archaeology has three masters: the academic world in which the rigours of the subject require credibility; the standards of a professional archaeological community as laid down by the Institute for Archaeologists (IfA); and the legal obligations that are tied into the complexities and processes of any crime scene operation and court room appearance. They are not always happy bedfellows. In fact, in the wider context of forensic investigation, the subject is not longer really about archaeology at all, although archaeology remains its theoretical core. Moreover, in 25 years of practice the forensic world has moved on, the role (and definition) of the 'expert' has changed significantly, controls are more rigid, and the range and types of evidence have expanded.

In pulling the various strands of this book together I have been aided immeasurably by my co-authors Barrie Simpson and Caroline Sturdy Colls; all three of us have different backgrounds and experiences and we felt that the volume would be more balanced and informative as a result. Time will tell. The first of the eight chapters is very much an introduction: it provides a broad overview of the subject area and will be particularly suited to students or the general reader interested in seeing the nature and breadth of the subject, and perhaps pursuing elements of it. The subsequent three chapters (Chapters 2–4) consider search theory (mapping, GIS and remote sensing), search application (geophysics, cadaver dogs, mechanical excavation and water search) and search design (boundaries, landscape interrogation and probabilities) respectively. Chapter 5 explores the less well-trodden route of longer-term 'no-body' investigations and the effects of both natural and cultural forces over time. This is also extended to urban environments (planning and building controls) as well as burials grounds and landfill sites. Chapter 6 (Stratification and Destruction) and Chapter 7 (Recovery, Sampling and Dating) are focused on recovery once the body has been located. The former includes fire scenes, formal exhumations and record systems, and the latter sieving, taphonomy, anthropology and scavenging. Finally, Chapter 8 reviews mass graves, not so much from a technical, practical perspective, but from the point of view of social history, and from the need to learn from previous experiences, notably the Holocaust.

The diversity of themes and interests covered by the book required us to seek external support and advice to ensure accuracy of content. Not least here was generous advice given by Colin Hope (National Search Advisor) who kindly commented on various search chapters, Cecily Cropper (formerly of EULEX) on various aspects including mass graves, Dave Cowley (RCAHMS) on remote prospection, Dr Dave Lucy (University of Lancaster) on statistics and probabilities, Dr Lucina Hackman (University of Dundee) on anthropology, and Dr Richard Wright (mass graves). We are indebted to their advice, and also to Dr John Manlove, Kathy Manlove, Dr Anna Sandiford and Sam Pickles (all from MFL Forensics) who advised on the entomology and pollen sections, Mick Swindells (Search Dogs UK) for his advice on the training and deployment of cadaver dogs, and Jon Sterenberg whose knowledge on the use of heavy plant and machinery on excavations is second to none. Brian Kerr (English Heritage) generously provided information on the archaeological work undertaken in the aftermath of the fire at Windsor Castle, and help on particular case studies was given by Julie Roberts (Cellmark), Corrine Duhig and Dr Karl Harrison (Cranfield University). In places we drew heavily on some excellent postgraduate dissertations/theses many of which are wholly underestimated in their forensic value; these included works by Vicki Gray (hair and fibres), Theresa Farren (geographical profiling), Nadine Ross (sieving) and Sara Turton (scavenging). Their efforts have all entered the mix and we trust we have not misquoted or misrepresented them. We have also taxed several of our colleagues about various issues and are grateful for their views and knowledge, notably Paul Cheetham, Rob Janaway, Geoff Knufper, Steve Litherland, Dr Barry Meatyard, staff of the Missing Persons Bureau (NPIA) and Alastair Ruffell.

Acknowledgements and permissions for specific images are noted in the individual captions, but the authors would like to offer specific thanks to Andrew Graham and Graeme Cavers from AOC Scotland for allowing us to use their LiDAR images, to both Stratascan and Malcolm Weale for their geophysics images, to Zoltan Czajlik for his aerial image, and to Duncan Staff for his research and images on the 'Moors Murders'. A number of line drawings have benefitted significantly from the work of Henry Buglass (formerly the University of Birmingham) and Rosie Duncan (Forensic and Crime Science Department, Staffordshire University); we are also grateful to Kevin Colls who supplied a number of images and also assisted in the proof-reading.

Any volume of this type that contains case studies requires permissions from various police forces and Senior Investigating Officers. Many case studies have been 'anonymised' in order to facilitate this and, although some elements of individual cases have been changed in order to prevent recognition, the thrust of the principle or lesson from each one has been left unaltered. Permissions have been gratefully received from the following Police Forces: Cumbria, Gloucestershire, Humberside, Metropolitan, Northern, Nottinghamshire, South Wales, Tayside, Thames Valley, West Mercia, West Midlands and Wiltshire.

Last, but by no means least, we would like to thank Fiona Seymour at Wiley and Sons for her tolerance, patience and understanding during the preparation of this book. We hope she likes the result.

John Hunter
Tysoe, Warwickshire
February 2013

The authors

John Hunter OBE BA PhD FSA MIFA FFSSoc was appointed Professor of Ancient History and Archaeology at the University of Birmingham in 1996. Apart from following an extensive scheme of research excavation and survey in Scotland, he began to develop forensic archaeology in 1988, He is involved operationally throughout the UK, has also worked in Bosnia, Iraq and the Falklands and routinely lectures to police and forensic professionals. He helped found the Forensic Search Advisory Group, was a lead assessor for the CRFP and was primary in setting up the current validation system for forensic archaeology. His publications, including ten books, cover a range of archaeological and forensic topics. He is a Royal Commissioner on the Ancient and Historical Monuments of Scotland, an appointee of the Cathedral Fabrics Commission for England at Worcester Cathedral and sits on several public and editorial committees. In 2011 he was awarded an OBE for services to scholarship.

Barrie Simpson BA MSc MSc MIFA MFSSoc is a former Senior Investigating Officer (SIO) and active forensic practitioner. He has a keen interest in landscape archaeology and holds MSc degrees in both forensic archaeology and forensic and biological anthropology. As an SIO he encouraged their use within the police service and became the Police Liaison with the Forensic Search Advisory Group (FSAG). He is a strong advocate of crime scene analysis and the use of interdisciplinary approaches. On retirement from police service he has worked for many years operationally within the UK, and additionally in the Western Balkans, Iraq, on Ascension Island and Thailand. He has been involved in the development of forensic archaeology, initially as secretary of the Forensic Search Advisory Group and, more recently, as the secretary setting up the current validation system for forensic archaeology within UK.

Caroline Sturdy Colls BA MPhil PhD AIFA is a Lecturer in Forensic Investigation at Staffordshire University, specialising in forensic and conflict archaeology. She is also a consultant forensic archaeologist, working throughout the United Kingdom and is a committee member of the IfA Forensic Archaeology Special Interest Group. Having completed her PhD at the Institute of Archaeology and Antiquity at the University of Birmingham in the area of Holocaust Archaeology she continues to research this area and has undertaken the first archaeological surveys of the former extermination camp at Treblinka (Poland), the sites pertaining to the slave labour programme in Alderney (the Channel Islands), and the former Semlin Judenlager and Anhaltelager (Belgrade, Serbia). Her other research interests lie in the application of forensic archaeological methods to the investigation of cold cases and socio-historic conflicts. She has a number of publications in these areas.

The three authors are consultants with MFL Forensics Ltd based in Wantage, Oxfordshire.

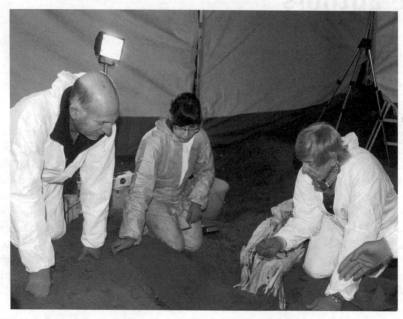

The authors seen here on a potential crime scene: John Hunter (left), Barrie Simpson (right) and Caroline Sturdy Colls (centre).

About the companion website

This book is accompanied by a companion website:

www.wiley.com/go/hunter/forensicremains

The website includes powerpoints of all figures from the book for downloading.

1 An introduction to buried remains

1.1 Questions of time

This is a book that deals specifically with buried remains of forensic interest – that is, remains which are germane to a modern criminal investigation; it is about finding these remains and recovering them. It is a book about clandestine burials and concealment, about what can influence search and recovery processes, and about what matters in a forensic sense. It is not a prescriptive manual or a set of standard operating procedures (SOPs) for the specialists involved. The Senior Investigating Officer (SIO) will not find a useful set of 'tick boxes' that will guarantee a successful enquiry; nor will the Crime Scene Manager (CSM) find a list of actions that a proper investigation ought to undertake. This book tries to examine how different subject areas interact when it comes to investigating the modern buried past. Successful forensic excavation requires awareness of the component evidential elements and what they signify, together with an understanding of formation processes and how to interpret them. Thus, this is a book about questioning, not about giving answers. This first chapter provides a general introduction to the chapters that follow.

Strictly, the word 'archaeology' is a misnomer in a forensic context because the subject of interest, although buried, is not 'ancient', which is the usual definition of the discipline. That said, the phrase 'forensic archaeology' appears to have become well cemented in forensic literature as well as within archaeological circles, and so this is the phrase used throughout this book. In any event, the approaches to studying 'ancient' (archaeological) buried remains and those used to investigate in a modern buried forensic context are largely the same. It matters not whether concealment in the ground occurred yesterday morning or in prehistoric times thousands of years ago. Not only are the processes of finding and recovering evidence from these two chronological extremes much the same, but the methods we use to make sense of that evidence are substantially the same too. It is not really the extent of elapsed time between then and now that is the issue (although it would be incorrect to maintain that it had no effect at all), but the critical difference that lies in the questioning or interrogation of the evidence recovered according to the answers needed.

Take, for example, carbonised grains discovered from a prehistoric hearth: they may tell us about crops grown and thus land use and clearance, while the weeds of cultivation from the same hearth have a direct bearing on harvesting methods and crop processing. Together these prehistoric grains enable us to enquire about a developing farming community and its

Forensic Approaches to Buried Remains, First Edition. John Hunter, Barrie Simpson and Caroline Sturdy Colls.
© 2013 John Wiley & Sons, Ltd. Published 2013 by John Wiley & Sons, Ltd.

impact on the landscape. Grains caught in the trouser turn-ups of a victim buried yesterday will identify particular crops in a specific habitat harvested recently or growing naturally; they enable us to take the enquiry to particular landscape locations at a particular time. The physical evidence is much the same in both instances, but we need to ask different questions because of the different purposes to which the answers will be put. Equally, when a small piece of clothing fabric survives in a prehistoric burial, archaeologists will seek to ascertain what the material was, how it was woven and what dye was used in order to learn more about early textiles and dress. A similar piece of fabric found in a grave caught in a victim's clothes may belong to the offender. The forensic scientist will look to define the fibre mix and colour, the type of garment from which it originated and the commercial outlets from where it might have been purchased. The evidence can lead investigators in many different directions according to the nature of the questions posed. In such cases, elapsed time is not a major factor compared to what can be gleaned from the surviving evidence.

1.2 Questions of interpretation

Remains lying under the ground surface – buildings, pits, walls and so on (including the human dead) – become buried according to a host of different processes and are surrounded by, and integrated with, different layers of earth that relate to their deposition and formation. These layers and their study (stratigraphy) are raw materials to the archaeologist; their analysis is the method by which our archaeological sites and ancient landscapes are excavated and understood; their significance is basic to all archaeological textbooks (Figure 1.1) (e.g. Greene 2002, ch. 3; Carver 2009, ch. 11). The majority of these layers are human-influenced – actions such as building, occupation, fire, demolition or abandonment

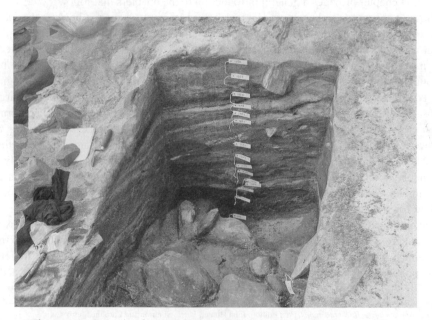

Figure 1.1 Example of an archaeological matrix of layers during excavation.

can all leave archaeological traces in the form of layers of differing magnitude, colour and physical character. Other layers are created by natural processes, for example, silting in river valleys, soil formation over abandoned buildings, sand blow or volcanic activity such as at Pompeii. The two types – anthropogenic and natural – can often occur together (see Case Study 1.1, also Section 6.1).

Take a simple forensic example – a grave that has been dug and left open for a period of time might accumulate a thin layer of silt from wind-blown soil and leaves. Later, when the victim is buried, the grave may become sealed by natural soil formation, hill wash and vegetation. This combination of natural and cultural events, together form a tangible sequence that is revealed in the ground. Archaeologists identify the actions in that sequence by interpreting the layers that reflect them. This is fundamental to field archaeology; the investigation of layers and their relationships enables us to reconstruct what happened in a given place during a past time. The stratigraphic evidence that the archaeologist records is empirical; it makes no difference whether the buried event occurred yesterday or 6,000 years earlier, the same principles apply.

Understanding layers, beyond their physical attributes, is about interpretation; there are no hard and fast rules as to what a particular layer signifies and each archaeologist will have his/her own idea about the significance of deposits (e.g. Case Study 1.2). Archaeologists tend to work in shades of grey rather than in clear black and white (see Section 1.7). They tend to temper their remarks according to the nature of the evidence and hedge their bets accordingly. Understanding layers is as much about interpretation as fact, about probabilities rather than absolute certainties, and this may create tension or conflict in a forensic environment. Archaeologists are trained to have deductive opinions as opposed to fixed assumptions about what buried evidence means; this applies not just to remains that are chronologically distant, but also to those from yesterday. Layers can be defined and recorded quite objectively, and most archaeological organisations have their own process-driven systems that allow this to be carried out (e.g. MoLAS 1994). Relevant pro-formas will require information on soil type, inclusions, colour, texture and so on, but this clinical data is meaningless unless interpretation is derived from it. The data set can always be returned to by future archaeologists. This process can be summed up in the phrase 'preservation by record' used widely in planning circles as a result of mitigating against an archaeological site threatened by building development (PPG 16 1990; PPS 5 2010; DCLG 2012). Once data has been recovered from the ground and recorded in terms of plans, sections, photographs and a written record, those data can always be reviewed. One curious thing about being an archaeologist is that one's interpretations cannot normally be deemed 'right' or 'wrong' and the evidence can be subject to continual reassessment; each interpretation has to be assessed against the data, and some will no doubt be considered more valid than others.

A famous experiment took place in the United States in the 1970s and involved the excavation of an indigenous Indian settlement known as 'Millie's Camp' that had recently been abandoned (Bonnichsen 1973). The archaeologists duly collected the material remains and, on the basis of the character, distribution and location of these remains interpreted what activities had gone on, and where. They were astonished, when confronted with the former inhabitants, just how wrong their interpretations had been. It was a corrective exercise that provided salutary food for thought, given that archaeology traditionally concerns itself with timescales well beyond living memory and contemporary society. But it also emphasises the caution needed in interpreting forensic remains that, like Millie's Camp, are also almost certain to be known to living witnesses. The following two cases illustrate this central issue.

Case Study 1.1

A small boy disappeared in the 1960s (Hunter *et al.* 1996, 54ff). He was subsequently found over 25 years later partly buried at the edge of a wood beside a collapsed dry-stone wall little more than half a kilometre from his house. Archaeologists excavated and recorded the scene, and identified that the wall had collapsed over the body but not before large stones had first been placed on the body in a probable attempt at concealment. The body had not been buried as originally thought by the police, but had been lying on the ground surface where it had become hidden by natural soil formation and organic matter over the intervening years. Moreover, the archaeologists were surprised to find that the skeleton was almost intact and had not been scavenged, even although it had been lying on the surface. As a result of their excavation the archaeologists suggested that the body must have been wrapped (hence the absence of scavenging) and laid on the ground below the wall. Large stones from the wall top had then been placed over the body. At some later point in time the wall collapsed and the boy's remains became further sealed by the wall rubble. The boy's stepfather, when arrested, was unaware of this interpretation, but when eventually charged with the boy's death he confessed to the murder. The confession matched the archaeologists' interpretation step by step. Apart from providing confirmation of the archaeologists' hypothesis, the case also demonstrates further the interaction of cultural and natural formation processes: the wrapping, the laying down of the body and the placement of stones reflect human activity, whereas the subsequent soil development and the collapse of the wall are natural phenomena.

Case Study 1.2

A pit was discovered in the flagged cellar of a house where two persons had gone missing, although their bodies were never found (Hunter *et al.* 1996, 53f). The pit had been cut through the levelling material under the stone flags, and then excavated deep into the natural clay that characterised the local subsoil. Some of the clay had been put back into the bottom of the pit, and the rest of the pit had then been filled in with rubble. The fact that the fill of the pit (rubble) was substantially different from the layers through which it had been cut (clay) suggested that much of the clay had been removed off site, and that rubble had been introduced from elsewhere. When archaeologists excavated the pit they found that various items of interest had been concealed at the bottom under the thin re-deposited band of clay. Their interpretation was that the pit had been dug and used as a temporary place of disposal: first, objects from the murder that the offenders wished to dispose of were thrown in and then sealed with some of the clay. The pit was then probably used to conceal bags of dismembered remains and then covered up. At some later date the bags were removed for permanent disposal; rubble was subsequently brought into the cellar to fill in the pit before the floor was reflagged. The offenders never admitted to this, but equally they offered no alternative justification for the presence of the pit, nor for the character of its fill. The presence of a human fingernail below the clay at the base of the pit suggested that the archaeological explanation may have been reasonably accurate. The case illustrates well how archaeological layers can be open to interpretation.

This first chapter introduces key elements that will be pursued in the chapters that follow. The elements are undeniably archaeological even although they do not deal with ancient times, and it is difficult to deny that this book has an underlying archaeological theme. However, the authors have deliberately omitted the word 'archaeology' from the title. Archaeological techniques and thinking may be central to much that is discussed, but the spectrum is much wider than that. The forensic recovery of buried remains encapsulates, *inter alia*, aerial photography, psychology, cartography, geophysics, landscape analysis, fieldcraft, cadaver dog handling, ecology, botany, entomology, palynology, anthropology, pathology and conservation; it is about interdisciplinarity rather than multidisciplinarity and, above all else, it demonstrates the extent to which seemingly different fields of endeavour meet up and rub shoulders under a forensic umbrella.

1.3 Forensic archaeology

The use of the word 'forensic', by definition, shifts archaeology firmly into modern, criminal scenarios, in which archaeological (i.e. buried) evidence may be presented in a court of law. Usually this will involve the investigation of clandestine graves by adapting standard archaeological techniques (aerial imagery, geophysics, field walking, etc.) in order to locate burial sites, and by employing excavation strategies to recover the human remains they contain. On occasions other types of buried objects/artefacts may be searched for and excavated, typically drugs, firearms, other weapons and, in one famous example, ransom money packed into a holdall (see Section 2.1). Archaeologists may also be asked to resolve issues of date when human remains are discovered during building operations, or when human disarticulated bones are encountered as 'stray' finds by members of the public. They may also be asked to take part in formal exhumations undertaken by the police in order for a post-mortem to take place. There have also been instances where archaeologists have been deployed in mass disaster recovery, or even in fire debris where stratigraphic investigation is required in order to ascertain sequences of events. In short, they may find themselves involved in any matter involving buried or sealed remains, or remains which may have been buried, and which become part of a criminal investigation, thus requiring expert operational input or opinion.

Although a relatively new discipline, forensic archaeology has become routinely accepted by police and courts in the UK and has now gained wider recognition in other parts of Europe, notably the Netherlands and Scandinavia (Marquez-Grant *et al.* 2012). The use of archaeological techniques at scenes of crime is now reasonably well established (see Hunter 1994 or Cox 2009 for history; Cheetham and Hanson 2009 for methodology; Hunter and Cox 2005 and Hunter 2009 for case studies). It also has a widely accepted role in the recovery of victims from mass graves where the scale of application has necessitated the development of new techniques and protocols (e.g. Haglund *et al.* 2001; Cox *et al.* 2007).

The breadth of involvement and the interdisciplinary nature of archaeology itself have generated novel research areas, notably in geophysics and remote prospection (e.g. Ruffell and McKinley 2008; Kalacska *et al.* 2009) and in taphonomics (e.g. Haglund and Sorg 1997, 2002a). That said, the discipline is still essentially 'hands on'; it adapts conventional archaeological techniques and involves fieldwork and excavation.

However, unlike more conventional archaeology, forensic archaeology is normally part of a much wider picture of evidence capture: it requires integration with other, often unrelated disciplines from which other types of evidence are drawn. These can include a wide range of forensic interests, some of which will be familiar archaeological territory (e.g. pedology, palynology and diatoms), some of which may be less frequently encountered (e.g. entomology and DNA) and others that will be novel (e.g. fibres, paint, blood and pathology). Indeed, some of the processes involved in the analysis of evidential materials will be little different from those encountered in the archaeological science laboratory, notably in the referencing of samples to host standards. For example, an archaeologist might take samples from a pottery vessel and endeavour to source the clay, and a forensic scientist might take soil from a person's clothing in order to demonstrate that they had been to a particular place.

However, the similarity largely ends there. In the more distant past the archaeologist who encounters human remains is dealing with an anonymous population and seeks clarification of generic factors, for example, disease, diet, trauma, longevity, mortality rates, etc.). In a forensic context, it is the determination of specifics which is necessary, not least of these being the identification of the victim whose remains have been recovered. Moreover, unlike the collection of evidence in conventional archaeology, the collection of forensic evidence normally relates to individuals recently deceased or still living, either as victim or as potential offender(s) respectively. As a result behavioural sciences are introduced (e.g. offender and geographical profiling), which archaeologists may need to understand and integrate into a larger evidential equation. The overall picture is a wide one: it draws on many disparate skills and areas of expertise of which archaeology is often merely one small element. Archaeology is an annoyingly connective discipline: while a science in its own right, it feeds upon, and integrates with, a host of other disciplines. As one eminent academic is reputed to have said 'being an archaeologist is like working in the hedgerows, it lies in neither one field nor the other'. It is an impure discipline that has few firm boundaries.

The closest forensic links, however, are likely to be those with physical anthropology, particularly in contexts where the victims are substantially, or completely, skeletal, and where matters of identification and specific trauma require expert interpretation (Figure 1.2) (Natfe 2000; Blau and Ubelaker 2009). In some instances, notably in the excavation of victims from mass graves (below), practitioners will need to be highly experienced in both fields. There is sometimes confusion between the terms 'archaeology' and 'anthropology' particularly in discussion between US and UK practitioners (Steadman 2005; Komar and Buikstra 2008). In the USA archaeology emerged as a secondary discipline under the umbrella of physical anthropology, whereas in the UK archaeology and anthropology both emerged as primary disciplines but with anthropology being more dominantly 'social' as opposed to 'physical', hence the scope for confusion. A working definition might be that forensic archaeologists are expert in field skills but with an awareness of physical anthropology, whereas forensic anthropologists are expert in the examination of skeletal tissue, but with a basic understanding of excavation field skills. As all forensic work is

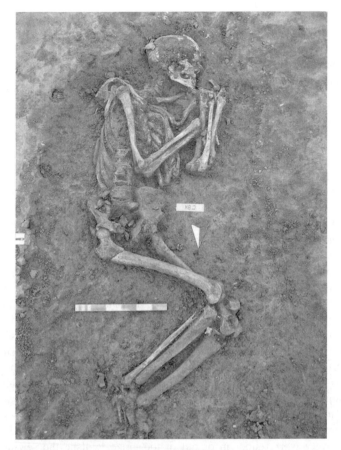

Figure 1.2 A grave requiring both archaeological and anthropological attention. Image by courtesy of K. Colls on behalf of Birmingham Archaeology.

open to cross-examination in Court, individual competence tends to be very skill-specific with practitioners taking care not to drift outside their field(s) of expertise. Staying within the limits of one's discipline competency (i.e. archaeology) is one of the pre-requisites of successful forensic investigation; as a consequence the former Council for the Registration of Forensic Practitioners (CRFP) in the UK held separate registers for the validation of both archaeologists and anthropologists.

Criminal investigation in the 21st century is properly concerned with protocol, quality, standards and accountability. In the UK the Office of the Forensic Regulator located within the Home Office is charged with oversight of these matters and is supported by other discipline-specific agencies. The Institute for Archaeologists (IfA) is one such body; this has peer validated levels of membership and specific codes of conduct for archaeologists. Under the IfA's wing forensic archaeology is a defined subject group (formerly 'Area of Competence') and has dedicated sets of standards and guidance to ensure appropriate practice (http://www.archaeologists.net/sites/default/files/node-files/Forensic2010.pdf). These cover, *inter alia*, standards and codes of practice for briefings, for search, for recovery, for reporting and presenting evidence at Court. The document is comprehensive and, apart from generic issues such as health/safety and continuing professional development, includes codes for specifics such as pre-scene attendance, search management, the recovery of exhibits, the taking of samples, recording, the retention of spoil from field excavations and the prevention of contamination. Many of these individual codes differ significantly from those used in more conventional excavations, and it is the specifics contained in the forensic archaeology codes that effectively define the character of the subject. The codes of practice were established *not* to say that there is only one way to conduct a forensic search or excavation, but to emphasise that actions which circumvent or shortcut defined methodologies need to be flagged up and/or explained. Archaeology 'by the book' is not normally a feature of forensic work (see also Section 6.1).

The Forensic Regulator is concerned with the quality of forensic services both at and away from the crime scene, and especially with the provision of forensic science. Since the effective privatisation of government funded forensic laboratories in the 1980s, the provision of forensic science has developed into a substantial industry in its own right. Both large and small players provide services, some very specialist (e.g. geoforensics), others deal with more commonly required services (e.g. fibres, blood marks or DNA), or with the evidence from volume crime (e.g. fingerprints). Police forces are obliged, as part of the current market process, to 'bundle' their requirements for key services with a single forensic provider for a period of three years before review. However, archaeology and anthropology are considered insufficiently mainstream to sit within the present bundling system and are commissioned independently. But this does mean, for example, that any evidence recovered during excavation is likely to have particular specialist services to which the police force in question is committed. This can be inhibiting in certain archaeologically-connected disciplines, notably in ecology (palynology, entomology, etc.) where many archaeologists would prefer to utilise their own specialists with whom they have worked before and who in their judgement may better understand any archaeological issues involved.

Key to recovery work, either in or out of the grave, will be the seizing of exhibits (the recovery of finds in archaeological parlance). Seizing kick-starts a rigorous chain of continuity which ensures that the life story of any exhibit, once seized, is fully documented and its location secured. Some exhibits will simply be maintained in store in case they are required as evidence in Court; others will undergo more complex processes of analysis or further investigation. Exhibiting covers *everything* taken or removed from the scene and includes bulk soils kept for further work and any samples taken, as well as individual objects such as fibres or even hair (see Section 7.1). All require the same degree of rigour in their collection, maintenance and record keeping. Without this guarantee of continuous control the evidence may be vulnerable in Court, and this extends also to the keeping of bulk materials, for example soil kept for sieving if it has not been maintained in sealed, labelled containers and kept in a secure location.

1.4   Legal issues and procedures

In the UK, criminal investigation is subject to tight legal constraints, and barristers are quick to identify even the slightest technical breach of protocol. There are several relevant pieces of legislation, but there are two in particular of which any archaeologist at a crime scene, or at a potential crime scene, will need to be aware, the Police and Criminal Evidence Act 1984 (usually known as PACE; HMSO 1984a) and the Criminal Procedure and Investigations Act 1996 (usually referred to as CPIA; HMSO 1996a) and the Codes of Practice issued under the Acts. Both are complex pieces of legislation that are explained in more detail elsewhere (see Dilley 2005; Ozin *et al.* 2010).

Briefly, and as far as archaeology is concerned, PACE primarily introduces an unwelcome time factor, although it also stipulates issues as to how a search can be conducted. Essentially, it requires the police, having arrested an individual, either to charge that individual with an offence, or to release him/her without charge within a specific period of time (Dilley 2005, 185, figure 7.3). In England and Wales that span has a minimum duration of 24 hours and a maximum of 96 hours, subject to approval of a higher authority, ultimately a Magistrates Court, providing that grounds for an extension can be proven and justified. In Scotland there is a single period of 6 hours only. Under certain circumstances, therefore, archaeologists may be required to search and/or excavate and to provide evidence sufficient for the police to make a charge within the constraints of the timescale defined by the 'PACE clock'. This might necessitate, for example, geophysical survey, focusing of target locations, use of machine stripping, or the physical investigation of aerial photographic features either at short notice, or within a defined time limit. Moreover, a crime scene involves a relatively large number of personnel, typically a Senior Investigating Office (SIO), a Deputy SIO (usually a rank or two below), a Crime Scene Manager, Crime Scene Investigators, an Exhibits Officer, operational support officers (trained searchers), uniformed officers to secure the scene and, *inter alia*, a press officer and others with different roles. The resource implication can be considerable and much may rely on the interpretation and findings of the archaeologist. This is a new and highly pressured environment for an archaeologist, and one which often requires the archaeologist to innovate in order to satisfy the demands of time and situation. Crime scenes are not arenas for either the faint-hearted or the *prima donna*. Issues can be straightforward, such as the examination of a small piece of disturbed ground, or the more complex search of a large garden or woodland. An investigation will normally have been the subject of briefings before the arrest was made, but there is still pressure on the archaeologist to perform on a landscape of questionable history and substrate using methodologies designed to either (a) discover in a manner which is evidentially respectable, or (b) eliminate confidently. The two are not easily reconcilable, and archaeological purism can be thrown out of the window early on.

The CPIA offers a different type of constraint. This Act stipulates that all participants at a scene of crime are required to make their evidence available to the Court. This means that whatever the archaeologist produces in terms of making a written, graphic or photographic record must be made available to both defence and prosecution authorities. The archaeologist, like any other forensic scientist or expert witness is deemed to be a witness of the Court, not a witness promoting the interests of the commissioning body, either the prosecution or defence agencies. Archaeologists are in Court to provide objective scientific opinion on the issues in hand, not to support a particular side. The Crown Prosecution Service (CPS), set up through the Prosecution of Offences Act 1985 (HMSO 1985), was deliberately established to allow prosecution to take place quite separately from police investigation and to demonstrate its independence from policing processes. The police will consult the CPS to ascertain whether they have enough evidence to prosecute, or indeed whether it is in the public interest to prosecute, but the two bodies otherwise work independently. Thus, the archaeologist will need to submit to the court all aspects of recording, including contexts sheets, primary plans and section drawings, sketches, tape recordings, photographs, daybooks, site logs, and the various lists of contexts, plans and images that characterise any modern excavation. Many of these, especially section and plan drawings, may typically be crossed out, erased, re-defined, or simply altered and amended as a customary part of creating the most accurate primary record. We all do this. But the Court may wish to know why these changes have been made, what levels of confidence or uncertainty are indicated by these changes, and how such alterations and revisions might reflect on the integrity, judgement and professionalism of the archaeologist concerned.

It is, of course, the tactic of the commissioning authority, usually the CPS, to bolster the credibility of the expert archaeological witness in Court. It is equally the role of the opposing side, usually the defence, to discredit the witness' evidence by identifying (for example) any perceived shortcomings in the work carried out, ambiguities in the statements presented or inadequacies in the previous experience of the witness. No matter whether archaeologist, blood spatter authority or entomologist, the expert witness tends to be a pawn in a much larger, essentially adversarial scenario. As such, his or her evidence is fair game for demolition, and the archaeologist needs to be prepared for that. The best preparation, of course, is at the crime scene itself, making sure that no questions are left unanswered, that every record is completed at a professional level, and that statements are produced that demonstrate competence. It is, however, also a salutary experience to have to present evidence to a jury whose members may be unfamiliar with archaeology and its terminologies, or whose perceptions of the profession (varying perhaps between Indiana Jones and the *Time Team*) may be misplaced. It is the jury that the barrister is attempting to convince; it is the jury that decides the verdict.

1.5   Decay dynamic

Conventional archaeology tends to deal with 'inert' materials of study, such as buried walls, ditches, pits, etc. However, forensic archaeology needs to consider the effects and timing of the human decay dynamic, particularly in terms of search methodology (and especially geophysics). This decay factor has implications for how and when a grave might best be found, and in what condition the body might be recovered. At death human bodies are subject to a decay process which follows a well-defined route – typically primary decay, putrefaction, black putrefaction, fermentation and dry decay (e.g. Clark *et al.* 1997; Vass *et al.* 2002; Galloway *et al.* 1989). The last of these (effectively skeletonisation) is the one most familiar to archaeologists, but is one which is rarely achieved in forensic timescales. The speed at which this complete process occurs depends on a plethora of factors involving both the physical characteristics of the individual (and clothing/wrapping), and the nature of the burial environment including, for example, depth, the pH of the soil, the moisture content, the presence of oxygen, temperature, the proximity of bacteria, and the accessibility of flies and scavengers, among others. This is a scientific process which is largely predictable, but not exact.

During the decay processes stages of temporary equilibrium can sometimes be achieved, such as is marked by adipocere formation (a greasy fatty state often caused by wetness, Figure 1.3), but decay is otherwise progressive and, unless the burial environment is particularly acidic, the process usually stalls at a stage of skeletonisation. Complete absence of

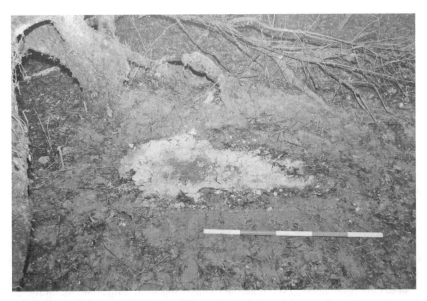

Figure 1.3 Example of adipocere formation permeating the ground after body removal.

skeletal survival, even over long archaeological timescales, requires very unusual environmental conditions. An interesting example occurred regarding the exhumation of Cardinal Newman, an eminent Catholic priest who died in 1890. His remains were exhumed from a private oratory in 2009 as part of his canonisation; this received some press attention (e.g. *The Daily Mail*, Tuesday 4 November 2008). At his own wish he had been buried in the same grave as his long term companion, Father Ambrose St John, who had died previously. To the apparent surprise of those involved no skeletal parts had survived, although pieces of metal coffin furniture and some fabric were still identifiable. The absence of human remains was ascribed to the nature of the soil, but tests on soil elsewhere in the vicinity (but not at the oratory itself) suggested that the burial environment was only moderately acidic and certainly not at a level that might cause a skeleton to vanish completely. Moreover, metal coffin furniture and textiles tend to be more susceptible to decay and are likely to have decayed first. There exists, therefore, some mystery surrounding Cardinal Newman's final resting place; it may possibly be due to Victorian attitudes to his perceived sexuality in wishing to be buried with his male companion, but equally there may have been other contemporary reasons. On the evidence available, however, the burial environment does not appear to have been the cause for the complete absence of any physical remains.

There are other taphonomic extremes, for example in the instances of 'bog bodies' where peat can provide an anaerobic preservative medium, or in dry, arid conditions where desiccation can occur, but such instances are rare (Brothwell and Gill-Robinson 2002; Steadman 2005). The presence of buried, soft decaying tissue, apart from being unpleasant to excavate, may also create other significant effects, but at particular time points in the decay process. These include the emission of heat, liquefaction, a propensity to attract scavengers and providing the impetus for surface vegetation change – all of which have implications for the types of techniques deployed to find a grave and the timescales at which those techniques can be optimised during stages of the decay process (see Sections 2.3 and 3.1). Many researchers have used observations based on buried pigs as human analogues under controlled conditions in order to try and create a more precise equation that may allow these effects to be better predicted (e.g. France *et al.* 1992, 1997; Powell 2010).

Decay, defined more broadly in terms of 'taphonomics', has become the focus of considerable interest. For example, in even more complex scenarios, Courts may require guidance as to how ambiguity between the time since death – the post-mortem interval (PMI) – and the level of decay state might accurately reflect the removal of a body from one physical environment to another. Determining the PMI is a key factor in forensic investigation; some experimental work has also been carried out to assess the extent to which human remains might be spread by seasonal ploughing (Haglund *et al.* 2002), in much the same way that similar experimental work has been started on localised pottery spreads (Reynolds and Schadla-Hall 1980; Reynolds 1989). Scavenging, for example by foxes, badgers and rats, has also played a part in determining PMI, both in terms of using spatial extent of the distribution of surface scatter as a coarse indicator of elapsed time since death, and also (as a corollary) the predicted extent of surface distribution after a given time (see also Section 7.4). In addition, forensic science is now also concerned with the impact of human decay on associated grave materials which might be either identification-bearing (e.g. textiles, clothing, jewellery or contents of pockets), or forensically-related (e.g. fibres, cigarette butts or projectiles) (e.g. Janaway 1996, 2002, 2008).

1.6   Search methods and adaptations

The search for shallow sub-surface remains is especially suited to archaeologists who have an evolved experience in noticing topographical nuances and vegetation differences brought about by the presence of buried features, as well as utilising, adapting and developing techniques of geophysics, aerial reconnaissance and other methods of remote sensing for these purposes (see Cheetham 2005). Some of these methods are now particularly advanced, notably the use of LiDAR, digital terrain modelling (DTM) (see Section 2.3), the use of Geographical Information Systems (GIS) and the advances in gaseous detection used by earth scientists (Chapman 2006; Kvamme 2006). The potential of earth sciences has yet to be fully explored for forensic relevance and Ruffell has provided an introductory definition of pedology, geology, geosciences, geoforensics and soils for clarification purposes (2010; also Pringle *et al.* 2012).

However, not least of the overall search weaponry is the humble map in its many types, scales and editions which mirrors land use and landscape change over time as well as helping define useful factors such as accessibility, solid/drift geology and geomorphology (Ruffell and McKinley 2008). Some of these aspects are discussed in more detail in Chapter 2. Although the search processes adopted may be similar to those used in more conventional archaeological survey there are significant differences: first, the forensic targets are both small and very specific, and second the individual locations will need to be fully eliminated as deposition sites before the search moves on to another area. The use of aerial and geophysical techniques often yields a plethora of anomalies or possible disturbances which, in conventional archaeological terms, can often be interpreted without invasive action. In forensic procedural terms, however, the SIO is committed to eliminating each one, either by trial trench or, more often, by venting the anomaly (i.e. probing the ground to allow gasses

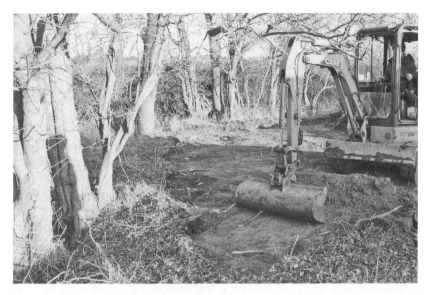

Figure 1.4   The use of heavy machinery in searching for burials.

to escape) to enable use of a cadaver dog. Forensic search normally operates its procedures sequentially from the non-invasive to the invasive in order to minimise potential loss of evidence. There is, however, often a 'trade-off' between method and speed which depends on the extent to which the SIO may consider one particular location to be of greater potential than another. For example, lower ranked sites might be stripped using machinery in order to eliminate them (e.g. Hunter and Cox 2005, case study 21), while higher ranked sites may be subjected to geophysical survey, cadaver dog attention and careful excavation in a defined sequence (e.g. Hunter and Cox 2005, case study 2). This is amplified in Chapter 4. The definition of relative site importance is a management decision, not an archaeological one, although archaeological opinion might be taken into account in identifying priorities. The use of heavy machinery in the search for human remains may offend some archaeological sensitivities but is usually a pre-requisite in the elimination of sites at the lower end of the confidence spectrum (Figure 1.4). Moreover, heavy machinery is sometimes an essential at the higher end of the same spectrum depending on surface conditions and geology. Archaeologists who have worked with experienced excavator operators will know just how subtly and cleanly a wide machine bucket can be used to strip thin horizontal spits of earth across a given area (see also Section 3.3). Under many circumstances machine stripping is equal to, if not better than, manual trowelling.

A key difference in the application of archaeological techniques lies in the decay chemistry of the buried human remains (above) in comparison to the inherently stable features that generally constitute more conventional archaeological targets, not least of these being the emission of heat during the active decay process itself. The rate of taphonomic change is not always predictable and can be affected by a host of natural factors (type of soil, climate, etc.); to some extent they can also be influenced by the actions of the offender (for example, the extent to which the body is wrapped, or the depth of the grave). Moreover, offender profiling (the psychological analysis of an individual's behaviour), geographical profiling (the use of mapping to identify a person's spatial movements), witness statements, evidence of last sightings and cognate information may also need to be brought into the equation. There are now behaviour databases covering many thousands of abduction/deposition scenarios which provide statistically-based starting points for search on the basis of previous crimes (Francis *et al.* 2004). These take into account factors such as vehicle access, relationships (age/sex) between victim and likely offender, and distances travelled/walked, as well as deposition probabilities according to offender habits.

The application of archaeological techniques in search scenarios makes good sense, but the framework within which the application takes place has to be heavily geared towards logistical efficiency (Section 2.1). The level of search reflects not only the constraints of legislation (above), but also the resource implication of manpower, time and costs in relation to the demands of other simultaneous enquiries being handled by the same officers. Not least of this resource implication is the presence of in-house role-based officers (e.g. for exhibits, press, crime scene management, photography, etc.), specialist personnel (e.g. for child protection, community relations, etc.) as well as external specialists (e.g. archaeologists, geophysicists, dog handlers, etc.) who may be brought in from different parts of the country. There will almost certainly be an Operational Support Unit (OSU) which will be working on a shift basis between a variety of scenes and duties, and Police Search Advisors (PolSAs) to direct search strategy. The whole exercise requires extreme coordination and timing, extensive briefing for all concerned, and extensive de-briefing afterwards. The smoothest, most efficient operations result from everyone knowing who is doing what, when and how. A typical search may involve archaeologists, dog handlers, an OSU led by a PolSA, a geophysics team, a Crime Scene Manager, and detectives, and the command chain and decision-making process can become blurred to the archaeologist. The search of a house and garden for a concealed body with a team such as this, often involving clearance of one room or part of a garden at a time, requires search sequencing in an exact manner. This ensures that the property can ultimately be eliminated with confidence, that the individual elements of search dovetail neatly in a manner that allows the search methodologies of one group not to inhibit or negate the efficacy of the next group, and that personnel are not standing idly kicking their heels for hours on end waiting for their turn. The archaeologist has a focal role in this under the coordination of the PolSA, initially in assessing ground surfaces for subtle disturbances, and subsequently supporting geophysicists in the interpretation of data, identifying targets for cadaver dogs and, as a result, determining priority locations for intrusive work and, ultimately, investigating those locations by excavation.

1.7 Recovery methods and adaptation

All field archaeology, whether forensic or conventional, is undertaken according to design in order to answer specific questions. In the forensic arena these questions are often very different from those an archaeologist might normally ask. Common questions, for example, will bear on the identity of the individual buried, the manner in which the grave was dug, the presence of evidence within a grave that may link the grave to an offender, or the presence of material which might link the body to a different environment. The over-arching question, and one probably never posed in conventional archaeology, is 'who was responsible for the murder and burial of this victim?'.

No two forensic excavations are ever the same and there is no 'by-the-book' solution to the recovery to the various types of potential evidence. Often it is not possible to define the spatial limits of the crime scene: unlike conventional archaeological graves, which tend to be sealed by subsequent layers, the forensic grave is normally cut into a contemporary ground surface which is likely to be part of the crime scene itself. It is here that the offender(s) stood and worked, that material may have been dropped, footprints or tyre marks left, and that the body may have been rested. In some mass burials the grave edge is known to have been used as the execution site, as witnessed by the presence and concentration of empty cartridges. Hence the area around the grave needs to be searched and cleared before any excavation commences; it is often best to treat the grave itself as a 'mini crime scene' within the framework of the larger crime scene.

As with search, there will be a range of different personnel offering differing skills and requiring coordination in the detailed examination of a crime scene, usually under the direction of the Crime Scene Manager whose responsibility it is to ensure that the record and collection of evidence (including the body) occurs in a manner which will allow the different strands to be processed (and/or analysed) and integrated into the larger evidential picture to provide the objective evidence that can underpin a prosecution case. At the same time a documented chain of actions will need to be maintained. Different cases sometimes require different weighting of evidence in order to prove specific points, thus briefings between all concerned are essential. Interested parties here will include the pathologist, entomologist, archaeologist, toxicologist and perhaps the anthropologist. One widely unrecognised role of the archaeologist is in providing a three-dimensional record of the grave into which the sampling of other specialists can be set and the location of exhibits defined.

Because archaeology is a destructive exercise and is not replicable in the same way as laboratory experimentation, there is always the need to make comprehensive records as the work proceeds, ideally using photographic, graphic and written methods. The type of photography used in conventional archaeology is well suited in that archaeologists normally use the camera to record specific 'events', i.e. changes in layer and visibility of features, or to reference staged processes during excavation. Crime scene photography is often more generalised and the crime scene photographer may need to be instructed as to when shots need to be taken, from what angle, and what the specific features of interest are. Photographic scales are essential for archaeological purposes, especially in detailed shots, but very few crime scene photographers seem to use them. Graves can be half-sectioned (i.e. one half removed first); this allows a vertical view of how the grave was constructed, how and with what it was infilled and where the body lies in relation to other layers (Figure 1.5). This procedure can be started when the grave cut is first identified, and can be concluded when the body has been removed. It would normally be planned at a scale of 1:10. The grave outline itself will also need to be planned, usually at 1:20 and tied into fixed points (e.g. fence posts or corners of buildings) in case the exact location of the site needs to be revisited at a later date. These procedures are evaluated in more detail in Section 6.2.

The precise removal of the grave fill is critical as it can contain the evidence that might link the grave and victim to the offender. In forensic cases burial fills are typically mixed and are best excavated in arbitrary 'spits' some 10 cm deep, unless clearly defined layers can be identified. Strictly speaking, it is the interface between layers that is critical for interpretation in conventional archaeology – that is the 'gaps' between stratigraphic events.

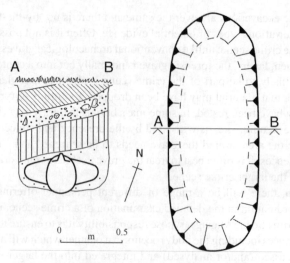

Figure 1.5 Typical scale plan of half-sectioned grave.

However, in many, but by no means all, forensic recoveries these interfaces are limited to the grave surface (usually the present ground surface) and the grave edges (i.e. the junction where the grave fill touches the cut edge of the grave). The latter is particularly important at the base of the grave as this is where evidence, for example for silting or footprints, might be found sealed at the bottom of the grave by the initial grave infill. The use of arbitrary spits provides some measure of control for re-locating the position of exhibits seized from the grave fill and provides some form of three-dimensional record, albeit a crude one. It also provides a more manageable measure of the former location of fills for any subsequent sieving of bulk spoil (see Section 7.1). More accurate three-dimensional control can be secured by using a total station system (electronic distance measurer – EDM) or a global positioning system (GPS). These would be the preferred choice of any archaeological purist, but archaeological purists tend not to work in the dense woodland, thick undergrowth or cluttered back yards where many forensic disposals tend to occur. Irrespective of limited sight lines, tree canopies, or the simple absence of space, which make electronic systems awkward to use, one might also question the level of accuracy required in any plan or record and how that might best be achieved. Under most circumstances, string, tape measures, local fixed points, a planning board and perhaps a dumpy level are the most effective (Figure 1.6). They always work, irrespective of circumstance. And they do not require batteries. In an age of increasing survey technology (see Chapters 2 and 3) they tend to be viewed as rather antiquated. However, one distinct advantage is that the image (plan) can be drawn up and checked at the scene without the need for later downloading and potential loss of data or, as experience has shown, confusion as to which way up the image should be, and which points should be joined up. Despite technological advances, field archaeology is still, thankfully, very much 'hands on' and visual.

Each spit is numbered uniquely and any exhibits (finds) that are seized (recorded) can be assigned accordingly. The exhibits will be different from the sherds of pottery, corroded

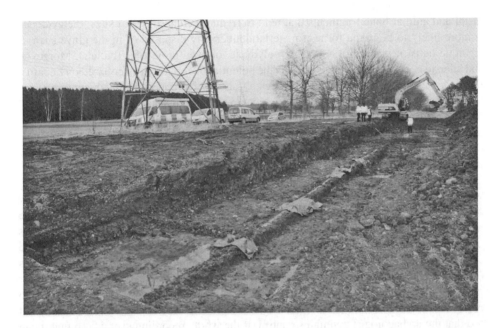

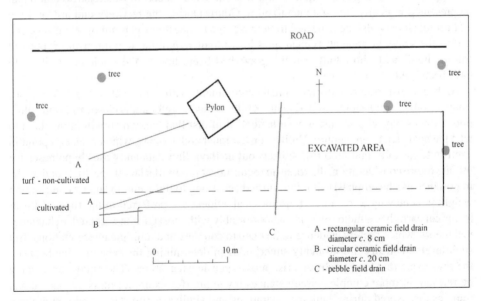

Figure 1.6 A site plan using local fixed points based on an electricity pylon and trees showing (top) machine stripping of site and (bottom) existing excavation plan to which this new cumulative stripping can be added as the enquiry continues.

metal and animal bone fragments that tend to frequent archaeological sites; the evidence is more likely to be in the form of material deliberately disposed of in the grave such as cigarette butts, newspaper, packaging, polythene, or even projectiles (bullets). Moreover, and alien to conventional archaeology, is the potential of contact transfer based on Locard's principle, namely that every contact leaves a trace, which underpins much contemporary forensic science (see Section 6.1). This includes evidence which has accidentally transferred from offender to grave, such as fibres, hair or even footprints. Equally, there may be material accidentally transferred from a vehicle to the grave with the body, or botanical evidence carried from a former location where the body had been kept. All this will provide intelligence for the SIO as to where further enquiries should be directed.

The nature of this trace evidence is such that (a) it can easily be contaminated by those working at the crime scene (which is why all work is undertaken wearing special suits or overalls and using new or sterilised equipment) and (b) it may not always be visible to the naked eye. The soil from the separate layers or spits may need to be sealed in large bags or containers to prevent contamination and taken to a controlled environment for detailed sieving and investigation. Moreover, in conventional work archaeologists pride themselves in having their excavated *in situ* remains, especially skeletons, clean and well defined for photographs. Such meticulous cleaning is avoided in forensic cases as it would serve to remove any contact trace evidence that might link the offender to the victim. It is important too that the archaeologist maintains control of the whole recording exercise so that it can be presented logically in a statement and in Court. During the recovery and at Court the archaeologist may also be expected to field a range of questions pertaining to these layers, and to the grave in general; typical questions might require an opinion to be expressed 'on the hoof' as to how long ago the grave had been dug, or the implements likely to have been used.

Archaeologists traditionally measure their comments with terms such as 'could', 'might', 'may' or other expressions of relative probability. Courts prefer a less elastic opinion, while police forces typically require a clear statement of distilled fact which will allow them to take the next step in an enquiry. Unlike conventional archaeology, which is an end point in itself in terms of a final report which sets out method, lists data and poses hypotheses for infinite future consideration, the forensic requirement is part of a larger spectrum of data. Its importance can be emphasised or diminished according to the scenario and its contributing weight in achieving a 'result'. Archaeological evidence is preferred in the form of linear historical narrative, a factor that sits uncomfortably with most current accepted archaeological theory, which prefers evidence to be open to complex and multiple interpretations. But such levels of theory are normally superfluous in determining the relationships between the few layers that tend to characterise most forensic excavations. They may conceivably be relevant in more complex circumstances involving (for example) mass graves, human remains discovered during building operations and similar circumstances, although these rarely approach the multiple-layered, multi-period types of site exhibiting vast data banks covering artefacts, ecofacts and stratigraphies. More awkwardly, the archaeologist may be drawn into unchartered waters in being required to comment as to whether a grave might have been dug hurriedly by a perpetrator, or whether it was more likely, or less likely, that a particular scenario occurred, in an attempt to fix opinion or likelihood into a particular spectrum of Bayesian probability. In short, the archaeologist can expect to be placed under some pressure to be specific.

1.8   Mass graves

Forensic archaeology has also found itself heavily involved in the investigation of mass graves resulting from genocide, particularly in South America and in the former Yugoslavia. These sites have been prominent not only in seeing the development of excavation techniques and strategies but also in providing experience for workers in a relatively infant discipline at the turn of the 20th and 21st century. There is now a reasonable literature on the excavation of mass graves; this has developed beyond the straightforward practicalities of methodology and logistics into less tangible concepts of social justice and human rights (Schmitt 2002; Skinner *et al.* 2003; Cox *et al.* 2007; see Chapter 8). Although the techniques applied are similar to excavating single graves, there are some significant innovations, for example the use of dedicated pro-formas and certain recording techniques. In addition, the way in which the interrogation of the remains is undertaken may differ: identification may be a less prominent factor in relation to human rights violations, particularly in some earlier work, where evidence was solely concerned with determining cause(s) of death. Each scene, whether a mass grave or an individual clandestine grave, will require its own set of questions and its own set of approaches.

The nature of the recovery exercise in mass deposits is usually made more complex by the intertwining and compression of victims, or by commingling of the remains in more advanced states of decay (Figure 1.7). Differential decay within the grave can also occur, caused by the differing taphonomic effects occurring in different parts of the mass of bodies. This can be exacerbated in secondary graves (i.e. where bodies have been moved from one buried location to another), a feature that characterised many of the burials in the aftermath of the Balkans conflict in the mid 1990s. There, most mass graves were originally created by mechanical excavators, which provided an easy method of concealing large numbers of victims in a short space of time. The largest were approximately 3 m wide reflecting the width of a typical excavator bucket and often over 2 m deep and 15–20 m in length with a ramp at one end to allow vehicle access. Mechanisation can also be extended to the interment of the victims, causing significant post-mortem injuries, especially in the case of bodies moved mechanically from one grave and shipped to another. Some bodies were also affected by the presence of vehicle movement above the bodies when the grave was subsequently infilled; this may create additional difficulties for the anthropologists and archaeologists at the point of excavation. These are circumstances when those involved in the recovery process will require both anthropological as well as archaeological skills (see also Section 7.4).

Mass graves are excavated for two main reasons: for humanitarian purposes in order to recover, identify and repatriate victims, or for forensic purposes in order to provide evidence to help convict a particular offender, for example a senior military figure whose orders were being carried out. In instances of genocide, when many thousands die and there are numerous graves, not all graves will necessarily carry the forensic potential, the viable witness accounts or other information available to implicate known individuals. For the majority of graves, therefore, the excavation process may have a more humanitarian focus and, given the number of graves likely to be identified, may take a considerable time, even if fully funded. The resources might be immense (archaeologists, anthropologists, pathologists, mortuary technicians, DNA sampling, storage facilities and security personnel); nor are investigations likely to be undertaken within the time frame expected

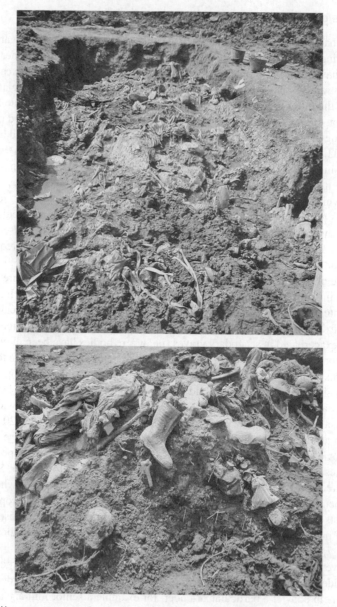

Figure 1.7 Mass grave excavation (top) and detail of commingling (bottom). Images by courtesy of Cecily Cropper.

by families and relatives desperate to have their loved ones returned and who may wish to embark on the process of excavation themselves (Hunter and Simpson 2007). Repatriation of bodies to families requires every bit as much attention to detailed excavation and recording as forensic work if the integrity of the process is to be maintained. This is especially the case with body parts as opposed to complete individuals. Presumptive identification (i.e. using clothing, documentation found on the body and similar evidence) is a last resort. The use of DNA is the preferred method, but this also requires community involvement, outreach programmes of DNA matching and all the resources thus entailed in order to be effective.

It is sometimes difficult to understand that the level of forensic detail afforded to each individual victim in a given mass grave is not commensurate with the level of detail afforded to the single individual in a criminal clandestine grave. The view is necessarily a more generic one: the Court needs answers to simple questions and may often assume, for time and resource reasons, that the victims represented in the grave can be treated collectively. The answers to simple questions such as likely date of death and the cause/manner of death, linked to the disappearance of presumed individuals from place X and their discovered burial in place Y, may well be adequate for prosecution purposes. To pursue this in more detail would be legally unnecessary and, no matter how much the personal ethics of each archaeologist and the dignity of each victim might demand it, would not serve to make any difference to the outcome of the judicial process. The issue is one of answering specific questions within a legal system where the end justifies the means. Archaeologists in these circumstances are witnesses of the Court, not followers of moral crusades. Purists may not find this to be the most satisfactory of processes, but it is not the purists who set the resource budget, frame the legislation, nor undertake the practicalities of exhumation in hostile environments. Archaeologists do what they are asked to do; rather than pose questions formed within a conventional research design they are obliged to play out a role in someone else's agenda. They may not be morally comfortable with that agenda, nor indeed with the political environment in which the agenda was drawn up, but they also have to ask themselves what might happen if their specialist skills were not incorporated, if the remains were excavated only in part by others, or by machine, or by a hostile faction, or if they were invited in the capacity as observers with no authority to influence the mode of recovery at all. These are personal decisions to which the archaeologist may be subjected. Forensic archaeology is no easy ride.

2 Search theory and the landscape

2.1 The theory

Searching for buried human remains is a complex and inexact science on which much has been written. Most literature concerned with search contains useful lists of the methods available and give a reasonable idea of both pedigree and chronology of development (e.g. France *et al*. 1997; Killam 2004; Pye and Croft 2004; Hunter and Cox 2005; Ruffell and McKinley 2008; Powell 2010). Individual searches may share some similarities but no two are ever identical – landscapes and buried soil profiles can differ as much as the knowledge and mindsets of the criminals who bury their respective victims. This chapter endeavours to explore the processes which constitute generally accepted practice together with the philosophies that underlie them. It also reviews some of the more frequently used techniques available.

One of the key issues in any search scenario is the need for a sequential and phased approach. In enquiries that present stratigraphic parameters (typically burial or fire) where essentially an archaeological input is required, the initial action is normally non-invasive, given that invasive methods may ultimately be destructive in recovering evidence. Primary search methodologies tend to be 'desk-top'; many have an archaeological pedigree and are used systematically in attempting to locate clandestine graves both in current and 'cold' case scenarios using, for example: documentary sources (including earlier maps, drawings, illustrations and photographs); site-use history and aerial imagery. Subsequent field-based actions (geophysical survey, fieldcraft, probing, etc.) lead to more invasive operations (test-pitting, machine stripping, excavation, etc.), and an evolving literature shows how all these techniques have been satisfactorily adapted to forensic purpose (Morse *et al*. 1983; France *et al*. 1992, 1997; Hunter *et al*. 1996; Killam 2004; Hunter and Cox 2005). Additional, non-archaeological methods (including cadaver dogs, offender profiling and applied behavioural sciences) have now extended the whole issue of forensic search into a more rounded discipline in its own right. In the UK, operational support for search has been developed through the establishment of the Police National Search Centre, and the creation of special Police Search Advisors (PolSAs), initially to deal with counter-terrorism searches (firearms, explosives, drugs, etc.), but now extended to missing persons.

In theory, the most efficient searches are seamless and coordinated and much effort will have been put into their planning. There are three key police operational manuals which detail this: *Practice Advice on Search Management and Procedures* (ACPO 2006); *Guidance on the Management, Recording and Investigation of Missing Persons* (ACPO 2010) and *Police Search Management – Missing Persons* (ACPO 2011a). All three are concerned with search in its many forms, targets and contexts; the first two are less focused on methodology and more on protocols and organisation, but the last, intended for PolSAs, has a much more practical outlook. Procedures normally assume that the missing person is still alive in the first instance; this is recognised in the recommended strategies, for example in ascertaining a missing person's level of risk and in pursuing a search design which takes this into account (see also Newiss 2005). It is difficult to ascertain the exact number of recorded missing persons nationally given that not all missing persons are formally reported as missing. A centralised record of those that are reported missing is held on the Police National Computer (PNC) by the Missing Persons Bureau in the National Policing Improvement Agency (NPIA). Last year the figure was around 240,000. For 2010/2011 the number of missing persons reported to the police in England, Scotland and Wales was 326,764 (ACPO 2011a); it is difficult to analyse from this figure how many of these result in homicides, given that the number includes 'returns', as well as suicides, accidental deaths etc. However, an analysis by the NPIA of 11 UK Police Forces on the 2010/2011 numbers indicates that the fatal outcomes amount to less than 1%; this repeats earlier research by Newiss (2006). Home Office figures record over 600 homicides in England and Wales in 2010/11 (Smith 2012, 30).

Persons of all ages go missing for a wide range of criminal, social and medical reasons, not least being depression and dementia, as well as children who become lost or abducted. Many cases are now held in data banks compiled from closed cases such as the Centralised Analytical Team Collating Homicide Expertise and Management (CATCHEM) database (dealing with children and young persons). The more widely-based *Missing Persons* document produced by Grampian Police analyses around 3,000 cases of missing persons of all ages. It provides predictive models of where a missing person might be located according to circumstances, on the basis of age, sex and elapsed time (Gibb and Woolnough 2007). By applying the trends evidenced in this type of data an enquiry can to some extent predict the potential location needed for search and the likely target points within it. However, the Grampian statistics deal with living persons who are mostly responsible for their own actions, not those who have been abducted, murdered and buried. By contrast, CATCHEM is homicide-centred and can provide data on deposition statistics, killer–victim relationships and a range of other critical factors which, like the Grampian models, can provide a search with starting points. CATCHEM, however, is concerned with children and young persons. While much of its underlying theory is transferable to the fate of adults, it cannot assume the same level of statistical probability.

Best search practice follows a well-trodden path: appropriate techniques (often known as 'assets') are identified and evaluated through briefings; the landscape is mapped; search boundaries are defined; specialists are deployed efficiently in an agreed sequence; the search is monitored and periodically reviewed; the whole process is recorded and logged, and the data subsequently archived irrespective of whether the body has been located or not. Although the key objective is to locate a clandestine burial or deposition site, there is an important ancillary objective in ensuring that the area of search can be confidently eliminated should the burial not be found. This is sometimes overlooked: elimination *per se* does not feature as a specific concern in either of the operational manuals referred to above.

Of course, search theory and application are two very different beasts and there is always a danger that field search can take place in a more disjointed way than is desirable. Sometimes, and for justifiable logistical reasons, it is not always possible to brief specialists together and devise sequential deployment. There are occasions when sensitive detection equipment functions ineffectively and provides false assurances in the squalor of a suspect's back garden or across a tussock moorland landscape. The weather may be adverse, the light inadequate, assumed access limited, and there may be time constraints imposed by legal sanctions (Section 1.4). There will be occasions too when shifts change, one cohort of search officers may be relieved and another arrives needing briefing, on-the-spot training and a fresh acquaintance with the landscape. At the most basic level, machines can break down, computers crash, batteries run out, and there is always the possibility of human error. Anyone with much in the way of search experience will be familiar with the potential for things to go wrong. Even with the best of wills and the best of Standard Operating Procedures (SOPs) these things happen because search is a hands-on, practical exercise at the mercy of landscape, climate, logistics and resources. Sometimes, through nobody's fault, the practical search ends up second best to the theory.

Search is a complex exercise which requires not only integration of skills and personnel, but also an understanding of the wider picture by all parties concerned. To operate otherwise is to introduce a blind man's bluff effect in which none of the cooperating parties are fully aware of what is going on, how their respective methodologies might impact on those of others, and how their findings might be weighted in the overall enquiry. Interaction between parties is important (Section 3.1). Moreover, search works best if there is a consistent, single individual to whom all can turn for decision-making and support. This is a position usually held by a senior PolSA (Search Coordinator) and is a key role recognised in all manuals for large scale or complex searches. Undefined leadership has the potential for creating an uncomfortable management hiatus between the different external groups and individuals descending on the incident – dog handlers, archaeologists, machine driver, search officers and forensic specialists, to name but a few. Somewhere within this melee of skill sets needs to be someone who is sufficiently familiar with the nature and limitations of the techniques being applied to be able to assess their findings, draw the threads together, and transform a multidisciplinary exercise into an interdisciplinary one. Only then is the whole outcome likely to be greater than the sum of the individual components.

Normal practice tends to separate the search process from the investigation process in as much as the search is managed by a PolSA and the investigation by the SIO, although the two processes are closely interlinked throughout (ACPO 2011a, 5). This has evolved as best practice, although separation inevitably runs the risk of useful intelligence or information not being fully transmitted by one of the parties to the other because it was not felt to be sufficiently important or relevant. Additionally, it is sometimes easy for a specialist to find him/herself in a confusing 'piggy-in-the-middle' position, not knowing to whom he/she is responsible. In the best searches the roles are clearly defined from the outset. Given the potential for dislocation it is perhaps worth remembering that there may be no such thing as a perfect search.

None of the various techniques (e.g. fieldcraft, cadaver dogs or geophysical survey) should be seen as 'bolt-on' given that the various buried features to which the techniques may/may not respond are in the interests of all. Every observation is key to a PolSA involved in the search, as well as the SIO or his deputy, as all responses or observations will possess some probability or likelihood. If a search is to commence from a non-invasive starting point (such as using maps or aerial photographs) then the process will involve grading areas of greater likelihood from those of lesser likelihood (see Section 4.2). There are issues of probability involved and also issues of interpretation: in the same way that a PolSA may offer various views as to the relative importance of a location defined from topographical change or distinctive vegetation, or a dog handler assess the level and significance of a particular canine response, so the geophysicist will be in a position to interpret the nature and relevance of sub-surface features. An archaeologist who is able to work through data with a geophysicist, or discuss the level of response with a dog handler is much more likely to be able to prioritise than if they are simply greeted with second-hand information or a set of spray-on markers on the ground.

Moreover, some techniques, and especially forensic geophysics, are very much developing disciplines and require feedback if they are to evolve more fully. If the location of a geophysical response is excavated then it is important to know what sub-surface attribute has caused that response to be made. Equally, if a buried body is eventually recovered in an area where the geophysics has proved negative, there is a need to learn or understand why that was the case. In all techniques there is some responsibility on the part of the practitioner to pursue a wider goal in the development of the discipline rather than to treat each scene independently as a 'one-off' job. As an example of how best practice might be developed, archaeologists worked closely with geophysicists in the examination of a concrete barn floor in the search for a potential burial (Figure 2.1). GPR data were reviewed jointly and targets were drawn out on the barn floor based on a common grid. Each target was excavated systematically and the results communicated to the geophysicists, who were then able to assess what had caused the responses and why, thus potentially honing their understanding of the technique's potential for future use.

Search methodology is designed to maximise the probability of finding the body and any forensic evidence in association. It does so by targeting areas of interest and then continues through a logical process of elimination until the body is found. It is how these target areas are identified and what methods are used to eliminate them that are the subjects of enquiry here. In order to find the body a search utilises a number of well-tried procedures and applies a series of techniques or assets according to circumstance. These techniques can range from the laborious and the manual (e.g. line searching) to the use of expensive hi-tech prospection equipment (e.g. GPR) and can now draw upon new aerial mapping techniques (e.g. LiDAR). Potential search methods are not listed or reviewed further here to any encyclopaedic extent, although some of the more commonly used methods are discussed elsewhere in this volume in terms of their relative merits of application.

Search usually tends to commence with a 'desk-top' analysis – that is a review of the available evidence from all sources which can then be given spatial context on a map. Every search needs somewhere to start. This can be generated by the enquiry from a variety of sources including witness information, recovery of items, knowledge of the victim's movements, knowledge of a suspect's habits and so on, or from a statistical database created from other disappearances which may have predictive elements. This information can be readily transferred into map form so that an operation can be planned and costed. This map constitutes the basis of any search, either in simple visual form, or in more sophisticated digitised mode (below). Maps are essential for large areas, plans for smaller areas. Depending on the information available the search area may be a large tract of

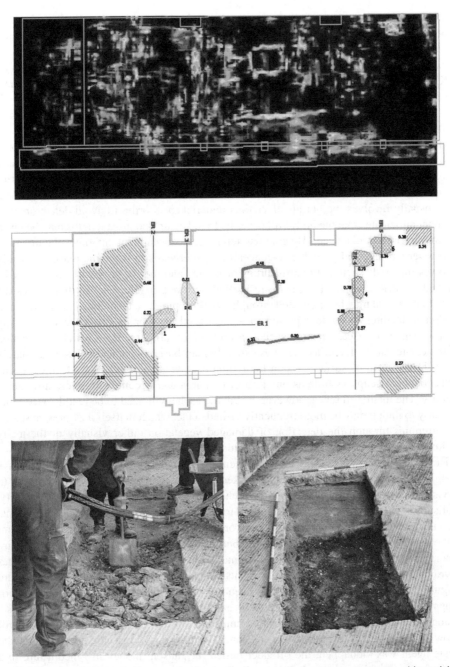

Figure 2.1 Excavation of the concrete floor of a barn marked out on a common grid resulting from GPR responses. The top image shows a horizontal radar slice at an estimated 0.5 m depth; the middle image shows the overall interpretation of radar responses at different depths, and the bottom images show the excavation of one of the potential targets. Geophysics images courtesy of Stratascan Ltd. (*For colour details please see colour plate section.*)

landscape that may be broken down into smaller units for search purposes. Conversely, it may be a relatively small area (a garden or a defined element of woodland). Some searches may be site- or scenario-based, that is, radiating out from a single point according to the place the missing person was last seen (place last seen – PLS) or to their last known position (LKP) (ACPO 2011a, 27). However, most searches for graves, and particularly those where the information is limited, will involve the investigation of wider areas without defined starting points and this places particular demands on search organisation and resources as well as on mapping.

Of course, some clandestine burials have nothing to do with human remains: they can also encompass items that are concealed temporarily and that can be recovered at a later date. The manner in which these items and buried bodies are concealed differs in terms of *intent* and they present different parameters for search. Concealment on a permanent basis usually involves the burials of victims undertaken in order to avoid detection. The offender anticipates that the body will never be found again and great lengths may be taken in order to prevent discovery. By contrast, temporary concealment embodies the intention of recovery, re-use and probable re-concealment afterwards in the same place; it usually involves materials such as firearms, drugs or money and the location will necessarily be marked in such a way that it can be re-located with reasonable ease. In these cases the route to the burial may be re-enacted through 'winthropping' – a technique that uses natural landscape features to guide a person to a specific place – or by reference to an easily distinguishable landscape feature such as a wall end or large tree from which the location of the cache can be identified. A clandestine human burial occupies, on average, barely more than 1 sq m of surface terrain (assuming a grave size of *c.* 1.8×0.6 m); a cache will probably occupy as little as one fifth of that area and is commensurately difficult to identify. The main difference, however, is that the cache will need to be readily accessible and easy to find; it may be more frequently visited, a fact which in itself may present search opportunities through the detection of damaged vegetation either visually or thermally (below). These elements will need to be factored into any search strategy.

However, the distinctions between permanent and temporary concealments are not always clear cut. Many clandestine graves are marked in a way which will allow a perpetrator to re-visit the scene for peace of mind, or to check for any disturbances or animal activity. Statistics demonstrate that offenders tend not to dispose of their victims in random locations, they invariably use places familiar to them, or to where return is possible. A case in point is the disposal pattern of Ian Brady, whose burials of children in the Lancashire/Yorkshire moors in north England in the 1960s were marked by photographs he took of his partner Myra Hindley standing or squatting on each site against a characteristic landscape feature (Figure 2.2). In cases like this marking need not be specific, but with buried firearms or drugs it is more essential to have the exact location marked. Marking can take many forms – a small pile of stones or a piece of wood embedded in the ground – something that will allow the individual to locate, recover and conceal again rapidly. In a case in which a female estate agent was kidnapped, the offender buried the ransom money in Lincolnshire in a fairly remote location surrounded by small shrubs. The location lay at the top of a railway embankment which he could justifiably access by means of his hobby (train spotting). The holdall containing the money was buried just out of view from nearby fields and houses, and was marked by a small heap of bricks.

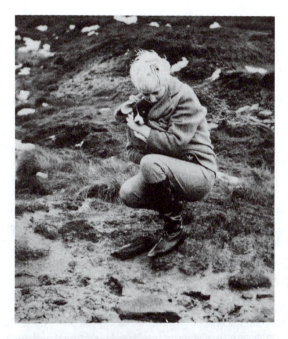

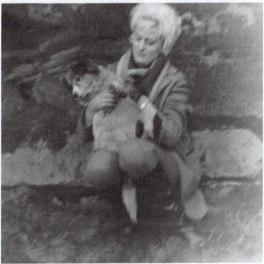

Figure 2.2 The so-called 'Moors Murders'. Top: a photograph taken by Ian Brady shows his partner Myra Hindley crouching over a landscape feature that later transpired to be the grave of John Kilbride. Bottom: Another of Brady's photographs possibly representing a further burial in a location as yet unidentified. Note the characteristic shape of the rock in the background. Images by courtesy of Duncan Staff.

The importance of *intention* in burying remains has an interesting history. The English law known as Treasure Trove, which was drawn up in medieval times and was replaced in 1996 by the Treasure Act (HMSO 1996b), was also concerned with intention, that is, whether a person in antiquity concealed or buried something in the ground for safe keeping with the intention of taking it out on some future occasion (e.g. a coin hoard), or whether the intention was to leave it there permanently (e.g. a gold torc placed in a grave or presented as a votive offering in a sacred bog). The implications were significant: if it could be proven that the intention was to recover, then the 'treasure' was deemed to belong to the Crown; if not, it went to the finder. This placed the Crown's agent, the Coroner, in whose jurisdiction these thorny matters lay, in the invidious position of having to read the intention and state of mind of an individual living several thousand years ago. In these present contexts, however, the issue of intention has ramifications only for how the concealment might be detected. The contents of any clandestine burial, irrespective of intention, will be of forensic value and require specific approaches in recovery (Section 6.1) – a requirement not always fully recognised in search experiments for non-human concealments (Rezos *et al.* 2010).

2.2 Landscape mapping

Landscape mapping is a formal process which is undertaken automatically by most search groups and individuals on the basis of intuition and experience. At the simplest level it considers landscapes from a variety of standpoints based on rational and practical search parameters, usually by allowing landscape division into workable search zones often referred to as 'domains'. In most cases these domains are defined by features of *linear* character: some of these features can be purely natural, for example rivers, streambeds or significant contour breaks such as ridges or plateaus; others can be quasi-natural such as woodland edges or hedgerows, or they can be cultural (man-made) such as fence lines, fields, roads or trackways (Figure 2.3). To some extent they can be tailored to suit: Ruffell and McKinley cite one example in which local watersheds were used on the basis that waterflow was important to the enquiry (2008, 29f). Essentially, boundaries constitute any feature which reflects discontinuity in the landscape and allow it to be divided into convenient units for search purposes. Their size may sometimes be determined as being an area that can be completed during the working day or shift allocated (ACPO 2006, 130), thus minimising areas being overlooked between shifts or not being recorded fully. Most searches will give each domain or unit area of search a reference number or code which will be used for cross-referencing date, weather, time, personnel and other records.

Reference to contours on a map is important in a number of ways: three-dimensional representation allows the terrain to be manipulated and interrogated more effectively using Geographical Information Systems (GIS); contours can present a more realistic understanding of landform to guide the strength, duration and deployment of manpower, and they also allows analysis and prioritisation of individual domains to be conducted at desk-top level. In instances of 'cold' cases these features can also provide controls for comparing historic maps and aerial photographs to record landscape change or evolution, or for providing reference points for the rectification of oblique aerial images.

The map is the basic tool of search (ACPO 2011a, 25–7) and comes in many forms and scales. Maps are usually treated as empirical in that they represent some form of absolute truth about landforms and features. In the UK, while the latest Ordnance Survey (OS) maps

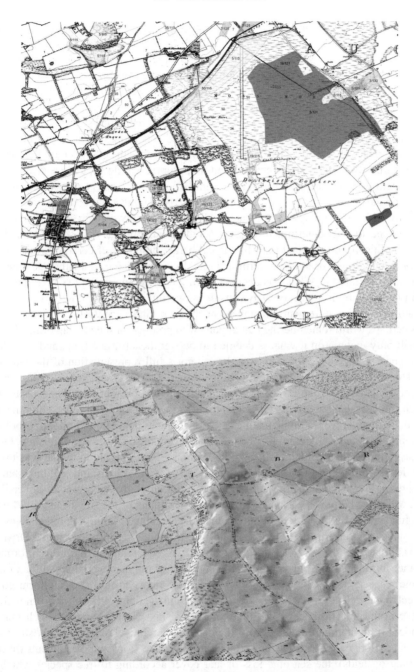

Figure 2.3 Overlying maps showing current and 'historic' landscape features for breaking down into domains. The top image shows area of shading for Historic Landscape Assessment purposes (HLA data from RCAHMS) and the bottom image shows the use of underlying contour. Image by courtesy of K. Colls on behalf of Birmingham Archaeology.

have been produced from aerial images since post-war times, the level of detail is only at the resolution that the mapping service considers appropriate for general need. It would be wrong to consider any map as being a wholly objective representation of landscape character. There is inevitably an interpretative or subjective element of record involved, and while this may be relatively consistently maintained in modern times through digital aerial recording which began in the later part of the 20th century, earlier maps exhibit a much greater degree of cognitive influence as a result of using more manual survey methods. In the earliest OS editions places and features were mapped according to contemporary criteria, and place names were recorded by sappers (Royal Engineers – the OS was initially set up for military purpose) in locations where they felt it appropriate to do so, and were logged in a form of spelling of personal choosing. The 'Name Books' or 'Parish Name Books' in which these field notes were kept are now part of national record collections and illustrate well the manner by which these maps were created. All maps probably contain some level of bias, which may be socially determined (e.g. by including inhabited as opposed to uninhabited houses), politically determined (e.g. by the deliberate omission of certain government or military installations), or tourist determined (e.g. by emphasising footpaths and amenities for hikers or motorists). What was deemed worthy of mapping in the OS first editions of the mid 19th century is not necessarily considered worthy of mapping now and *vice versa* – time, attitudes and requirements change as much as the landscape itself.

It is perhaps worth remembering that anyone who produces a sketch plan or hand-drawn map will only include on it what is deemed to be significant at the time, and is included for the purpose for which the map was drawn, not a full representation of the landscape in question. That has important ramifications in search terms. Maps reflect only what the cartographer chooses to depict, not necessarily what is fully present on the landscape, either through choice, the nature of the technique used, or the level of detail reflected in the scale of the map. In other words, some features are drawn out as being more important (or basic) and, hence by definition, the importance (or value) of other features is diminished. One of the illustrations below (Figure 2.4, top) shows a large scale digital map that was used to find a deposition. It shows basic features such as roads, field lines and buildings but will not represent the steep slope down from the road to where the body was discovered, the bog in which the body was located, nor the dense scrubland of the site itself – all of which are of fundamental importance to both planning a search and identifying target areas. The same applies to urban areas (Figure 2.4, bottom). In search terms (and in a true Orwellian sense) all aspects of the landscape have to be treated as equal until such time as information and other introduced criteria suggest that some aspects might be more equal than others. In some respects, it is wisest to use maps only as primary spatial and landform guides, irrespective of scale: they are no substitute for being in the field, although this is not always possible in the first instance. Also, there are often 'historical' elements which may not be evident from map-based data even if the disposal is relatively recent. Many short-lived historical factors can affect feasibility including land use (for example the cultivation or ploughing of fields), the seasonal loss of leaf cover according to tree species which can affect concealment factors, or the changing hours of darkness/lightness during the year.

The 1:50,000 (2 cm to 1 km) OS map series is the one most commonly available commercially (marketed as the 'Landranger' series) and contains reasonable spatial information for general geographical purposes. It shows contours at 10 m intervals, roads, woods, tracks and buildings but is inadequate for dividing up an area for search purposes other than to

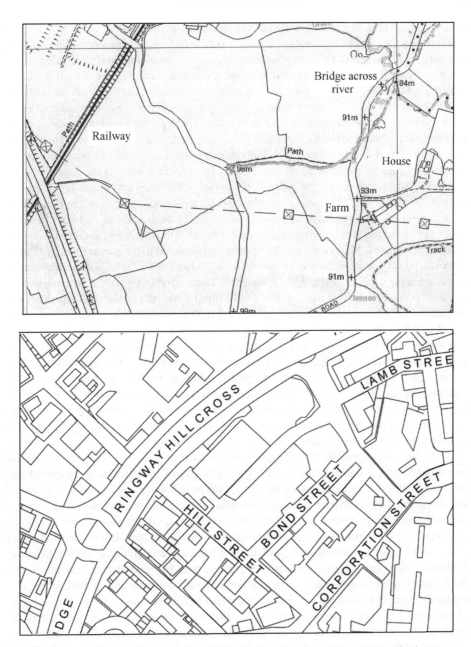

Figure 2.4 Large scale maps of (top) a rural area and (bottom) an urban area used in the recovery of missing persons. Although they depict key fixed points they lack contours, inter-visibility, points of concealment, or other useful landform features and are best used for primary planning purposes than for detailed searching. © Crown copyright 2013 Ordnance Survey.

present a broad idea of exposed, concealed or inhabited landscapes. Better is the 1:25,000 (marketed as the 'Explorer' series, 4 cm to 1 km), which shows greater detail of fields, boundaries and trackways together with increased resolution of contours, which are marked at 5 m intervals. Both the 1:50,000 and 1:25,000 series of local areas are normally available from bookshops and outdoor specialist suppliers; alternatively, maps for all areas can be ordered centrally from the OS or from any of a number of specialist map outlets. These outlets will also be able to supply what many consider to be the optimum scale of paper map for field purposes – the OS 1:10,000 series (marketed as 'Landplan') – which provides even greater detail at a size that can be workable in the field; the scale is especially useful in more complex town and suburban landscapes. The 1:10,000 series is the largest to show contours. Larger scale maps are particularly useful when a search area is localised and most police forces have access to, or subscribe to, digital mapping services that enable them to print out detailed maps at a specified scale. The scale chosen, however, needs to reflect the size of the area being searched, the character of the landscape in question and the methods being used. Maps will need to be of sufficient detail to be able to identify defined reference points for work on the ground; they will also need to be at a scale that can be annotated in the field, shaded and scribbled on. In large searches two scales of maps may be needed – a smaller scale to cover the whole area and a larger scale for detailed aspects. Some examples of different scaled maps emphasising differences in detail and content are shown in Figure 2.5.

It is also worth emphasising that Britain is relatively well served cartographically, as are most other parts of western Europe, but many other countries do not possess similar levels of structured mapping service other than perhaps through military agencies. As a result, searches can become much more complicated and less easy to define, organise and record. For example, when working in parts of the former Yugoslavia, where large scale maps are lacking and where smaller scale maps are of limited access, the value of the UK's OS resource can be fully appreciated.

Most maps are available digitally and can be used at desk-top level to provide the background for GIS manipulation and analysis (for a general introduction see Burrough and McDonnell 1998). GIS is now an everyday tool for just about any task that requires spatial understanding, from land management and planning to mountaineering and archaeological fieldwork. For the purposes of this particular application, GIS is no more than a digital representation of the present landscape based on the humble map; it can be made as simple or as complicated as the search requires, and it can be manipulated according to needs. It allows, for example, geographically referenced data to be managed, interpreted and displayed in order to investigate relationships or to provide a simple, visual image of a landscape that can be understood by all concerned. Digital maps come in two types – vector (coordinate-based) or raster (pixel-based). Both have different properties and potentials, their relative merits are discussed at length in the relevant literature (e.g. Chainey and Ratcliffe 2005) and a number of applications can be demonstrated (Ruffell and McKinley 2008, ch. 5). At a simple level, it allows the search to overlie or 'drape' various attributes that may be relevant, such as land use, type of soil, geology, distances from vehicle access points and so on. Orengo (2008) has demonstrated its application as a predictive model for locating disposal sites in Leicestershire using similar criteria; he used colour trends to weight more heavily areas further away from urban centres, and emphasised roads as being key to body transportation. Also factored into the model was the importance of the passenger side of the

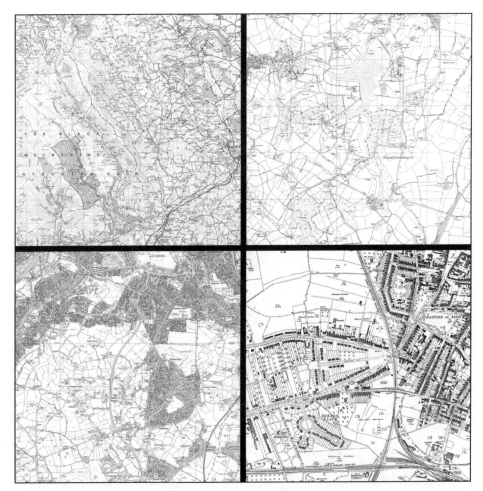

Figure 2.5 Examples of different scaled maps illustrating differences in detail: top left scale 1:50,000; top right scale 1:25,000; bottom left scale 1:10,000; bottom right scale 1:5,000. © Crown copyright 2013 Ordnance Survey. (*For colour details please see colour plate section.*)

vehicle (for removal of body) and the downslope side of the road (for dragging purposes). At more complex levels, data such as these can be manipulated and integrated with other data, and the landscape recreated as a three-dimensional digital terrain model (DTM) enabling it to be rotated and viewed from different aspects. DTM is sometimes confused with digital elevation modelling (DEM), which is more strictly concerned with a more comprehensive elevation view of features which include the ground. DTM is used throughout here as reflecting the value of the ground surface proper as being the main subject of interest.

DTM is an advancement of simple mapping in that it allows the contours, which show height on a map, to be generated three-dimensionally on a computer screen (Figure 2.6). This presents a much clearer understanding of the topography and allows the landscape to be viewed from any chosen angle or aspect. It also enables the viewer to 'fly through'

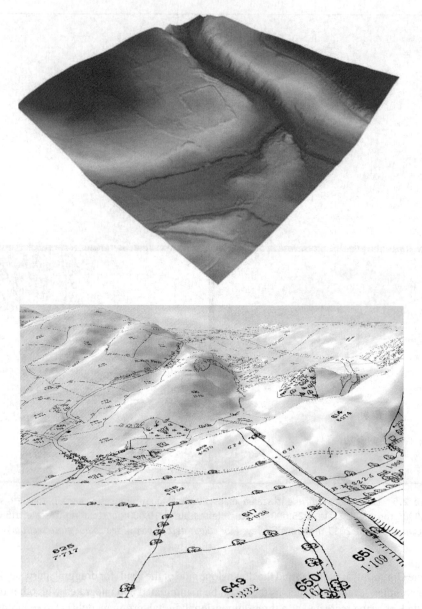

Figure 2.6 Examples of computer-generated digital terrain models (DTMs) of the Trent Valley. Image by courtesy of K. Colls and P. Breeze on behalf of Birmingham Archaeology.

the three-dimensional model on screen, changing direction or altitude as appropriate. An experienced reader of maps can probably carry out the same process mentally, but one significant advantage of DTM is that it presents all viewers with a much clearer illustration of the main elements of a landscape including roads, tracks and slopes, and the relationship between each. At a preliminary search stage this can enable the logistics of a search to be planned more effectively, and without visiting the site. But its real forensic advantage lies in its three-dimensional capability in allowing areas of concealment from roads and buildings to be more easily identified, vehicle access points to be better understood in relation to potential disposal sites, and severity of slope and ease of movement to be better evaluated. Other elements can be incorporated, including draping of features such as current land use, viewsheds (an area of the environment visible from a fixed vantage point), domains searched/not searched, aerial images and geophysical survey results, all scaled appropriately. It can even be viewed in shadow by altering the position of the computer-generated 'sun' to show landscape in shade at different times of the day. Used creatively, GIS provides potential for both planning a search and for assessing the value of particular target areas.

Earlier maps can also contain different information from more modern maps and are often a useful asset in assessing landscape or land use change and showing earlier access routes, abandoned buildings, wells, mine shafts and former watercourses which may have been known to an offender. Using GIS these can be imported in digital form and superimposed over modern maps to enhance the spatial data historically (see Figure 2.3). Earlier editions of maps are probably available in most county record archives, as well as on some internet sites, notably the Edinburgh University *Edina* site, which has a full range of maps dating from the early 19th century available at various scales that can be used for comparative purposes. Edina's *Roam* series enables the user to view a landscape at 12 pre-set scales (1:50,000 down to 1:1,250), although the largest scale with contours is only 1:25,000). Geology and land use maps can be used to provide complementary information regarding what strata are likely to exist below ground and what vegetation can be expected above ground respectively. In short it is possible to research general landscape history quite comprehensively without leaving the office and, in urban areas, this can be supported further by reference to planning history (see Section 5.7).

2.3   Remote sensing

Complementary to mapping is a range of other resources that fall under the broad heading of 'remote sensing'. This involves the application of techniques such as aerial photography, satellite imaging and some methods of geophysical survey; these can provide information about a landscape in a completely non-invasive manner. Of these the use of aerial photography is perhaps best known and can be exploited, either by using existing aerial images or by commissioning new ones, according to need. Existing images can illustrate landscape changes over time and are particularly useful in ascertaining the (pre-crime) character of domains in terms of buildings, open spaces and relevant concealment features in relation to the current (post-crime) character of the same domains (for a recent example see Ruffell *et al.* 2009; also for war graves see Albicht 2010). These are especially helpful in cold cases where it becomes necessary to understand how a landscape of deposition may have changed over an intervening 10, 20 or even 30 years (see also Section 5.3). Woodlands or scrub growth may have expanded, quarrying moved, buildings created and, for example in moorland environments, peat exposures may have eroded or shifted significantly over time. The landscape available for disposal may have been very different than it appears today.

Aerial photographs taken since the last war provide a valuable resource and a remarkably wide coverage of both urban and rural landscapes in the UK. Images have been taken for a wide range of planning, land use and commercial reasons by both central and local governments as well as by commercial and military users. Most of these photographs are in the public domain, and although altitudes differ and usefulness varies, they are normally all of high quality and can usually be depended upon to provide a range of images spread across the last 50 years. Sometimes complementary or overlying images taken at different times can increase an understanding of a potential deposition location. Collections of aerial photographs are normally housed within local authority planning departments or archives where they can be consulted. There is also a central facility located in Swindon, Wiltshire under the curation of English Heritage. Other important collections are held in the Unit for Landscape Modelling at the University of Cambridge (formerly the Cambridge University Committee for Aerial Photography) and the National Collection of Aerial Photographs (NCAP) held by the Royal Commission on the Ancient and Historical Monuments of Scotland, Edinburgh which includes a global collection of several million aerial images taken during World War II (see also Cowley *et al.* 2010a; Ferguson 2011). Further information regarding the history, theory and usefulness of aerial photography in the detection of shallow sub-surface remains has been outlined by Bewley (2006).

'Google' images, particularly 'Google Earth', may have an underestimated part to play here: these images can be freely downloaded from the internet and depict landscapes at scales to suit the viewer, although resolution can vary. Their main advantage lies in the viewer being able to perceive spatial relationships and land use at the time of image capture, but they are 'flat' and require the third dimension supplied by DTM to be of optimum value. The integration of landscape mapping can be further enhanced by exploiting aerial photography, either by drawing on existing images taken over the last 50 years by the military or local authorities, or by commissioning new images of specific areas. If required these can be ortho-rectified to remove distortion to provide a true-to-life 'flat' image and imported into a GIS analysis (Figure 2.7).

The commissioning of new aerial images can serve several purposes, the most obvious being an overview of a target area in order to assess the nature of the landscape, obstacles and potential difficulties not evident on maps. This is particularly relevant if the approach is necessarily covert, for example in a house garden or small-holding where a single aerial sortie can provide the required information (e.g. the presence of paving, hard standing, lawns, trees and sheds) without arousing suspicion. In other circumstances aerial photographs may detect buried features, which manifest themselves as anomalous vegetation growth or plant succession from shadows and soil marks. The construction, the deposition of a body and the backfilling of a clandestine grave can result in a differential growth pattern with the ground level vegetation cover, and a basic knowledge of the first plants to colonise a freshly disturbed area can be extremely useful in locating the grave without stripping away the ground vegetation and assist in dating the burial. These are the stress resistant ruderals, which quickly colonise freshly disturbed ground, for example: Common Nettle (*Urtica diocia*); Broadleaved Dock (*Rumex obtusifolius*); Creeping Thistle (*Cirsium arvense*); Spear Thistle (*Cirsium vulgare*); Welted Thistle (*Carduus crispus*), and Bramble (*Rubus fruticosus agg.*).

These phenomena are well documented (e.g. France *et al.* 1997; Hunter and Cox 2005, ch. 2; Powell 2010, ch. 3) and need not be amplified here (see also Section 7.3), although Powell's additional observations on the value of upcast as a vegetation modifier, as well as a longer-term indicator of ground disturbance, is worthy of additional mention (2010, 96 and 98–101). Suffice it to say that the mere disturbance of the ground, especially in a

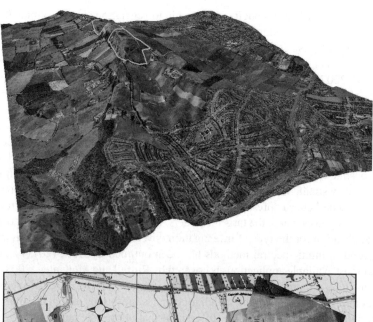

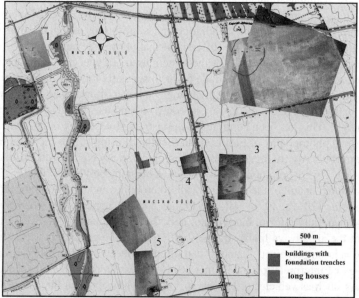

Figure 2.7 Superimposition of aerial photographs: top, full coverage over a DTM at Barr Beacon. Image by courtesy of K. Colls and P. Breeze on behalf of Birmingham Archaeology; bottom, partial coverage over a simple contoured map of a Hungarian landscape. Image by courtesy of Zoltán Czajlik. (*For colour details please see colour plate section.*)

relatively undisturbed area, may have a distinct impact on the immediate surface vegetation or on the manner in which the nature of the disturbed soil may exhibit change. These can be long-term effects but may only be evident according to angle of light, growth season or land use. Change may also be exacerbated by the human decay products present in a burial. Human decay itself has been the subject of much research (e.g. Haglund and Sorg

1997, 2002a; Vass *et al.* 2002) but its relationship to vegetation change, although observed (e.g. France *et al.* 1997), continues to remain a neglected source of research. Some recent experimentation suggests its effects are minimal (Powell 2010, 91; Caccianiga *et al.* 2012), although recorded changes in both microbial activity and pH resulting from decomposition (Wilson *et al.* 2007) might be expected to have some vegetation impact.

The use of specialised imaging, notably deploying the infrared (IR) and near infrared (NIR) parts of the spectrum, has been used to determine differences in vegetation growth stages to be observed as well as in identifying disturbed ground through stressed vegetation reflecting discrete biological or physical changes (e.g. Ruffell and McKinley 2008, ch. 4); these have obvious implications not only for individual burials and mass graves, but also for other clandestine activities including buried firearms, drugs and contraband, although the scale here is very small. Though not within the visible wavelengths, these differences have the potential to be better expressed through the NIR part of the spectrum, particularly in relation to mass graves where the target is larger. Although relevant, NIR is felt to be of less practical application for the type of investigation covered here and is not discussed further. A background to multi-spectral methods has been outlined by Beck (2011) and a useful analysis of most available applications is covered by Ruffell and McKinley (2008, 110–14).

What has to be remembered, however, and in common with most remote sensing techniques that have been applied to the search for clandestine burials, is that the area of interest is frustratingly small and the level of differential that allows the anomaly to be observed often lies outside the detection limits of the system used. Targets can simply be too small to be detected accurately from high altitude flights (especially military photographs) or can be hidden by obstructions according to flight angle at lower altitude (see also Powell 2010, 101). Crop marks and shadow marks rely not only on land use, but also on season and on angle of sunlight. This has been admirably demonstrated by Cowley in his analysis of the systematic aerial photography of East Lothian (Scotland) using sorties recorded from 1977 and later, from 1992. Approximately 160 archaeological sites were recorded in total, but less than 10% of these were common to both sorties, a phenomenon he ascribed to, *inter alia*, differing moisture content of the ground, localised cropping and methodology, all of which can cause biasing (2011a, 49 fig. 4.7; see Figure 2.8). A single sortie, whether historical or commissioned, may inform, but will not necessarily eliminate. Moreover, a landscape viewed from the air always looks strangely different on the ground, not least in contour and in scale, and its perceived 'flatness' can often be deceiving (for wider discussion on knowledge-based interpretation see Palmer 2011). Unless there are features that can act as scale markers, such as vehicles or houses, it is easy to misrepresent the nature and extent of a search area. In one of the authors' cases the interpretation of a commissioned aerial photograph by police identified a search area as being 'about the size of a tennis court'. A strategy (including deployment of a small mechanical excavator) was devised on this basis but was found to be wholly inadequate on arrival at the scene. What had been interpreted as hedges were in fact lines of large trees, and what had been interpreted as a dry ground surface was substantially waterlogged. Given the equipment and personnel deployed, the operation took several times longer than anticipated.

More useful, but harder to define in temporal terms, is the phenomenon of heat emitted from a corpse during the decay process. This has been recognised for some time (e.g. Rodriguez and Bass 1985; Millar *et al.* 2002). This temperature level in the grave, which can be significantly higher than the temperature level of the surrounding ground, occurs

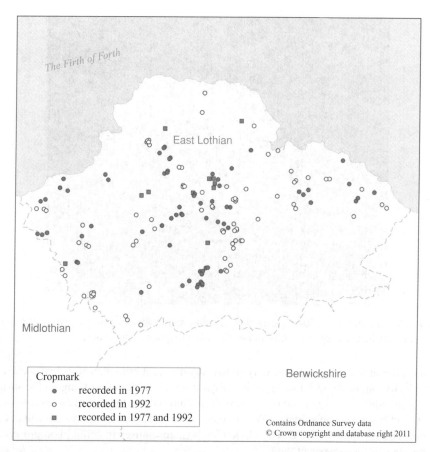

Figure 2.8 Plan showing discrepancy between sites identified under different conditions (Image courtesy of RCAHMS. © Crown copyright: RCAHMS. Licensor www.rcahms.gov.uk). (*For colour details please see colour plate section.*)

only when the body reaches a specific stage of decomposition. The point at which this commences can be accelerated or hindered by a range of environmental and contextual factors such as clothing, depth of burial, soil type, temperature and climate. The actual duration of the main heat emission depends on similar factors, and typically continues in terms of days rather than weeks, although longer-term temperature changes have also been observed (Wilson *et al.* 2007); indeed, there is some evidence to show that the soil temperature of a large burial ground or cemetery is *consistently* higher than surrounding soils as a result of high levels of bacteriological activity (Prangnell and McGowan 2009). However, detecting this window of opportunity in a single clandestine grave depends on as much knowledge of the burial as possible and, on the basis of daily temperature changes, might involve persistent flying in order to obviate false assurances of landscape elimination. In addition, freshly disturbed ground, particularly during hotter months, may lose its heat differentially to surrounding undisturbed ground during the cooling part of the day, typically in the early hours of the morning (Scollar *et al.* 1990). This differential can be detected using

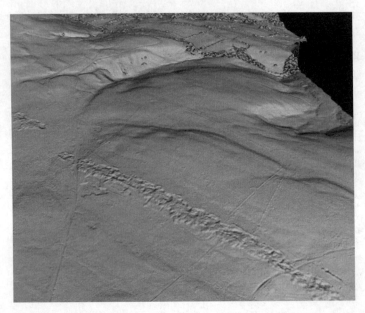

Figure 2.9   Example of a LiDAR image that captures subtle topographic change on the ground surface. Image by courtesy of K. Colls on behalf on Birmingham Archaeology.

thermal photography, but unfortunately so will any innocent ground disturbance caused, for example, by gardening or building, or quietly rotting domestic refuse lying on the surface. The cooling differential may be observable until such time as the disturbance ceases to be 'fresh' and becomes consolidated. Police forces in the UK have access to the Joint Aerial Reconnaissance Intelligence Centre (JARIC) which specialises in aerial photography and interpreting all these types of data.

A further airborne application, based on laser scanning, is a light detection and ranging system (normally abbreviated to 'LiDAR') which has the ability to present a three-dimensional model of the ground surface within which topographic change can be identified (for detail see, for example, Wehr and Lohr 1999) (Figure 2.9). This is a relatively new technique as applied to forensic investigation and merits some evaluation as it offers a considerably more enhanced resolution of surface topography than that of OS contour mapping. It operates by transmitting laser pulses from an aircraft and measuring the time taken for the reflection pulse to return, thus calculating the distance between the aircraft sensor and the points at which the pulses hits the ground surface. Accurate measurement of the aircraft's position by using a Global Positioning System (GPS) attached to the aircraft's sensor array, or by reference to fixed points on the ground, allows each point to be given full x, y and z coordinates. By transmitting thousands of pulses it becomes possible to generate a point cloud that can be converted into a three-dimensional model of the ground surface to create a digital terrain model (DTM). This then allows the model to be imported into GIS software for shading, simulated lighting/shadow angles and other enhancement techniques (Figure 2.10). The greater the number of points measured across a given area, the greater the resolution that can be achieved. LiDAR has the ability to collect vast quantities of data at high speed and has considerable application in viewing archaeological landscapes or

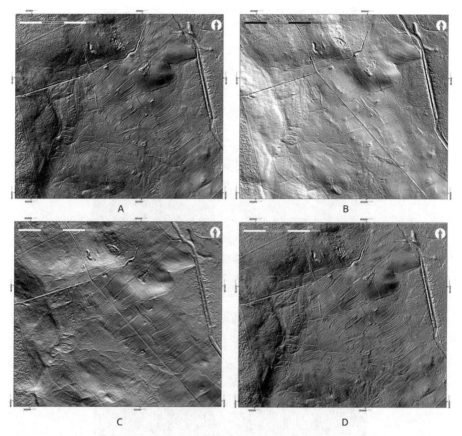

Figure 2.10 Four LiDAR images of the same landscape showing the effects of different computer-generated lighting angles. Images by courtesy of AOC Archaeology.

large areas of ground cover for military, land use, infrastructure planning or environmental application, such as flood risks. A useful overview and outline of applications, particularly in archaeology, has been compiled by Crutchley and Crow (2009); more broadly-based applications of laser scanning can be found in a sister English Heritage publication (Jones 2011; see also below).

LiDAR scanning is mostly used for wider landscape coverage and can present a number of problems in locating smaller scale features such as individual graves. It assumes in the first instance that the grave, or spreads of spoil and disturbance caused by digging the grave, will have some form of measurable topographic expression. A main issue is one of size, in that the typical number of points taken per square metre (normally averaging between one and four) that is adequate for large linear features such as buried ditches and field systems, might fail to meet the resolution required to identify a grave measuring, say 1.75 × 0.75 m, as a clearly detectable landscape feature. In theory this can be overcome by increasing the point density or by repeated and overlap flying. Archaeological work in Ireland, for example, has successfully used up to 60 points per metre to produce high

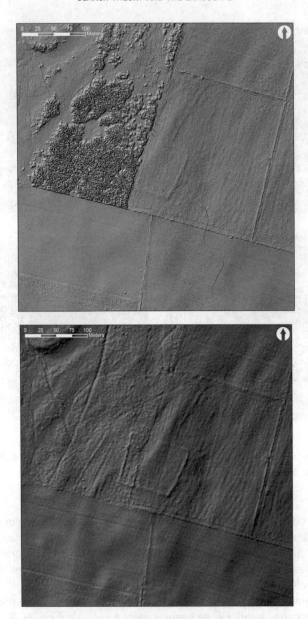

Figure 2.11 LiDAR images showing an unfiltered (top) and filtered (bottom) landscape. Images by courtesy of AOC Archaeology.

resolution mapping of an archaeological landscape by using a helicopter, which allows the point density to be increased by flying at a slower speed (Corns *et al*. 2008; Jones 2011, Case Study 11). In doing so it was possible to see the footprint of an excavation undertaken some 50 years earlier (Shaw and Corns 2011, 81 fig. 6.6). The LiDAR images reproduced here (Figures 2.9, 2.10 and 2.11) were recorded at approximately seven points per metre. On the downside, increased point density also serves to increase the already huge quantity of data requiring processing and storage and thus causes an expediential increase in expense. Although some compensation for this can be made by covering smaller areas (i.e. narrowing of the search area), it assumes that the likely location of the grave can be fairly well targeted, whereas in many cases even the general location of the grave is unknown and necessitates the coverage of more substantial tracts of landscape. Identification of large (i.e. mass) graves (typically *c.* 15–20 × 3 m in size) is less of an issue in that the relative scale of the topographic expression is substantially greater and the need for higher resolution commensurately less (see Chapter 8). LiDAR's effectiveness also relies on there being a recognisable topographical distinction between the (sunken) fill of a grave, or the slumped part of a grave edge, and the surrounding land surface that is measurable within the limits of the technique. Here experimental observations by Powell are discouraging in noting that her research graves only exhibited visible depressions after two years (2010, 98), although topographical change caused by animal scavenging and burrowing was fairly persistent throughout the recorded history of the sites (*ibid.*, 62–69). The LiDAR limit is normally around 100 mm in a depth/height dimension, although the measurements are relative and this figure can be slightly reduced. This may sound an unrealistically large differential for a grave, but one which might easily be met or even exceeded if one takes into account piles of spoil and a partial consolidated slumping of a grave fill which together might present a specific signature. Existing archaeological LiDAR surveys would suggest that it is the physical size of the grave as opposed to its topographic expression which is the main difficulty to overcome. A LiDAR survey of the landscape around Stonehenge, Wiltshire using a point density between only 0.5 and 2.0 m was able to detect low banks that were not evident visually (Bewley *et al.* 2005); this demonstrates LiDAR's effectiveness in defining even subtle features at low resolution that are visually apparent neither in the field nor from the air. In terms of length and width these banks were substantial features, but Crow *et al.* (2007) were able to detect much smaller features – individual charcoal pits around 5 m in diameter – under tree cover in the Forest of Dean using a similar point resolution.

The presence of tree canopy is a further issue: laser pulses can be inhibited from reflecting off a solid ground surface ground by leaves, branches and trunks, not to mention undergrowth such as brambles and scrub. Waiting until a season of minimal leaf cover and low vegetation will lessen this problem but is not normally an option under forensic circumstances. However, a more accurate terrain model can be achieved by filtering out the initial pulses that reflect from the canopy and measuring only the residual pulses that penetrate the canopy and return from the ground (known as the 'last return'). The benefits of this have been recognised in an archaeological context (e.g. Devereux *et al.* 2005) and algorithms can be used in order to filter out unwanted targets allowing the 'true' or 'bare' ground surface to be modelled, effectively biasing the type of small features required. The effects of this can be seen on Figure 2.11, which illustrates a comparison between an unfiltered and a filtered image, the latter allowing the true ground surface to be seen below the vegetation. Because tree trunks are solid and will reflect in the same manner as the ground surface, these will also need to be stripped out later. LiDAR will only detect what is there, and that includes background 'noise' from other landscape elements, including geology, tree hollows and artificial elements, which will all need to be interpreted and, if necessary, removed from the collected data. A more recent development of LiDAR records 'full wave form' to allow more sophisticated processing, effectively dealing with vegetation issues (see Doneus and

Briese 2011), but with potentially more complex data manipulation and software issues. Existing work has shown its ability to 'strip' away ground vegetation and expose badger setts at even relatively low point densities (*ibid.*, 63 fig. 5.3), indicating the way to more appropriate forensic application.

Initially, the technique sounds less than promising in forensic application, but it appears to work well in some archaeological contexts where relatively small features are being detected. Moreover, unlike conventional aerial photographs, the method is not dependent on season, light and shadow. It produces a model of the terrain surface, subject to the impact of vegetation, snow or leaf litter. Additionally, it is also possible to measure the *intensity* of the reflected pulse as well as its speed. This has the potential to identify different expressions of ground surfaces and might, for example, be used to determine differences in ground moisture retention on the basis of reduced intensity of signal on return indicating wet ground, and some assessment work has been carried out in attempting to identify surface waterlogged deposits (Challis *et al.* 2008). In theory, therefore, this might also apply to ground that has been disturbed in the digging of a grave and which has become water retentive as a result. In addition, measurement of intensity data can also be used to identify certain vegetation differences that are not evident visually. Alteration to the soil chemistry in a grave brought about by human decay processes can affect the way vegetation growing above the grave will reflect light. LiDAR uses wavelengths within the infrared range and, as chlorophyll in plants is a good reflector of near infrared radiation (NIR), any changes in chlorophyll content resulting from localised change to the soil chemistry might be interpreted through its reflectance properties. This has already been the subject of successful research into locating mass graves (Kalacska *et al.* 2009) although not at the reduced level of scale required here. However, observations that experimental individual graves remained vegetationally distinctive for several years (Powell 2010, 98–101) may encourage further research in this area.

In short, LiDAR has the potential rather than the attested application for finding clandestine graves – a potential that depends more on the limitations of surface expression through size and subtlety than on the principles which underlie the system. In its favour is the opportunity for the investigator to make a speedy record and analysis of large tracts of landscape, including woodland, for ground disturbances without a physical presence in the field. This offers a good covert advantage as well as maintaining evidential preservation. The derived images, normally in DTM form, can be imported into a GIS package together with aerial photographic images for comparative purposes, and manipulated and enhanced accordingly. Targets can be earmarked in a cost-effective way for further investigation on the basis of either topographic or vegetation criteria. On the downside, the survey will need to be commissioned and may have a significant cost implication, although this can be balanced against the costs of deploying large numbers of search officers in the field (including access, transport, equipment, etc.) with the relative ease of desk-top analysis. Many areas in the UK already have LiDAR coverage (for example, see the coverage provided by the Environment Agency: http://www2.getmapping.com/Products/LiDAR), but unless the scanning took place since the victim was last seen, and to the appropriate resolution, then it will need to be repeated. Nevertheless, even existing scans have their uses as they can provide a ready-made DTM for determining search domains and organising logistics. The key difficulties in using LiDAR to find graves, as opposed to simply viewing landscapes, are the size of the target and the distinctiveness of its landscape expression. But even here LiDAR provides an opportunity to provide a remote analysis of an entire landscape and provide a terrain model that can be investigated on the ground, target by target, in a consistent and systematic way.

There may also be occasions when a relatively small area of land needs to be surveyed for more subtle changes in contour, below that of airborne LiDAR capability, which reflect ground disturbance, for example if a witness is insistent on a burial location within a defined given area. Automated laser scanning can also be undertaken from non-airborne platforms and has a range of applications in recording buildings and even artefacts where a static position allows tens of thousands of points to be collected every minute (Jones 2011). Known as terrestrial laser scanning, its application in landscape modelling is limited to relatively small areas and ideally requires a series of elevated positions, but the level of resolution can be considerable in compensation. Research suggests that a 1 cm topographical distinction on the ground would require a 0.5 mm point density to have a 95% certainty of visibility in the data; a 10 cm topographical distinction would require a 5 mm point density to have a similar level of certainty (Jones 2011, table 2). This lies within the capabilities of the technique but may require severe delimitation of boundaries according to topography and position of platform.

In relatively small search areas manual terrestrial methods can also be deployed, most often a differential global positioning system (GPS) which can be used to take a series of

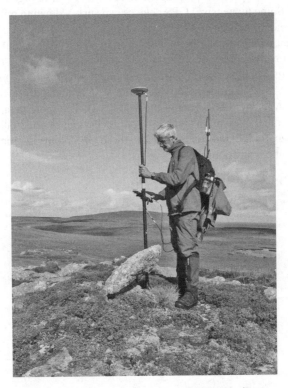

Figure 2.12 Surveying using GPS. Image by courtesy of RCAHMS. (Image courtesy of RCAHMS. © Crown copyright: RCAHMS. Licensor www.rcahms.gov.uk).

close-set traverses (less than 0.5 m) to create a local terrain model. There are various systems available that allow appropriate accuracy but which involve the presence of a fixed base station receiver and a carried mobile receiver (Figure 2.12) or connection via a mobile SIM card. The fixed base station makes simultaneous measurements to satellites and rectifies or minimises many of the errors encountered using (cheaper) hand-held devices giving x/y coordinate accuracy of within 1 m. More pertinently, providing the mobile receiver can be carried or pulled along the ground at a consistent height, it also has the potential to provide high resolution measurement of the z coordinate (height). This in turn enables a three-dimensional model of the ground surface to be created. Although manual and relatively slow it has the advantage of not requiring reference points (these are provided automatically by the GPS) and can be undertaken by one or two operators in relatively small locations. Areas of anomalous contour that may not be visible to the naked eye, as a result of vegetation growth, shadow or light, can be identified providing that the ground surface can be followed by the operator; these anomalies can subsequently be logged and investigated invasively.

The same instrumentation can be used to 'fix' reference points for a geophysical survey area enabling it to be imported into a GIS model in the absence of any other map-based reference features, or to locate peripheral points of a crime scene, items of recovered evidence, or even the grave itself before any excavation commences. This level of accuracy (<1 m) is more than adequate for plotting on most of the paper or digital mapping systems likely to be used. Some (expensive) GPS devices can survey down to millimetre levels and are widely acclaimed. Accuracy, however, is a relative factor – on a 1:10,000 map even a pencil mark indicating a particular point will cover an area with an actual diameter of about 10 m. Surveying to an accuracy of <1 m is more than adequate for these purposes as well as for the spatial record of scattered surface remains (Listi *et al.* 2007) which has similar GIS applicability. A useful guide as to which GPS system to deploy according to task and scale is given by Ainsworth and Thomason (2003, 12). The more detailed survey that is required in the eventual excavation and recovery process can be undertaken using different techniques (see Section 6.2) but can be tied into these GPS points in order to obtain a fixed position and absolute map coordinates.

3 Search application

Searching for human remains terrestrially can include many 'hands-on' methods. The most common of these are discussed in this chapter, not so much in terms of how they work, but in terms of how they can be misunderstood and the practical problems they can pose. The techniques reviewed here are those that, in the experience of the authors, are most likely to be employed: geophysical survey, cadaver dogs and mechanical excavators. A section on bodies in aqueous environments is also included. These tend to be overlooked in the literature; they pose a number of different issues which merit drawing together here.

3.1 Geophysical survey

The importance of an integrated forensic search strategy can be illustrated best by the use of geophysical survey techniques. There is now widespread acceptance of the value of shallow sub-surface geophysical analysis in finding graves, although there is somewhat less understanding of how the various systems operate and of their relative advantages and disadvantages. There are some valuable general texts that offer an archaeological focus (e.g. Clark 1996; Gaffney and Gater 2003) as well as those that are more forensically dedicated to the history of the techniques (Cheetham 2005), to their underlying theory and application (Fenning and Donnelly 2004), and to the comparison of their effective methodologies in forensic enquiries (France *et al.* 1992, 1997; Davenport 2001; Buck 2003; Killam 2004; Pringle *et al.* 2011). The use of forensic geophysics is not restricted simply to clandestine burials but has a wider forensic application that includes environmental controls, hydrology, contaminated ground, waste and landfill (see Ruffell and McKinley 2008, ch. 3). It is worth emphasising that individual techniques (typically electrical, magnetic and electro-magnetic) all respond to different physical properties of the buried environment and are not substitutes for each other. Geophysicists divide them into 'active' and 'passive' methods. Put crudely, the former stimulate the ground into response, and the latter measure what is there already. Some key factors regarding their feasibility are discussed below, but they each essentially depend on the ability to identify *differences* in the buried environment: these can be, *inter alia*, infilled ditches or pits, tree roots, foundations, cables and drains, buried rubbish, changes in the depth of bedrock, or a clandestine burial. The more subtle the differences, the harder they are to identify and the easier they are to miss. Individual techniques can discriminate between them only in as much as the operator is able to interpret the data generated. He/she may be able to identify a disturbance but it will not be possible to determine exactly what that disturbance represents, only that it represents something

Forensic Approaches to Buried Remains, First Edition. John Hunter, Barrie Simpson and Caroline Sturdy Colls.
© 2013 John Wiley & Sons, Ltd. Published 2013 by John Wiley & Sons, Ltd.

different from the surrounding sub-surface and is of a certain general size and orientation. Geophysics only presents to the operator what is there according to the techniques used; it is selective only in terms of physical properties, not of anything else. For example, if the foundations of a medieval building lie directly over a Roman villa, the survey will not necessarily respond to the medieval remains simply because they are nearer the surface. It may well be that the properties, or the range of materials to which the particular technique responds, lie more strongly within the Roman walls immediately below, in which case the result is not a fine geometrical image of either the medieval or the Roman, but an incoherent blur that encapsulates elements of both according to the levels of response of each.

In most instances a grave will be recognisable only as an anomalous sub-surface feature, not as a buried body. It is the effect resulting from burying of the cadaver (i.e. the disturbance) that may cause the response, as Powell's research has intimated (2010, 112), not necessarily the presence of the body itself, although the human decay factor will also have some part to play in this process (below). Moreover, the gradual natural compaction of a grave is itself a dynamic and is also likely to have an effect. Irrespective of the method used to find them, burials do not have an idiosyncratic geophysical signature that can be instantly recognised in the data, although some worthwhile modelling has been carried out in order to locate graves in specific local environments, both in historical contexts (e.g. Watters and Hunter 2004) and in current operations (Fiedler *et al.* 2009; Pringle and Jervis 2010; Novo *et al.* 2011).

All geophysical survey methods hold in common the need for a relatively consistent set of background readings against which any unusual or anomalous measurements might stand out. Ground which has been heavily disturbed will provide a very varied set of geophysical responses or 'noise' caused by other buried features or disturbance events within which the effects of the burial may not be readily recognisable. Forensic geophysics has developed substantially from archaeological geophysics where targets are generally both small and shallow, and are distinctive from the magnitude of target in which geologists are interested, or the intensity of target (e.g. concrete reinforcement bars) often required by engineers (see also Reynolds 2011 for a comparison of applications). Identifying the subtle difference between the consolidated disturbance caused by digging a grave many years ago and the surrounding ground into which it has been dug is one that pushes these techniques to their limits. Variation in response can also fluctuate even within a small locality, as Powell has demonstrated through experiments with buried donor cadavers as well as pigs and kangaroos (the research was conducted in Australia) (2010, ch. 6). Consequently, geophysics should not be seen as a one-off search method, but as part of a carefully chosen sequence of methodologies based on local environment and investigation circumstances.

Geophysics has the greatest potential of success if a burial is cut into otherwise relatively undisturbed or sterile ground. All of the discussed main methods are most effective on flat terrain without the encumbrance of trees, buildings, surface clutter or differing ground materials – an unlikely environment in most gardens or woodlands where scenes tend to occur. Unfortunately, many new developments in geophysical surveying are based on covering large areas and on speed of survey (Gaffney and Gaffney 2011). Using geophysical survey also effects a commitment to investigate, or at least review, all appropriate responses, not just those in areas of high interest, although these may be given priority when excavation is implemented. This means that the skill of the geophysics operator in being able to interpret the data is critical in taking the search further and in prioritising targets. The depth, shape and size of any target identified needs to be interpreted against a background of local geology, land use and site history. Experience suggests that in most cases background data will not necessarily have been evaluated before the survey commences, and thus the interpretation will be that much less viable. This is understandable if the preparations for an operation need to be carried out covertly, but it may mean that the operator will not be in a position to know which technique will work best and which to deploy. In order to avoid the 'blunderbus' approach (i.e. the indiscriminate throwing of all available techniques at the search area in question) noted by Reynolds (2011, 6), there are often resources in the public domain that can be drawn upon to provide at least some of the appropriate information, such as maps or aerial photographs that can provide basic information (for example, land use, buildings, likely tree roots, grassy areas, or compacted vehicle access surfaces) which might allow an initial choice of technique to be made.

It is worth outlining here the three key methods used in the UK and their strengths and weaknesses in a forensic context (for more detailed theory of the various techniques see, for example, Fenning and Donnelly 2004). Not all methods are equally applicable to all parts of the planet on the basis of geology, climate, terrain and land use (not to mention disposal culture). For example, Cheetham (2005) has usefully explained the limited use of resistance survey in North America compared to its more widespread application in the UK. The three techniques listed here are those which, in the authors' experience, have been the most commonly used, or the most effective in UK situations. There are many less common techniques which may be used in specific circumstances, for example seismic, gravimetric and radiometric systems (see Ruffell and McKinley 2008, ch. 3) or others that present theoretical application but may fail on practical grounds. All methods depend on the nature of the target and the environment in which the target is assumed to be located. No single method has been devised specifically for locating clandestine graves; those that are used are adapted from other applications. As Pringle *et al.* have demonstrated in a series of experiments undertaken over a three-year period, the relative effectiveness of different methods can depend on both time since burial and whether the individual was wrapped or not (2011). As will be evident below, techniques that work in controlled laboratory contexts do not necessarily offer practical effectiveness in the less controlled environment of moorlands, brown field locations, dune beaches or unkempt inner city gardens.

The three main methods are ground penetrating radar (GPR), magnetometry and resistivity. Of these, GPR is probably the most well known with the greatest number of case studies recorded (Ruffell and McKinley 2008, 79). These three methods tend to accord well with the type of data acquisition required in UK contexts; they also fit relatively neatly into systematic search routines in that the survey areas can be given defined boundaries for mapping and for elimination. Police forces have access to the Centre for Applied Science and Technology (CAST) based in the Home Office, which has expertise in these techniques. As with all methods of geophysical survey, work needs to be carried out systematically – usually by using a grid system, although single traverses can also be helpful over larger areas. Whatever system is deployed there is an essential need for the setting up of fixed points so that the survey can be repeated, or a different technique deployed, or the site revisited for excavation purposes (Figure 3.1). The use of differential GPS systems (see Section 2.3) is also useful for this purpose.

The use of complementary techniques not only provides better insurance against not missing the target, but also allows any identified target to be assigned greater confidence

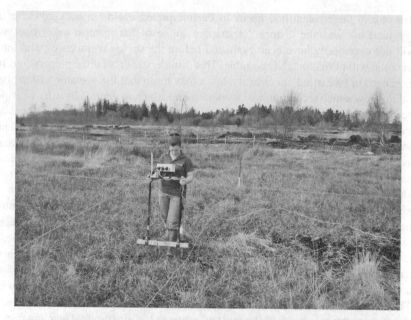

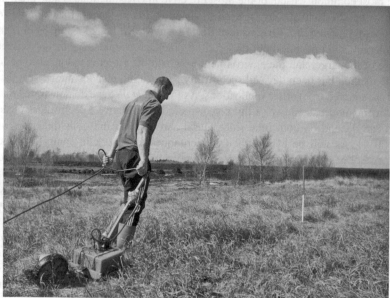

Figure 3.1 Two geophysical survey systems operating within a grid system: (top) resistivity survey; (bottom) ground penetrating radar (GPR). Unfortunately, crime scenes are rarely found on wide-open flat landscapes such as these. Images by courtesy of Stratascan Ltd.

(Case Study 3.1). Geophysicists sometimes refer to this a *conjunctive* approach (Ruffell and McKinley 2008, 57) where the respective methods identify different characters of material in the same location.

Case Study 3.1

In a garden search for a victim in the West Midlands the only knowledge of the terrain was a single aerial photograph taken covertly a week before the search. It showed a long, thin garden containing two wooden sheds, a concrete patio, flower beds, a few small trees around the perimeter and an open grassy area. On this basis three techniques were deployed: ground penetrating radar (GPR), resistivity and a cadaver dog (Section 3.2). The GPR produced some responses that the resistivity did not and the resistivity produced some responses that the GPR did not, but both techniques produced a small number of responses, or points of interest, in common. The degree of commonality noted here resulted from the identified targets containing mixtures of materials, the respective components of which responded to the two techniques applied. Every single response generated was then vented for the cadaver dog, which failed to react to any of them. All were then excavated, the targets identified including an animal burial, a soakaway and a ceramic drain.

Ground penetrating radar (GPR) has the advantage over all other methods of being able to penetrate solid materials, and is therefore of particular value in searching patios, swimming pools, house floors and walls or driveways, which may have been constructed to conceal remains. As such it has the benefit of minimising re-instatement costs which would otherwise be incurred by excavation or other intrusive work. It also has the benefit of being able to penetrate to a depth of several metres if required. That said, it can encapsulate a number of difficulties. First, interpretation of the data requires a skilled operator, one who can distinguish between 'artefacts' (i.e. large responses given by individual objects or spurious reflections) and more substantial real changes that may be relevant in an investigation. Second, there is also a trade-off between depth of penetration and resolution, that is, the deeper the electro-magnetic waves travel, the harder it is to define the character of the features which are causing them to respond. Different antennae with frequencies between, for example, 100 MHz and 500 MHz can be used to vary the depth penetrated and obtain a range of complementary responses (see Ruffell 2005), but the operator will need to be advised on the likely depth of remains in order to set the system up appropriately. Fortunately, most graves are dug in from near the current surface and relatively shallow GPR penetration may identify the disturbance. However, if the burial has been superimposed by other levels and features then an antenna of different frequency might be required. Pringle *et al.* (2011) have demonstrated that a single antenna of fixed frequency will not necessarily offer the flexibility that forensic work requires.

GPR works on a system of sending high frequency electro-magnetic waves into the ground and measuring the speed and energy by which they return. They reflect differences in the electro-magnetic properties of whatever lies below the ground surface in terms of layers, features or buried objects (Figure 3.2). Some materials respond better than others; some, notably heavy clays, can attenuate the signal and make the technique unviable. A freshly buried body is likely to constitute a significant change in density to the surrounding soil whereas a skeleton will not, and this needs to be taken into account. However, the disturbance caused by the grave cut may provide sufficient difference to effect a response, even if the victim is skeletonised (e.g. Powell, 2010, 102). There are numerous permutations to this scenario: for example, a victim buried in peat with the grave filled in with peat may provide a detectable target in its own right. However, the actual disturbance caused by digging the grave may not be detectable once the infilled peat has become consolidated. This is simply because the character of the consolidated disturbed peat and the character of the undisturbed peat would be much the same. Had the grave been dug through different substrates then the difference between the mixed infill and the undisturbed surroundings would be that much greater. Once skeletonised, however, the victim *per se* is unlikely to be detected in either instance unless voiding has occurred from the collapse of the body structure (see also Davis *et al.* 2000; Schultz 2008; Pringle *et al.* 2011).

In common with the other techniques, GPR work is normally conducted systematically across a grid using a series of traverses, and the strength of any response is likely to be affected by the angle at which the radar traverse passes across the line of the buried body. The maximum response would be if the traverse ran directly along the long axis of the individual concerned; the least observable response would be made by a traverse across the short axis (for illustrations of comparison between traverses across both the long and short axes, see Powell 2010, figs. 6.63 and 6.64). Given that an average cadaver/burial is likely to be some 1.8 m in length and approximately 0.6 m wide, traverses need to be less than 0.5 m apart in order to guarantee that the target is not missed. Moreover, given that the alignment of any burial in relation to the grid is unknown, traverses need to be carried out along *both* axes of a defined area at (say) 0.25 m to ensure that areas can be properly searched (see also Schultz and Martin 2011). Targets that emerge and that grow in definition through repeatability of response through different axes of approach, also grow in credibility. Multiple responses of this kind enable specific targets to be given greater priority in the investigation.

Traverses across larger targets (e.g. mass graves) can be carried out at wider intervals in order to identify grave edges (Watters 2003); these intervals can then be narrowed down in order to define the grave more fully. Machine-excavated mass graves can occur in a range of shapes and depths according to the types of machine used, and traverses taking in and extending over a suspect area need to be deployed accordingly. Large mechanical excavators either of a wheeled or tracked variety tend to have bucket widths of 1–2 m. The majority of these types of machine are used for building work in the main, but have been used to construct mass graves; the reach and depth of the excavator arm are sufficient to dispose of human remains at considerable depths. Several of these types of grave have been excavated in East Timor and Bosnia. Mass graves have also been constructed and backfilled by large wheeled front-end loaders. These types of machine have a front bucket width of between 2.3–3 m. This particular type of grave was well established by the use of military engineering equipment and was found to be the main type of mass grave related to the Balkans conflict of the 1990s. Front-end loader graves have a ramped base created by the machine as it excavates a pit. The depth of these types of grave varies but is commonly

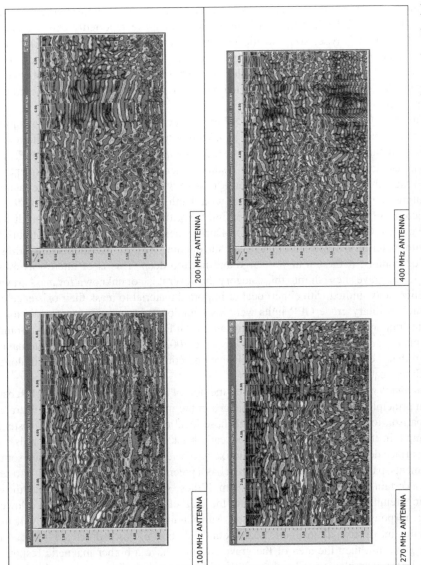

Figure 3.2 Typical radargrams (vertical slices) across known grave sites showing the effects of different antenna frequencies. The brightest responses at approximately 1.5 m depth indicate the presence of graves. Images by courtesy of Stratascan Ltd. (*For colour details please see colour plate section.*)

2–3 m in depth at the lowest point. This variable depth may have implications for the level of response during GPR survey. Graves dug with a JCB-type back-actor will be somewhat narrower (less than 1 m wide) but long and possibly with a u-shaped profile reflecting the arm movement of the machine. This type of mass grave has been excavated in Bosnia by the International Criminal Tribunal for the Former Yugoslavia (ICTY) and tests using GPR equipment were undertaken by the International Commission on Missing Persons (ICMP) in 2003 in an area where this type of grave reportedly existed. Three sites of differing soil type, size and location were chosen to test an array of differing frequency antennae. Initial results were good but also proved that GPR is completely ineffective in saturated clays and moist soils, the unit being unable to discriminate between very heavy clay sub-soils and the compacted nature of the backfill material in the graves (Watters 2003).

As with other techniques it must be remembered that GPR is only effective as a mapping tool in certain environments. GPR is not an effective tool when operated in certain soil conditions, in particular those that absorb the radar signal. Earlier applications of GPR on British archaeological sites achieved poor results, either because the antenna frequencies were too high or because the sediments had excessive water content, both of these factors contributing to a rapid attenuation of signal with depth (Sellers and Chamberlain 1998). A detailed list of buried features and the feasibility for the use of GPR has been produced by Conyers and Goodman (1997, 197–200). During their research they found that burials filled with material that was different to the surrounding matrix gave moderate readings with good contrast if the burial was large and not too deep. This is of interest as most contemporary grave sites fall into this category; however it is not unknown for mass graves to be deliberately infilled with either local or imported material to mask their existence on the surface. Military grade GPR units were also employed in an attempt to locate mass graves in Iraq and, under optimum circumstances, GPR was found to penetrate through approximately 15 feet (c. 4.5 m) of sand (Wessling 2003). However, testing of anomalies indicated that the use of GPR was inconclusive and could not be used as a 'stand alone' approach to location.

Magnetometry is not normally a favoured method of detection owing to its high sensitivity. In principle it relies on detecting changes in the magnetic strength of the substrates in comparison to local magnetic effects. If these local effects are strong or inconsistent, for example in the presence of wire fences, cars, brick buildings (i.e. fired materials) or ferrous surface debris, then the method is unlikely to be effective. However, there are some environments, particularly rural ones, where it has a potential role. Most soils and substrates possess a certain consistent level of magnetism. If these soils are disturbed by burial, those magnetic strengths can become diluted and the area of the grave site will have a lower magnetic response than the undisturbed soils surrounding the grave. Alternatively, if the grave is dug into a strongly magnetic bedrock and elements of this bedrock are introduced into the grave fill, then the area of the grave site may have a higher magnetic response as a result (for examples, see Cheetham 2005). Magnetometry will also respond to buried ferrous materials, but not to non-ferrous items. If, for example, a victim is known to have been buried wearing boots with steel toe-caps, or if the grave contains a spade, then the method may detect them, but a simple metal detector would probably perform equally well and may also detect other metals and alloys.

Resistivity, the final method to be discussed here, involves passing a small electrical current through the ground's sub-surface and measuring the resistance to the current (Figure 3.3). The current is passed between two probes and the effective depth penetration is roughly half the distance of the separation between the probes, although in reality a little more can be assumed. Because water is a good conductor of electricity, buried soils offer a lower resistance to the current than stone-rich substrates, which tend to be drier and therefore offer a higher resistance. Concentrations of readings that are different to the background (either higher or lower) stand out as anomalous and therefore may require further investigation. Exactly what these anomalies signify is another matter entirely. Higher readings may relate (for example) to tree roots, projecting bedrock planes or building foundations; lower readings may reflect former flower beds, gaps in the bedrock or robbed building foundations. In conventional archaeology, higher resistance readings typically reflect buried walls and lower resistance readings typically represent buried ditches. Resistivity is a technique well suited to detecting linear features, but it may also detect a grave fill by virtue of its disturbed, more water-retentive character (lower resistance) or by an infill which is stonier than the surrounding undisturbed landscape (higher resistance). The decay dynamic of human remains at the point at which compositional fluids occur will serve to enhance the likelihood of lower resistance detection (Hunter 1999; see also Pringle *et al.* 2011), whereas the initial burial and compression of backfill may offer the reverse (Powell 2010, 119). The eventual reduction of the cadaver to a skeletal state will not affect 'detectability' as such using resistivity as it tends to be the disturbance to which the technique responds, not the body itself.

Widening the probe separation will serve to increase the depth of current penetration but, like GPR, increased penetration brings with it lowering of resolution. One useful development is that of electrical resistivity tomography (sometimes referred to as electrical imaging); this is essentially a resistivity technique, but instead of just two probes it uses a set of inter-connecting probes set in a line. The current is passed between them in combinations of different probe separations to give a whole range of higher and lower penetration depths along the line, effectively providing a section (sometimes referred to as a pseudo-section) across the transect. For a single grave of estimated base depth 1.0 m and approximately 0.75 m wide, the probe line distance, using a probe spacing of 0.5 m, would need to be at least 10 m long; for a mass grave of estimated depth 2 m similar spacing would be needed over a line distance of approximately twice that in order to image both the grave base and sides effectively. Altering the probe spacing from 0.5 to 0.25 m would serve to increase the resolution of the section; this is more useful perhaps in the case of the mass grave in that it may be able to depict the location(s) of body mass (see Case Study 3.2).

A single transect can provide valuable information, but a series of parallel traverses taken at 0.25 m intervals along both the long and short axes, then converted into a three-dimensional plot using AutoCAD or similar software, can provide a rotational three-dimensional image allowing the grave to be studied and the data interrogated. This has potential for both single and mass graves, particularly the latter in that it can be used to identify grave volume, hence likely victim numbers, in turn providing information on the number of archaeologists, anthropologists, pathologists, mortuary technicians and crime scene staff likely to be needed, not to mention requirements for storage, security and overall resourcing.

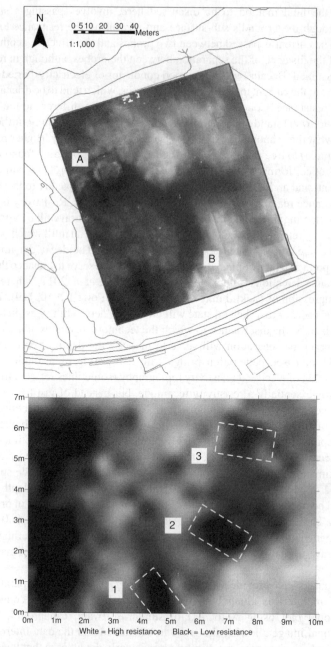

Figure 3.3 Resistivity plots showing areas of higher (lighter) and lower (darker) resistance indicating harder more compacted ground and cut features such as ditches and pits respectively. The top image shows a surveyed area *c.* 160 × 120 m draped over a map and illustrating a likely collapsed circular structure (A – lighter) and a larger circular ditch-like feature (B – darker). The bottom image is at a larger scale and illustrates three likely graves (darker) from experimental pig burials (after Lynam 1978; Cheetham 2005, 74).

Case Study 3.2

In the mid 1990s, during the civil war in the former Yugoslavia, thousands of Bosnian Muslims were brought into the town of Srebrenica as a 'safe area' under the monitorship of the United Nations. The murder of thousands of Muslim males of fighting age undertaken over a few days at the hands of the Bosnian Serb Army in Srebrenica has been well documented (e.g. Honig and Both 1996). The sheer number of victims resulted in the construction of mass graves in mostly uninhabited areas that had been effectively 'cleansed' by the Serbs, the majority lying in eastern Bosnia close to the border with Serbia. For various political reasons the bodies were exhumed from these primary graves and transported to many different locations where they were re-interred within secondary (or even tertiary) mass graves, also in eastern Bosnia. The largest of these secondary mass graves were located intermittently along a valley floor track known as the Cancari Road. A few witness sightings in conjunction with some important aerial photographs taken by the USAF were enough to establish that several areas of disturbance required investigation. The ICTY undertook several large-scale excavations in order to recover forensic evidence for prosecution purposes and the human remains. The repatriation of recovered remains to surviving families was undertaken by the ICMP who continued to work with local government missing persons commissions to undertake recoveries and further collection of forensic evidence.

Part of the research associated with this repatriation programme, set up under the auspices of the ICMP, successfully used GIS in order to provide a predictive model that might locate additional grave sites along the same route (Hunter *et al.* 2005). A number of factors were considered, including distance from main roads, elevation of sites, visibility and geology (Reddick 2005). The data were combined with satellite imagery, which was used to pinpoint characteristic vegetation changes known to be created by ground disturbance. Variation in vegetation attributes could be added to the GIS data and a set of possible sites created. These sites were then assessed on the ground and a number subsequently eliminated. The remaining sites were then subjected to geophysical survey (resistivity transpired to be the best method) in order to identify more precisely the grave footprint. This footprint was typically some 3 m wide (the width of the front-end loader machine bucket with which the grave had originally been created) and anything between 10–20 m in length. Once the footprint had been defined, it was also possible, by using more elaborate methods (electrical resistance tomography – ERT) to produce sections through the grave at set intervals, typically every 0.25 m, across both axes of the grave. Once these sections had been generated they could be amalgamated digitally into a three-dimensional image and rotated using appropriate software. This marked a useful advance in forensic geophysics in that it allowed the grave to be visualised in three dimensions, the depth and profile could be identified, and the ramp defined (Figure 3.4). Greater resolution might even have allowed the concentrations of body mass to be interpreted. Information of this nature enables the degree of necessary resources to be estimated before any work commences. More strictly on the forensic front, it means that the total physical profile of the grave is known before any excavation commences and that recovery can start with minimal loss of evidence.

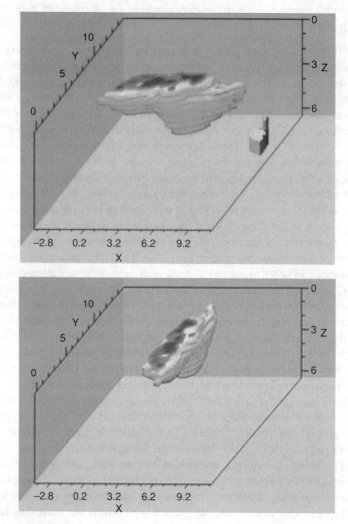

Figure 3.4 Three-dimensional view of mass grave generated using electrical resistance tomography. Image by courtesy of the International Commission on Missing Persons. (*For colour details please see colour plate section.*)

3.2 Cadaver dogs

Dogs are increasingly being employed in the search for buried materials, particularly in attempts to locate human remains; they play a significant role in many search sequences (ACPO 2006, 40; ACPO 2011a, 42–3) and are readily available to UK investigations. Body scent dogs (cadaver dogs) now tend to be maintained and trained in-house by only a small number of police forces; they are made available on a 'mutual aid' basis or for a daily fee. There are also a number of commercial dogs available, usually trained and maintained by ex- or retired officers. Since the beginning of the last decade (2000s) there is a licensing procedure that effectively validates dogs for operational work, although this is not mandatory for private handlers. The majority of dogs used for body search are trained uniquely to that end, but some are dual purpose and are also trained to scent blood (below). The characteristics of the dogs best suited for these types of work have been outlined by Rooney *et al.* (2004). Literature on the use of cadaver dogs is somewhat limited and tends to be restricted to case studies in the USA and Canada, where climate, seasonality and landscape types bear little relevance to the determiners affecting search in the UK (Komar 1999; Rebmann *et al.* 2000; Lasseter *et al.* 2003).

Cadaver dogs are best deployed as part of a sequence of search techniques, as many of the cited case studies demonstrate (Case Study 3.3). However, in certain circumstances they might be deployed as the *only* asset, for example in the search of woodland where human remains are thought to be scattered on the surface, or where a shallow burial might be expected but where other search techniques such as geophysical survey are impractical (Case Study 3.4). In general there are two types of use for cadaver dogs, 'free roam' and focused. Handlers differ in the manner of their approach to this, but generally in the former the dog is directed by the handler to run freely but led in a systematic manner across a defined area; in the latter the search location is smaller or more specific and the ground will be systematically 'vented' by the handler in order to release any gases. Venting involves pressing a narrow metal probe (about 2 cm diameter) into the ground, usually to a depth of 30–50 cm. This can be carried out across a grid, typically at 0.5 m intervals depending on target size and information, or along a single line laid over a specific surface feature. The venting needs to be effective enough to release any gases, but not so excessive as to damage what is buried. There is a waiting time of about 10–15 minutes which allows the ground to 'breathe', and the dog is taken, with any wind blowing from behind, from one end of the grid or line to the other, being directed to each vent hole. The following two case studies give an indication of the type of contribution made by cadaver dogs.

Case Study 3.3

An area measuring some 30×15 m of overgrown shrubs and brambles had been identified through intelligence as the possible burial site of a victim several years earlier. The area was cleared of vegetation and inspected for ground disturbance and change. Three potential target areas were identified. A line was positioned across each, extending well beyond the apparent edges, and vented at 0.5 m intervals in order to allow gases to escape for the dogs. The dogs were then introduced to each hole down the line, but failed to respond. The whole area was then gridded systematically and vented at similar intervals until the dogs had scented every vent hole. Absence of any further response suggested that no buried human remains were present. However, in a relatively small area such as this it was possible to strip the surface using a machine in order to eliminate the area completely.

Case Study 3.4

Police received information that a known missing person had been murdered and buried in a particular woodland covering several acres. The use of criminal statistics (distances from pathways, vehicle access, concealment, etc.) and likely disturbed ground allowed certain locations to be targeted ('red' zones in a RAG system), but the remainder of the wood still needed some level of search. This was carried out using search officers, but supported by free roaming dogs that complemented officers' observations in order to locate any surface, near-surface or scavenged human remains. As it happened, none were forthcoming. This did not entail *elimination* of the majority of the woodland; this could only have been achieved by a massive deployment of manpower and excavation, but it provided the SIO with some reassurance that he had done all he could with the techniques and resources available to him. Geophysical survey was impracticable owing to the nature of the vegetation, and aerial photography was inhibited by the tree canopy. Manual foot search and the deployment of cadaver dogs were the only options available.

Cadaver dogs are trained to detect and react to particular scents; they do not detect human bodies *per se* – they detect the gases produced by the body during the decomposition process as well as bodily fluids that leach into, and alter, the chemical composition of the surrounding soil. Unlike geophysical survey or aerial photography, dogs can be trained to discriminate between types of target, for example between live and death scent, as well as human and animal scents, hence their usefulness in searches for deceased individuals. Venting the soil releases any such scent into the air in a so-called 'scent cone'. Given the nature of the dog's olfactory system, they are able to detect both the source of a scent, which lies at the tip of the scent cone, and its presence more widely, given the broader dispersal of scent molecules in the air (Rebmann *et al.* 2000).

Although the scent presented by human remains changes from the point of death through to the complete skeletonisation of the corpse, cadaver dogs appear to be largely unaffected by the length of interval since death. Their ability to detect remains years after deposition has been recorded by many handlers, although there appears to be little consensus about exactly how long after burial cadaver dogs remain effective, given the lack of dedicated research. Some handlers have suggested a 20 year window, others 35 years, and some have demonstrated the ability to detect remains in 17th century cemeteries (for examples see Rebmann *et al.* 2000; Rebmann undated; Komar 1999; France *et al.* 1997). The authors here, in partnership with an experienced dog handler, undertook an experiment using archaeologically recovered human bone from an Anglo-Saxon cemetery. The dog was able to detect the bones, which were concealed in a vented container placed on the ground surface in a line of identical empty containers. Mummified remains are also recorded as having been detected (Lasseter *et al.* 2003; Rebmann *et al.* 2000). Experience suggests that it is more likely to be the nature and circumstances of the context (including climate) as opposed to either the state of the remains or the extent of the post-mortem interval (PMI) that is likely to impact upon successful detection. However, while the use of cadaver dogs is now a recognised search asset, it does not mean that the dog is always right. Like people, dogs have moods, good days and bad days, and can be distracted. They are not pieces of machinery. They respond only to what they are trained to respond to. As such it is usually deemed best practice to have two dog handlers and two dogs present at any scene to provide a control check and to facilitate the observation of the dog's behaviour (Oesterhelweg *et al.* 2008).

The use of cadaver dogs has increased steadily over the last few decades and they are increasingly called on in both domestic and international searches. The issuing of the ACPO *Police Dogs Manual of Guidance* (2011b), which contains specific guidance on the use of search and recovery dogs, has cemented their role in the investigative process and provides Standard Operating Procedures (SOPs) for cadaver dog handlers, as well as outlining the legal process within which the dogs operate (*ibid.*, section 7.29.3). Figure 3.5 outlines the various phases that might ensure a 'thorough and efficient search'. Adoption of

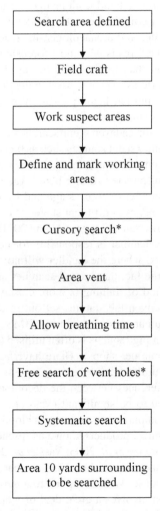

Figure 3.5 Recommended phases of search for cadaver dogs (adapted from ACPO 2011b, 7.29.3). Asterisks indicate optional tasks.

the *Guidance* effectively provides some level of validation; adherence to it better protects handlers against 'litigation, scrutiny of welfare issues and evidential challenge' (ACPO 2011b, 1). A 'licenced' dog is one which, together with handler, has passed a series of training exercises defined by ACPO (*ibid.*). Key requirements of the process include the ability of the dog to identify and indicate the presence of human remains, the ability of the handler to advise an SIO on the appropriateness and value of use, and some recognition of the rapport that the handler possesses with the dog, both in training and in operation. What is less well-defined, however, is the need for the handler to possess fieldcraft skills, i.e. the ability to recognise subtle changes in vegetation, animal spores, topographical expression and an underlying appreciation of landscape. The need for this ability is acknowledged (see Figure 3.6) but not pursued as far as it might be. Handlers and dogs work as a team. Often their remit will be vague, for example in being given instructions to 'search a garden', and the handler may need to prioritise certain locations in order to get the most out of the dog. Cadaver dog handlers, like archaeologists, develop fieldcraft skills over time; there can be a strong affinity between handler and archaeologist in 'reading' ground surfaces and in understanding landscape change. This is why most forensic archaeologists prefer to work in harness with handlers, rather than finding the dogs used independently as a 'bolt-on' asset. Fieldcraft is also recognised as a specific asset in the PolSA guidance (ACPO 2011a, 29–30). The value of dogs lies in their being part of an integrated search strategy and in being complementary to other techniques.

Dogs may be trained solely for cadaver scent searches or they may be 'cross-trained' which enables them to detect other scent sources such as blood. The benefits and disadvantages of cross-training have been frequently debated (e.g. Lit and Crawford 2006; Cabalk and Sagebiel 2011) but are not pursued further here. Training usually involves building up the dog's search abilities slowly, stage by stage and by repetition; ideally it involves the introduction of decaying remains at different stages of decomposition, clothing or soil containing bodily fluids, and different soil types (ACPO 2011b, 7.24). Training will consist of a number of tests where the handler is responsible for depositing the evidence, and a number of so-called 'blind tests' where the handler will not be aware of its location. The benefits of the latter relate to the fact that 'actual searches are essentially blind problems to the handler', thus this method of training is more closely related to operational work (Cabalk and Sagebiel 2011). Given the statutes set out in the Human Tissue Act in the UK that prevent the use of human flesh in training (HMSO 2004a; HMSO 2006; HTA 2009) a substitute in the form of pig remains is often utilised (dried pigs' ears, for example, are readily purchased from some pet shops). There have been various criticisms of this, particularly from researchers in the USA where it is possible to utilise human material in research, given that the differences between the decomposition chemistry of pigs and humans has been demonstrated to be significant (Vass *et al.* 2004; Cabalk and Sagebiel 2011). In view of this, certain human materials such as blood or decomposition fluids have been used, not to mention chemical products known as 'pseudo-scents' designed to mirror the scent of decomposition (Lorenzo *et al.* 2003; Vass *et al.* 2004). Not all dogs are trained the same way; it is often important to know how, and on what, a dog has been trained as this will have implications for response. Will it respond to a buried cat or sheep, or to human faeces? Training a cadaver dog involves a great deal of work and the development of an animal able to undertake operational work is not easily achieved. Handlers are justifiably

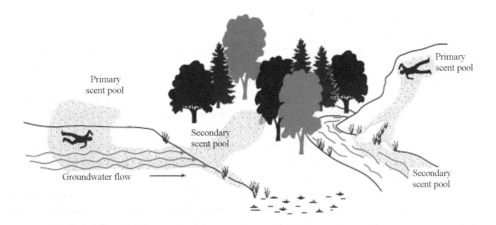

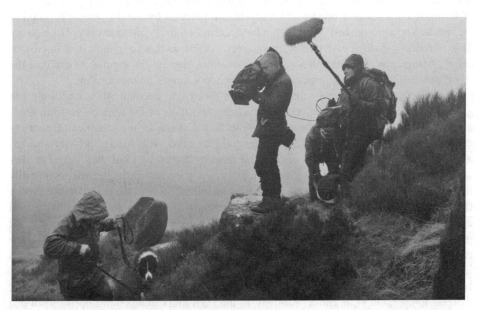

Figure 3.6 Top, examples illustrating the potential travel of scent according to landscape and water coursing (based on Rebman 2003); bottom, a dog at work in heavy rain following a line of vent holes at the base of a slope as part of a training film.

defensive of their dog's ability, particularly in process-driven search routines where an SIO may be impatient and expect black and white outcomes.

On detection, dogs are trained to present either an active or passive response, something that differs according to the dog's natural instincts and the preference of the handler. Active responses include digging and scratching in the location where the scent of decomposition is detected, whilst passive responses are less destructive, usually in the form of 'freezing', sitting still or pushing their nose into the vent hole. The benefit of the latter is that it prevents disturbance to the ground, and therefore any evidence being damaged. The method of response reflects the way the dog has been trained: for example, a dog that 'freezes' may be rewarded by the handler with a ball or tit-bit; a dog that digs may be allowed to eat the 'find' (in training) – in other words, in the former the dog is working for the handler, whereas in the latter the dog is working for itself. There are implications here in that a dog working for a handler is more likely to give a 'false positive' in order to please, whereas a dog working for itself is not.

Responses are not always clear cut. At one extreme there may be no response at all, at the other the dog may scrabble wildly in the ground, bark loudly or adopt the perfect response posture required by the handler. However, there are equally likely to be less extreme responses where the dog 'shows interest' rather than showing a full blown response. This 'interest' is sometimes only recognised by the handler through a change in the dog's body language (e.g. the movement of the head, ears, eyes, tail and its stance), but it is a response nevertheless and one which merits interpretation. Some handlers prefer to rate the level of response on a scale of one to ten: a full blown reaction by the dog might be rated at ten, while 'showing interest' on a particular occasion might be rated at only six or seven. This introduces a degree of interpretation very similar to that in geophysical survey or aerial photography. In consequence, it puts some pressure on the handler to evaluate the significance of the response, especially if further work hinges on the outcome.

There are various inhibitors that need to be taken into account: soil conditions and ground temperature can impact on both the decomposition of the remains and the dog's ability to detect the scent – in peat environments, for example, the presence of methane can mask or mirror human remains (Hunter and Cox 2005, 40). Animal activity also has a bearing: not only can animals disturb the remains themselves but they can also alter scent dispersal through burrowing activity and mask the scent through their own bodily fluids (ACPO 2011b). Some animal scents may be intimidating to the dog, notably the fox (M. Swindells pers. comm.). Climate and temperature are also factors. There is general agreement that a moderate temperature (c. 4–16 °C) is ideal, with a slight breeze and moist ground conditions optimum (Lasseter et al. 2003). However, almost all studies regarding the effect of temperature have been undertaken in the USA and Canada, thus these assertions in the UK are largely based on anecdotal evidence acquired during operational experience. However, UK temperatures generally fall within this range for most of the year. More extreme temperatures can cause problems: in the USA and Canada it has been shown that temperatures in excess of 29 °C can decrease detection rates (France et al. 1997; Komar 1999). There has also been some debate concerning the affect of colder conditions (e.g. below freezing) with a study by Komar (1999) suggesting that, contrary to popular belief, dogs were able to successfully detect concealed remains at −30 °C. Wind can also offer a considerable impact on scent dispersal: too much wind can cause the scent to be dispersed over a wider area and away from the source, whilst too little wind can prevent the scent molecules being dispersed into the air, in both situations making it more difficult for the dog to detect. The direction of the wind can also affect the detection distance, depending on the environment being searched. Poor weather is otherwise not an inhibitor (Figure 3.6).

A particular problem encountered by handlers (and not always recognised by others) is that the source of the scent does not always lie directly in the ground where the dog responds (see Case Study 3.5 and Case Study 3.6). The source may lie further away uphill or on a sloping geological stratum from which water carrying the scent is draining. Water can move the scent away from its source, and barriers to water flow can cause secondary scent cones in places away from the original source. The dog may pick up the scent as it was trained to do, but any excavation in that spot will not find the victim there (Figure 3.6). The dog is not 'wrong'. The pressure is now on the handler again to work out where to go next. The following two case studies illustrate the difficulties of this.

Case Study 3.5

Information had been received that a body had been disposed of in the concealed corner of a field, which had not been cultivated for many years. The ground sloped down to a stream at one edge and was consistently waterlogged every winter. Search was undertaken in spring using a machine to strip off the topsoil down to yellow natural clay. As a result of persistent rain at the time the lower third of the field was still waterlogged and it was only possible to strip the upper two-thirds at that time. During the machine operations a faint dark linear feature was seen running downhill through the clay, together with some small dark patches of disturbance. The linear feature was almost certainly a field drain and was vented together with the dark patches. The dog showed interest to the extent that the handler undertook further probing upslope in order to try and pinpoint the source, but the dog failed to respond further. Two months later, when the lower part of the field had dried out the stripping continued; the body was found some three metres *downslope* of the point where the dog had displayed interest. The grave had been cut through the same field drain. The dog had scented it upstream, not downstream, presumably because the drain had 'backed-up' as a result of the higher winter water table.

Case Study 3.6

A search for a victim in a moorland environment had identified a possible target using geophysics and depth profiling. A cadaver dog responded well to the location and a small trench was excavated. No remains were found even when the search area was widened, although the dog continued to show interest in the spoil. The location was near the bottom of a grassy gully which contained a small boggy stream at the base. On a subsequent date the dog was re-introduced and the whole area gridded and vented systematically. The dog responded at a number of points upslope of the original target area and these were logged. The exercise was repeated some weeks later; the dog continued to show responses, but at different places within the same general area. The interpretation was that the changes in the water table were also causing changes in the way that underground water was moving through the local substrates, thus causing the scent to be transported differently. Using the same grid, ground penetrating radar (GPR) was introduced and a three-dimensional model of the shallow subsurface produced that showed the nature of the water coursing (Figure 3.7). The grid was extended further uphill to follow the underground water courses and the dog continued to respond until a point at the top of the hill where logic suggested the body must lie. Frustratingly, excavation failed to find the grave. This case, which is still ongoing, emphasises the complexities that can be encountered in attempting to 'chase' waterborne scents.

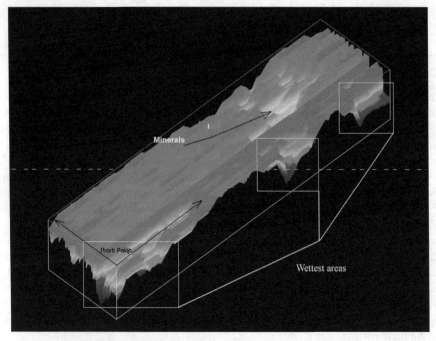

Figure 3.7   Three-dimensional model of moorland landscape from a ground penetrating radar survey showing wettest areas and underground water-coursing. Area covered is approximately 12 × 3 m and depth 2 m. Image by courtesy of Malcolm Weale. (*For colour details please see colour plate section.*)

3.3 Mechanical excavation

Despite the widespread use of mechanical excavators in commercial archaeology, police forces are often reluctant to use them as an asset in a buried body search. This stems mostly from unfamiliarity with the nature of stratigraphic formation processes and the extent to which a machine, directed appropriately, can remove soils in a constructive and systematic manner. Of all the different forensic professionals deployed in searching, archaeologists are the ones most familiar with, and trained in the use and limitations of, mechanical excavation; as such they shoulder much of the responsibility for ensuring that the equipment is appropriate and utilised effectively. Despite their growing role in searching there is no literature that allows their input to be evaluated for forensic purposes, and there are no guidelines as to the optimum type of excavator required for specific tasks.

To many people the use of heavy earth moving equipment is incongruous with the sensitivities (both physical and emotional) in recovering human remains. The popular perception of mechanical diggers is that they 'dig holes'; in actual fact their main strength is not in excavating vertically into the ground (which they can do perfectly well) but in the rapid horizontal stripping of soil surfaces across wide areas. Machines are far more flexible and efficient than manual labour, for example in moving excavated materials from one place to another, or in fragmenting and shifting hard surfaces such as tarmac or concrete. From a search point of view their benefit lies in removing large volumes of soil in order to encounter deposits which are archaeologically sensitive. This tends to be carried out by horizontal stripping under a careful archaeological watching brief enabling, for example, vegetation and topsoil to be skimmed away to expose the surface of the substrates below (see Case Study 3.7).

Machines come in many different shapes and sizes; there is no universal model that will satisfy every demand of terrain, difficulty of soil, depth, access or time factor, in the same way that there is no single geophysics system that is universally effective. Key features depend on the extent to which the arm (actor) can rotate (typically either 180° or 360°), whether the machine has wheels or tracks, and the width and capacity of the bucket. For forensic work, the authors have found that the most effective models are those equipped with tracks and with a 360° rotation facility. The tracks lead to stability, and the full rotation of the main machine body allows for greater movement and placement of spoil in different places according to local circumstances. Any machine used in forensic work should be equipped with a wide 1–2 m flat edged batter or ditching bucket. Excavation buckets equipped with 'teeth' are good for breaking rocks and hard ground, but they also scarify the layers below and damage the clean exposed surfaces that forensic work requires. These should be avoided if possible. Machines range from mini-versions – these are designed specifically to pass through standard doorway widths allowing them to access back yards and gardens which have no rear access by travelling through the house itself – to the multi-tonne excavators used in road construction. A small garden may require only a narrow 'bobcat' type machine, while an open field would benefit from a more substantial machine, probably one weighing eight tonnes or more with a bucket up to two metres in width. All these excavators can work equally effectively, but at different scales, using different techniques, and at different speeds according to size and bucket width. Access is often a key parameter.

Mechanical excavators need to be used as part of a systematic search strategy. Typical examples would include incidents where a witness has pointed to an area of land where a victim is alleged to have been buried, or where a garden needs to be eliminated from an enquiry. Depending on the confidence the SIO has in the particular area in question, the machine can be used as part of a sequence of assets (for example after geophysical survey and cadaver dogs have produced no responses). Equally, if there is an allegation that a person has been buried in a specific place and the SIO feels there is little credibility in the allegation, a machine can be used as a single method of elimination. A machine might also be used as a primary approach in an area which may not be conducive to either geophysics or dogs on the basis of environment or specific hazards. There are sometimes instances where informants may be taken to a site and point to a specific grave location. Unless there are features visible on the ground surface, there is a high probability that the information, although given with the best of intentions, is inaccurate due to the passage of time and changes to the vegetation and landscape (see Section 5.3). SIOs often show great enthusiasm in wishing to commence digging where 'X marks the spot', but in such instances, and in the experience of the authors, the grave (if there is one) usually lies several metres away from the point indicated. Controlled surface stripping across a wider area is the

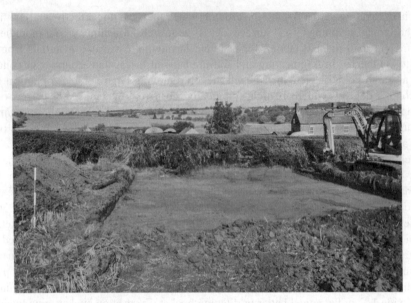

Figure 3.8 Careful machine stripping of surface layers in order to identify disturbances cut into undisturbed substrates. No disturbances are evident – compare with Figure 3.9.

method best suited to identifying the disturbance and, conducted carefully, can minimise any loss of evidence. Using a machine always presents a risk factor in this respect, but this has to be balanced against time (especially in view of PACE factors – see Section 1.4) and manpower resources.

The effectiveness of machine excavation relies on the fact that naturally formed buried layers tend to lie horizontally. These need to be identified before work starts; and intelligent searching will normally include the manual digging of a small number of test pits before machine work is deployed. A single test pit informs the search as to the depth and character of buried layers in a particular place; multiple test pits indicate the extent to which these layers are consistent across a larger area.

Not many burials are obvious from the ground surface unless they are very recent or have distinctive vegetation or surface indications. The majority will be evident when surface layers have been stripped away (e.g. Case Study 3.8); this allows the disturbance caused by the burial to be visible as a defined, darker intrusion cutting through cleaner undisturbed layers (e.g. Figure 3.8 and Figure 3.9). The clarity with which the grave can be distinguished depends on the age of the burial and on the nature of the substrates through which it has been cut. The edges of an older burial are likely to be more diffuse than those of a recent one; this is the result of weathering and interaction between the disturbed and the undisturbed soils. Possible extremes would be, for example, a recent burial dug through black topsoil into yellow clay, and a 20-year old burial cut through a brown field surface into made-up or disturbed ground. Once the surface has been machine-stripped, both graves should be evident to an experienced archaeologist, but the former would stand out and be easy to define, while the latter would be more difficult to distinguish from the surrounding soils. A good machine operator will be able to work the machine bucket horizontally to remove

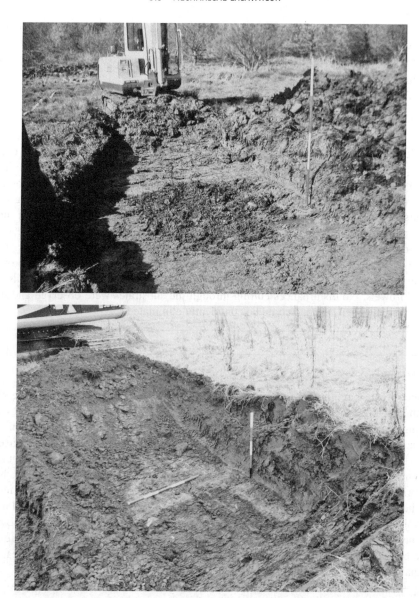

Figure 3.9   Removal of surface deposits clearly illustrates (top) the badly concealed burial of contaminated waste and (bottom) the remains of an earlier regular-shaped excavation for similar comparative purposes. Compare also with Figure 3.8.

as little as a 10 cm 'spit' of material in a single sweep, or follow a single layer, and leave a cleaned surface exposed as a result. Good operators are able to read the ground they are excavating and can usually overcome the problem of dipping into the soil by manipulating the height of the bucket as it strips.

Case Study 3.7

Intelligence had been received that a person had been killed and buried at the edge of a particular field some years earlier. There was a known missing person who had been associated with the informant, and this gave the information some credibility. The place of deposition at the field edge was unspecific other than within given limits. Boundaries were established but neither search officers using fieldcraft, nor free roaming cadaver dogs, were able to identify any likely targets. A machine was introduced which then systematically stripped away the field turf and the topsoil at the edge of the field to a depth of about 0.2 m. This exposed the undisturbed light brown natural soil beneath. Any questionable or discoloured areas were investigated using hand trowels. No disturbances cutting through the substrates were observed and the area that had been stripped could be confidently eliminated.

Case Study 3.8

Police were searching for a missing pensioner. It was known that during the time she went missing a local stream had been contaminated by a sewer pipe fracture and was being cleaned. A wet pasture field adjacent to the stream was being used by mechanical excavators for burying the non-sewage debris that had been collected. The sewage itself was to be taken off site and disposed of appropriately. Local residents believed that the contractors had not taken all the sewage away but had buried some of it with the other debris in the field. The SIO was concerned that the pensioner might have fallen into, or have been disposed of, within these excavations. Search was straightforward and involved systematic stripping of the field down to the natural clay substrate. Deposits of buried sewage were readily apparent cut into the clay and the local residents fears were confirmed. The pensioner was later found to have been drowned in a nearby canal.

One of the underestimated factors in using mechanical excavation equipment, especially in restricted environments, lies in the logistics of operation. Once soils are stripped they have to be removed and the landscape or garden re-instated. On larger sites the use of a second wheeled front loader to move soil can be advantageous, especially if the undisturbed soil is at depth. In most cases, for example within the confines of a domestic garden, the use of a skip to take the spoil off site is unnecessary; it also presents further problems of transport and access. The most practical solution is to use the excavator to clear one strip of ground at a time (typically one or two bucket widths wide), allow any features to be manually investigated on the exposed surface, then strip away the adjacent area dumping the newly removed spoil on the investigated strip. This process can then continue until the whole area has been completely exposed and investigated strip by strip. It is a process that requires careful planning, recording and a defined method of clear communication with the machine operator. A significant problem with this method is that the spoil from the very first strip needs to be cleared to a different part of the site in order to be re-deposited in the final opened strip. From a forensic point of view, the removed spoil is of little value: being disturbed it will be effectively contaminated and has to be 'written off' evidentially. As the potential depth of any burial is unknown, the process requires the removal of the strips of spoil to be under continual watching brief by an archaeologist or anthropologist in the event that grave material might be dragged up by the machine bucket. This may particularly apply to graves that may have been subjected to agricultural damage in plough soil (see also Haglund *et al.* 2002). Each case has to be considered on its merits in order to minimise the risk of losing evidence. The ultimate advantage of using a machine is that once an area has been exposed and investigated it can be immediately eliminated from the search with total confidence.

3.4   Bodies in aqueous environments

Given that the UK is a relatively small, sea-locked island with a dense river system, remarkably little has been written on the location and recovery of human remains lost in, or recovered from, water. Water provides a convenient and rapid point of criminal disposal as well as a source of potential for accidental death by drowning. From a search perspective the most useful contribution (and necessary reading material) is by Parker *et al.* (2010), which draws together the various search technologies together with summary case studies and reviews of the various methods available. As in terrestrial search there is a wide range of options according to environment, depth and nature of target in which seismic, sonar, ground (water) penetrating radar and magnetometry all offer relative advantages and limitations. These are specialist areas, but in brief: seismic methods rely on the reflection or refraction of acoustic waves in identifying changes or anomalies on the waterbed; sonar effectively maps the sea/riverbed using similar technology but in a more focused way; radar sends electro-magnetic pulses through the water and measures reflectance properties, and magnetometry can detect magnetic change (i.e. ferrous materials). The last two of these are essentially floating versions of their terrestrial counterparts. All are effective only in as much as detected anomalies can be distinguished from their backgrounds, that is that the seabed or riverbed is sufficiently consistent in character for the target to be identifiable within its local environment, and that the target is large enough either physically or in character of response to be recognised by the method being used. Moreover, the success of magnetometry will be limited by the (not uncommon) presence of unwanted ferrous material conveniently disposed of in water, and the GPR energies are severely attenuated by salt water, effectively making the method unviable in marine or coastal contexts. All methods are limited by depth (more strictly on the effect of depth on resolution) and the need to provide floating platforms for the equipment in question; in the case of magnetometry this needs to be non-magnetic or towed at a distance behind a vessel. Sonar systems, which have other uses in navigation and fishing, are the only ones that are likely to be built into existing vessels. Another issue, which is often overlooked, is the difficulty of providing a comprehensive survey across an area of water which, by definition, has no fixed reference points. Rivers are relatively straightforward in that positions can be fixed using the banks and total coverage achieved in single or multiple sweeps depending on technique and width of water. However, lakes and seas offer different challenges, now slightly ameliorated by global positioning systems (GPS).

Literature on the taphonomics of human remains in water is more diverse (see for example Sorg *et al.* 1997). Bodies entering water behave in very different ways from those buried in the ground: not only does water provide an additional dynamic in the decay process, but it also presents different types of predator. Under most circumstances, a body entering the water will float until such time as the lungs fill and cause it to sink. This can be accelerated by saturated clothes or slowed down by air trapped in the clothing. It will surface again when putrefaction has created sufficient gas in the corpse to overcome the weight of water overlying it; thus in deeper water this process may take longer as the weight of water over the body is greater. Sea (salt) water is denser than fresh water and will have a similar effect. Weighting down the body helps, but not always permanently; it also has the effect of producing a more substantial target for detection purposes. The body tends to float face down with the head, being heavier, slightly lower than the rest of the body.

As well as this vertical movement within the water, the body is almost certain to be subject to horizontal movement or drift according to environment. This occurs in maritime contexts through tide and currents, in rivers according to direction of flow and seasonal rainfall, and even in lakes where movement is restricted owing to feeder streams and annual circulation patterning as the water warms up. Only in canals is there likely to be minimal movement, but even here boats and propellers cause a degree of disturbance. To varying degrees these movements cause the body to travel, irrespective of whether it lies on the surface or the bed. In the process it can bump or rub against, or become snagged on, underwater projections, or even become dredged by sea-bed fishing. Transport will occur more rapidly, and the body moved further, in faster streams or tides, but more slowly where there is less movement where, for example, the body may be gently moved around the same general area. Either way, the process of transport and friction will enhance the speed of disarticulation.

The problem is, of course, that not only can bodies disarticulate differentially as a result of this movement, but also that once disarticulated or part-disarticulated, the individual elements can be transported at different speeds. Haglund and Sorg have produced a suggested trend as to the general order in which the skeleton disarticulates in water – hands and feet first, followed by limbs, with the skull and mandible separating somewhere between the two (2002b, 210, figure 10.2). Disarticulation depends too on the level of clothing and the susceptibility of the clothing fabrics to decay under aqueous conditions. Once separated, however, a process of sorting might occur according to transport conditions: the heavier skeletal components logically tend to be slower in transport and become deposited first, while the lighter bones move faster and become deposited last. The skull appears to be the element that travels furthest, partly because of its potential buoyancy and partly because of its roundness, which inhibits tendencies to catch or snag during movement. Skulls that exhibit extensive scuffing, scratching and/or facial fracture tend to be indicative of extensive transportation (Brooks and Brooks 1997; Nawrocki *et al.* 1997). The effect, therefore, can be in body parts being spread over a large area, sometimes in discrete assemblages and often following different taphonomic routes as a result. Slower moving or stationary body parts are more prone to adipocere formation (see Section 1.5; also Kahana *et al.* 1999), especially if clothed (Notter and Stuart 2012). Adipocere is characteristic of soft tissue decay in wet environments resulting in the formation of a white, greasy, lard-like substance. In rivers that possess significant bends, the lighter components are likely to travel in the faster moving, deeper water around the outside of the bends, whereas the heavier elements may drift more slowly along the inside shallows. When the water level drops, those on the inside may become deposited and only become transported again when rainfall causes the water levels to rise. Equally, once static, they may become completely buried by natural agencies. Nawrocki *et al.* (1997) have pointed out that any investigation resulting from the discovery of a skull in a river might be usefully directed upstream, given that the other major body parts may not have travelled as far, with particular emphasis being placed on the shallower banks lying on the inside of the bends.

The variables are such that when body parts are found it is virtually impossible to calculate with any accuracy how long they may have been there since the time of immersion (assumed to be equivalent to time since death) or how far they may have travelled to reach the point of recovery. At sea, a skull may become lodged in a rock crevice as the tide ebbs but is likely to be dislodged by the next incoming tide, whereas a skull caught in branches or weeds along a river bank may sit there for months until the river next floods. Local factors appear to apply in all cases, each river or tidal region being likely to possess its own characteristics. The only viable benchmark for estimating the PMI may be through creating local models by collating data from previous discoveries where the individual has subsequently been identified, the date of disappearance known and the local marine or riverine conditions recorded. But even this will only allow a rough estimate. The same applies to bodies or body parts washed up on the sea shore: local fishermen or coastguards will know where flotsam tends to land and how far jetsam thrown overboard tends to travel before coming ashore. But again, this can only be used as a guide. That said, in one instance knowledge of local currents and tidal conditions has been used to calculate roughly how far a murder victim had been transported before being washed up on a tidal estuary on the Humber. A broad area for probable deposition was identified higher up the river in which there were few vehicle access points, and the crime scene was identified at one of them.

Waterborne remains are also subject to different levels of scavenging, both as surface remains and underwater, and even between different aquatic environments (e.g. Hobischak and Anderson 2002). Moving water tends to minimise scavenging, as does clothing, but naked remains or remains where the clothing has become damaged are more susceptible. In both environments the body is prone to fish scavenging. Below water, and especially on the seabed, bottom scavengers such as crabs are active, and on the surface the exposed back of a floating body can be prone to both bird attack and insect infestation. Some work has been carried out on attempting to estimate the PMI from the succession of midges and gaddis flies (Haskell *et al.* 1989) and with bacterial succession (Dickson *et al.* 2011), but with limited results. Under laboratory conditions the succession cycle is both measurable and predictable, but it is harder to calculate in the field given many of the unknowns.

4 Search design

4.1 Search design

As Chapter 2 has shown, a mapped landscape of roads, fields and buildings can be given greater forensic status by the introduction of various factors. These can include simple elements such as geology (both solid and drift) which has an implication for the ease by which concealment can be undertaken in the ground, or access points, which are important if a body is being transported by vehicle. The additional use of GIS can, for example, show which areas are visible from roads, buildings or public places and which might therefore facilitate or obviate a clandestine disposal.

However, these are clinical parameters in the sense that they can be used to breakdown a landscape by means of a logical process. In combination they provide objective criteria which will allow a search to be undertaken systematically using manpower and other resources efficiently; they may enable certain areas to be given greater priority, but at this stage the process is entirely objective and requires a defined framework. In setting up the search structure, there are three key elements that need to be incorporated. The first is the *definition of search boundaries*, which enables geographical parameters to be delineated within which search can be undertaken, concluded and logged and, if necessary, which can be revisited and/or extended at a later date. The second is *recording and archiving*, which is important, not only for reasons of accountability, but also because it allows the methodology to be reviewed or the area returned to in the future. The third is the *extent of thoroughness* or comprehensiveness of search. Higher levels of thoroughness increase the probability of finding a burial; they also allow the area in question to be eliminated with increased confidence if the body is not found. This issue of 'confidence' is explored further below. These three key elements merit some amplification.

4.1.1 Definition of search boundaries

The actual definition of search boundaries is probably one of the most critical decisions to make but is often not recognised as such. The decision is a management one but, in the authors' experience, often becomes delegated to PolSAs or Crime Scene Managers or, rarely, is never identified as a serious consideration until the search is about to commence. Defining boundaries is a strategic decision and requires input from all sources, not least the SIO who is uniquely aware of the appropriate intelligence regarding circumstances and context, and the PolSA who is more familiar with landfall and search feasibility.

Forensic Approaches to Buried Remains, First Edition. John Hunter, Barrie Simpson and Caroline Sturdy Colls.
© 2013 John Wiley & Sons, Ltd. Published 2013 by John Wiley & Sons, Ltd.

Definition of boundaries will affect the subsequent stage of an enquiry if the search fails to find the target. The overall area selected will (a) include priority or target domains and (b) encompass areas wider than the priority or target domains in order to allow for latitude. Boundaries need to be agreed upon by all concerned from the outset, and the decision as to why those boundaries have been selected will be accountable. There is always the temptation, should the search not find the body, to extend the area a little here or there according to whim or landfall, or time available. This is unsystematic, difficult to monitor and usually unloggable, not to mention unprofessional. Each search should be followed by a review. If there is the feeling that (for whatever reason) the burial might lie 'just outside' the domain boundary, then the decision can be made to apply the same level of search to other adjacent domains, not parts of domains. A good search will sometimes overlap boundaries as insurance in order to ensure that no part of the landscape has been overlooked simply because it lies near the boundary edge (ACPO 2006, 26).

4.1.2   Recording and archiving

Anyone who has worked on a cold case review will recognise the importance of inheriting good clear records after a search has been concluded. Reviewing a search without them or with only minimal documentation inevitably requires search to be conducted from scratch again if integrity is to be retained. There is sometimes an unhealthy reliance on memory and anecdote on remembering, for example, which parts of a woodland were searched, or whether dogs were used on all allotments in an area or just some, or how far up the valley the line search progressed before the light faded. Recording this information is just as important between successive days as it is between successive decades, in fact probably more so given that there is always the temptation to believe that what happened one day can easily be remembered and continued the next. Weather and light can change, staff can become redeployed to a more pressing incident elsewhere, and a new shift will need to know who has done what, or where to start. The creation of daily records is paramount.

A detailed log will include date, time, extent of manpower, names of officers in charge, comments on the vegetation, weather, light, wind direction and method of search, all cross-referenced to maps. The annotated maps are probably the cornerstone of the record; they define the spatial components of the search and illustrate the daily progress and distribution of the various techniques deployed. They can also be used to cross-reference observations by search officers regarding locations at which they encountered specific difficulties, or where they noted points of interest which might benefit from repeated investigation. The maps can also outline zones where specific techniques such as dogs or geophysics were deployed, where a particular type of geophysical survey (e.g. GPR) was used in one location and another method (e.g. resistivity) in another, or where points of interest could be defined. At any time the data can then be applied to a GIS model incorporating the various techniques used. Records of this nature mean that any subsequent review can hit the ground running knowing exactly which areas have been searched, by what method, by whom, and the conditions prevalent at the time. Complementary or repeat techniques can be deployed with full awareness of what has already been carried out, and where, and future new technologies can be introduced as appropriate.

4.1.3 Thoroughness

This is a subjective term which has different connotations to different people; it is a term recognised in the ACPO 2006 manual, which notes that 'the officer in charge of the search should consider how thorough the search has been' and in doing so recognises the subjectivity that may be involved (*ibid.*, 132). There is a list of example criteria that may have affected 'thoroughness', including weather conditions, lack of appropriate equipment and searching in poor light. There is no 'by-the-book' method to search a given area and the best search leaders will take advice from specialists in different fields. Search is inevitably landscape dependant: what is deemed to be 'thorough' in one location may be totally inappropriate in another on the basis of landfall, geology, undergrowth or accessibility. Nor will the various techniques available necessarily all be viable. For example, aerial reconnaissance may be hindered by tree canopy or land use, certain geophysical survey methods are likely to be ineffective in woodland as a result of tree roots or may not work effectively in certain soils, and machines for soil stripping may not be able to gain access to confined spaces or gardens. Each search domain may contain a series of elements that allow some techniques to work, but not others; in other words it is not always possible to have consistency of approach. Conventionally, searches are carried out in a sequence using methods which are non-invasive in the first instance but become progressively more invasive thereafter. This minimises loss of buried evidence; it is also efficient in terms of use of manpower in that a large part of the work can be carried out away from the search area. Typically, this process might be defined as a series of four stages, each one becoming progressively more invasive than the one before. Larger areas may require all stages to be followed, but smaller targeted areas such as gardens may start at later stages. The stage at which input commences can depend not just on the physical nature or size of the search area but also on other circumstances which may surround the enquiry, not least being covertness. Each scene is different and will require different balances and strategies. Search theory is all very well, but is rarely straightforward in application and often needs to be implemented creatively.

4.2 Interrogating landscapes

We can outline a simple four-stage model of how a search strategy might be designed. It needs to incorporate information from the enquiry that can be transferred to a map, landscape features that characterise areas of interest, search techniques that will be relevant to those areas of interest, and sequences of actions that can be deployed subsequently. This might normally start with the most non-invasive actions in order to minimise any potential loss of evidence, thus:

- *Stage 1*. Desk-top: e.g. maps; aerial imagery (existing and commissioned); GIS.

- *Stage 2*. General field survey: e.g. field walking; line search; free roaming cadaver dogs; vegetation clearance.

- *Stage 3*. Focused field survey: e.g. geophysical survey; cadaver dog venting; probing.

- *Stage 4*. Excavation: e.g. test pitting, formal excavation, machine stripping.

Ruffell and McKinley provide a similar model, but with more points of potential discontinuity (2008, 276). Both models, however, show how different techniques can be used sequentially to narrow down the focus of the search area. The following of these stages is procedural, but they can only be defined as 'thorough' on the basis of the questions being posed to the landscape and according to the levels of confidence of the techniques being applied. Landscapes are invariably inconsistent in surface expressions such as open fields, woodland, water and domestic housing, and therefore can require the application of several different techniques. The same can occur on the micro-level, for example in a garden where features may include patios, lawns, flower beds and domestic out-buildings. The only way to ensure complete elimination of a search area for buried remains is to excavate it completely. This is clearly impracticable on a large scale if only through reasons of sheer cost, but is not uncommon in domestic gardens and there are numerous case studies to illustrate this (e.g. Case Study 4.1). Normally, however, search thoroughness is a compromise between the perceived importance of an area of land and what is practicable. A search might, for example, be considered 'thorough' even at Stage 2 if it was felt that the area in question was not of prime importance.

In this case the strategy was substantially defined by the level of confidence exercised by the SIO. His interpretation that the garden, on the balance of probabilities, was more likely than less likely to contain the girl's remains was the driver for a careful approach. If his level of confidence was lower it might have been more prudent to commence at Stage 4 in the first instance and use the mechanical excavator straightaway. If his level of confidence was higher, or the area larger, then aspects of Stage 2 might have been implemented initially. Search is often a balance, on the one hand between deployment of resources (i.e. costs) to find remains and, on the other hand, ensuring that as much evidence as possible is recovered. Had the presence of buried human remains been indicated at Stage 3, careful excavation could have ensured their proper recovery together with any associated evidence. This would have justified the approach taken. Had the investigation commenced at Stage 4,

---

Case Study 4.1

A particular example concerned the garden of a semi-detached property in western England where a cold case review had produced new evidence for disposal of a young girl. The garden consisted of lawns, a concrete terrace and some narrow flower beds. Briefing and discussion between the relevant parties agreed on a strategy that would effectively start at Stage 3 (focused field survey) on the basis that the area in question was sufficiently small to enable this to happen. The strategy involved using ground penetrating radar (GPR) across the whole of the garden, which was sufficiently flat. Responses, of which there were six (although relatively small), were then vented for the cadaver dog (Figure 4.1). Those under the concrete terrace were drilled in order to allow this. The dog responded to none of the GPR targets. Stage 4 was then implemented using a mechanical excavator under an archaeological watching brief to strip away the garden soils horizontally in order to expose carefully the undisturbed strata below. This was conducted across the whole of the garden, no human remains were found and the garden could be eliminated with the highest level of confidence after two days of work. The six GPR responses transpired to be small rubbish pits.

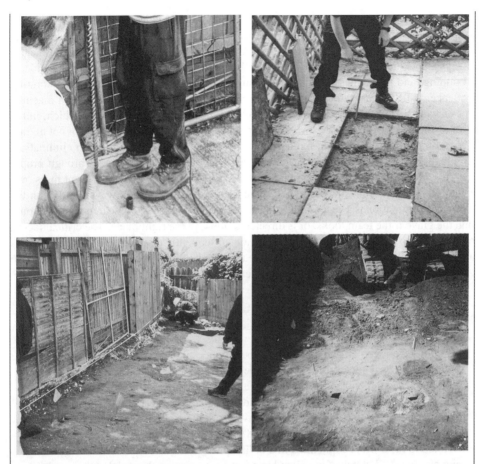

Figure 4.1 Top left, venting, drilling through concrete in order to vent a GPR response for cadaver dog attention (Stage 3); top right, venting below a paving slab (Stage 3); bottom left and bottom right, ultimate stripping by machine exposing innocent rubbish pits (Stage 4).

any human remains would have been exposed by machine and evidence lost in the process. The approach would not have been justified. In a small garden such as this, the body is likely to have been located by either approach but it depends on the questions the enquiry needs to address and the value placed on any evidence associated with the body. These are issues that will be paramount in the mind of the SIO who will need to balance them against levels of confidence in the site in question and the use of resources. 'Thoroughness' was easily achievable in a search area this size; it was the process by which it was achieved that mattered.

Other scenes may require a different stage of input according to circumstance. There are some cases, for example, where the SIO's level of confidence in a site is justifiably low. Many of these have a common theme, namely that a member of the public arrives at a police station and claims to have witnessed a disposal in a particular place. The event in question invariably occurred many years earlier, often measured in decades. The victim is unknown to the witness, no missing person is recorded in police files, but the location is absolute and identifiable within a few square metres (Case Studies 4.2, 4.3 and 4.4). There is nearly always a specific landmark involved, typically a tree, the corner of a fence, or the side of a building, and the witness is adamant throughout. In the absence of other corroborating evidence, the SIO can safely enter the search process at Stage 4, often using a machine to excavate the site, preferably with archaeological supervision. Such cases which, in the opinion of the SIO, present low levels of confidence – i.e. where the likelihood of not finding a burial is more probable than finding one – become effectively exercises in elimination. Elimination can be an important aspect of search. A location eliminated through proper search serves to narrow down the real burial location and is an accomplishment in its own right. When asked how successful our searches are, the answer is always '100%' on the basis that elimination is a successful element of the search process. A search team will only find the grave if the team looks, or is directed to look, in the right place. The critical factor, of course, is to make sure that the burial is not subsequently discovered in an area that has already been eliminated. And this is why search needs to be, wherever possible, thorough as opposed to cursory. Three relevant short case studies are described below.

Case Study 4.2

A middle-aged woman had come into a local police station in a fairly distraught state. She wished to provide information that she had witnessed two small boys being buried in a patch of woodland and shrubbery on a local golf course (by the 17th green) some 25 years earlier. The boys, she claimed, had been abused at a care home when she was a child in the same home. She claimed to have heard them being tortured before all went quiet, and their 'bodies' carried away and buried in woodland at the golf course. She claimed to have watched them from a hiding place behind some trees and was able to pinpoint the small patch of woodland in question. Enquiries showed that the care home did exist at that time and that the lady in question was recorded as being a resident there. In common with many such cases, no missing persons were recorded at that time.

It was difficult to establish the original extent of the woodland and shrubbery some 30 years earlier, but the trees were mature and would have provided root difficulty in digging at the time. However, there was a ditch running through the woodland, which had mostly silted up and no longer provided drainage for the course. On advice, the SIO agreed to vent the whole area, including the ditch for cadaver dog attention (Stage 3) and excavate only those parts of the ditch that offered the greatest concealment (Stage 4). Excavation was undertaken archaeologically and showed that the ditch had been re-cut on at least one occasion (unrecorded) and had become filled with a clearly-defined series of silt layers. The dogs were unresponsive to the venting and the excavations in the ditch proved unrewarding, although they did expose a stratified series of golf balls. The work took less than two days. The SIO's view was that the area could be eliminated with confidence. No missing persons had been recorded, no dog responses had been identified and covert lengths of the ditch had been fully excavated. In practical terms, other than digging out all the trees, nothing more could be done.

Case Study 4.3

Information was received from a person who claimed to have witnessed the burial of a murder victim several decades earlier. The witness was a child at the time but he was specific in terms of the location of burial which he said took place next to a small bridge over a stream in a very rural area. The witness claimed to have been hiding behind a hedge. He was also specific regarding the time of the event which occurred during the laying of a concrete drainage system, and that the body had been buried directly under the concrete pipe during the construction process. Enquiries were able to establish the time of the drain laying, and also that a missing person had been recorded at roughly the same time. This gave a reasonable degree of credibility to the information, despite the age of the witness.

The nature of the potential scene was such that the SIO wished to proceed carefully but was required to deploy heavy machinery in the first instance (Stage 4) in order to gain access below the concrete pipe. Once an appropriate length of pipe had been removed the suspect area could be trowelled over in order to identify any disturbances cut into the natural clay deposits (Figure 4.2). Even when the exposed area was extended, no disturbances were identified and the enquiry ceased. In cases such as this, an archive record of the exact length of pipe removed and the dimensions of the area investigated is essential should further work ever be necessary.

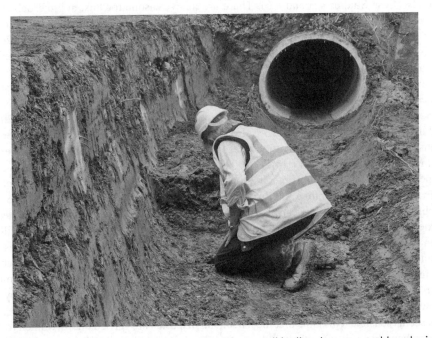

Figure 4.2 Careful trowelling in order to identify a possible disturbance caused by a burial during the construction of a pipe line.

Case Study 4.4

A lady in her late 30s appeared at a police station and recounted an event from her childhood many years earlier. She remembered her father fighting with a woman upstairs before carrying a large bundle downstairs and burying it in the back garden of their terrace house. Police checks ascertained that the lady giving this information had a history of drug abuse, but equally that her father (since deceased) was known to frequent prostitutes. As a result the SIO decided to commission a geophysical survey of the rear garden which was flat and grassy (Stage 3). The work was carried out discretely, and no responses were obtained. On the basis of the SIO's level of confidence in the allegation, this was considered sufficiently 'thorough' to enable the site to be eliminated.

Some of these older cases are more complex in that they concern neonatal or stillbirths where there is a direct relationship between the witness (often the mother) and the child, and where there are often psychological complications (Isser and Schwartz 2001). In view of the nature of the relationship, the SIO may have no alternative other than to assume that a burial *did* take place and that there is a body to be found. In other words the primary action is to locate as opposed to eliminate.

The case files of most forensic archaeologists will contain incidences of alleged illegal neonatal burials or disposals and it is worth dwelling on the issues in a little more detail (see also Case Studies 4.5 and 4.6). There are many reasons for this, and the deliberate concealment of neonatal remains can be traced back through archaeological timescales as recognisable aspects of ritual and cultural protocol in various societies (Mays 2000; Jackson 2002; Lewis 2007). However, in modern times concealment tends to reflect unwanted pregnancy, stillbirth or illicit abortion usually connected to matters of social stigma (illegitimacy), prostitution (accidental pregnancy) or illicit sexual relationships (incest) and can involve a range of offences, for example concealment of birth (Offences Against the Person Act 1861; HMSO 1861), rape (Sexual Offences Act 2003; HMSO 2003) and infanticide (Infanticide Act 1938; HMSO 1938), as well as deaths occurring under the terms of the Infant Life (Preservation) Act 1929 (HMSO 1929) or the Domestic Violence, Crime and Victims Act 2004 (HMSO 2004b; HMSO 2012) depending on the parties concerned, their age, relationship and circumstances. In all cases disposal of the remains poses little difficulty in that, unlike the disposal of adult remains, they are easily portable and unobtrusive in carriage. They can also be disposed of quickly, even by burial. Police interest in these cases tends to vary according to circumstance: at one extreme an enquiry will be keen to pursue and prosecute cases of suspected incest where child protection issues are at stake, but at the other extreme are less likely to prosecute, for example, in a case where a middle-aged woman admits to burying a stillborn infant when she was a teenager many years earlier. Although an offence may have been committed, it is not always seen by the Crown Prosecution Service (CPS) to be in the public interest to apply the law.

It seems sensible to assume that most neonatal disposals are carried out by women (often the mothers themselves), although there appear to be no statistics available on this. These will probably account for stillbirths or self-inflicted abortions and may even be located in a place that can be returned to for memorial purposes. Factors of conscience in a mother's later years may provide sufficient pressure for an admission in order to have the remains recovered. While this admission may not be worth pursuing from a prosecution point of view, it may well be worth following up in order to obtain better closure for the mother for psychological reasons, as well as satisfying 'duty of care' under the terms of the Human Rights Act 1998 (HMSO 1998) (Case Studies 4.5 and 4.6).

The disturbance caused by digging a clandestine neonatal grave is unlikely to be much larger than one or two spade widths in each direction and probably not much deeper than two spade depths for practical reasons alone. Such a relatively small target size is almost certainly beyond the sensitivity of most geophysical survey systems. The burial may not even penetrate bedrock (the 'C' horizon) making the disturbance almost impossible to distinguish from the topsoil into which it has been cut even by surface stripping. Search areas need to be defined carefully, but their locations tend to rely almost wholly on witness information (usually the mother). In instances where the time span between disposal and admission is great, the precise location may be difficult to pinpoint. However, landscapes change as vegetation develops, properties change ownership and domestic gardens become revamped over time. Features present at the time of the disposal may no longer be extant, levels may have changed and soils and materials imported. A new owner may know nothing of previous events which may have taken place on his/her land decades earlier. It may not be possible for a mother to revisit the scene for emotional reasons, or it may not be advisable to alert the new owner. As a result the witness account will be purely verbal, probably inaccurate in terms of distance (in paces or measurement) from fixed points (e.g. distance from the back door, at the bottom of the steps, or at the base of a tree). Moreover, those fixed points may no longer be there (see Case Study 4.5). The definition of search boundaries will have to take into account a number of factors: the mental state of the witness; the likelihood of the incident being 'real' according to the information available to the SIO; the probability of the area being 'right'; and the extent of the resources likely to be needed in order to excavate or sieve the soils. This will be a decision that is likely to be made jointly by the SIO and the Crime Scene Manager, supported by the archaeologist.

Case Study 4.5

An elderly lady on her death bed wished to confess to burying a stillborn neonate in the garden of her terrace house some 60 years earlier. The house was no longer standing and the area had subsequently been landscaped as part of a community centre. Reference to planning details and maps made it possible to identify exactly where the 'footprint' of the house and garden had been (Stages 1 and 2) and this was marked out on the ground with a fair degree of accuracy and was sufficiently small to permit careful machine stripping of the surface soils (Stage 4) (Figure 4.3). A small trench was also excavated in order to ascertain the nature and survival of the buried soils. The foundations of the house were exposed but the topsoil had been removed during the landscaping and had been deposited elsewhere. The neonate was said to have been buried in a shallow grave near a tree in a corner of the garden. The tree cavity was found but, despite careful excavation, no other disturbances were identified. The burial had either been removed during the redevelopment, or was never there in the first place. The enquiry had done all it could, and the search design had been deployed efficiently.

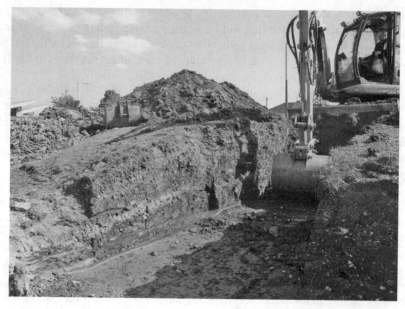

Figure 4.3 The use of a machine (Stage 4) in the search for the garden subsoil of a demolished building. Note the exposed section on the left which shows the present made-up soil landscape overlying the compacted rubble demolition. The level at which the machine is stripping is the surface directly underlying the rubble.

Case Study 4.6

A woman had secretly buried a stillborn neonate during darkness at the edge of woodland. Several years later she confessed this to the police who agreed to implement a search. There were two difficulties: the first was that the location was imprecise, and the second that the ground was heavily waterlogged. After due discussion, three target areas were identified, each measuring about 5 × 3 m, based on the information given and the woman's accompanied re-visit to the site (Stage 2). The wetness, the extent of overgrowth and the fragility of the target were such that search could only be undertaken by manual digging in the first instance (Stage 4): the turf was removed in a line across each area in question with careful breaking down and checking of the topsoil in order to expose the natural clay beneath. Each strip of clay was then cleaned in order to identify any disturbances and then eliminated before the next strip was exposed. This continued until the whole of the area had been covered. The neonate had been buried in a small heavy-duty plastic bag and this was discovered cut partially into the natural clay in the second area of interest (Figure 4.4). The witness had identified the general location successfully and the search design, although implemented at Stage 4, was conducted sufficiently carefully to identify the target.

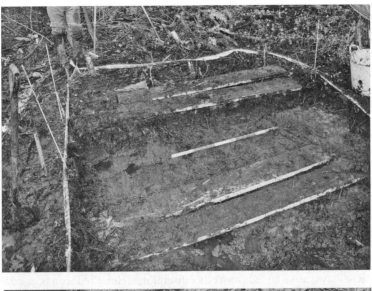

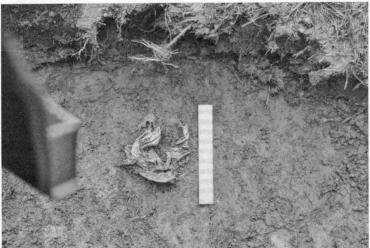

Figure 4.4 Careful excavation at the edge of woodland (top) in difficult wet conditions resulting in the recovery of a plastic bag (bottom) containing neonatal remains (Stage 4).

Some searches will require significant input at Stage 1. These are the cases where the location of disposal cannot easily be narrowed down and where the SIO's level of confidence has not yet been set. A hypothetical case (mirrored many times in real life) might involve a missing person (wife) and a suspected offender (estranged husband) who have argued over a matrimonial settlement. The husband is believed to have disposed of her body locally. Analysis of available evidence, witness information and reference to statistical data point to a disposal location in a particular direction from the suspect's house covering an area of roughly two square kilometres. This is the only starting point available and the SIO decides to implement a search. The proposed search area is identified, defined, sub-divided into domains and analysed at desk-top level. This analysis might include trawling through early Ordnance Survey maps to identify obsolete mine shafts, quarries and wells that might be known to an offender, and examining later maps for vehicle access points, trackways, patches of woodland and water courses. Geological maps and land use maps will be an important resource, as will aerial photographs. The Joint Aerial Reconnaissance Intelligence Centre (JARIC) may be commissioned to take new photographs and interpret them accordingly. The whole package of data can then be integrated and analysed, perhaps using GIS.

There is an important transition here when the acquired mapping and landscape data become analysed and interpreted; this is the point at which the search moves from objective to subjective mode. As all aspects of landscape theoretically carry equal weighting there needs to be justification for prioritising some areas over others, for example on the basis of landfall, geology, visibility, access distances, witness sightings, etc. Prioritising defines areas of greater likelihood, but by definition also relegates non-priority areas to a category of lower likelihood. A useful technique has been developed by Donnelly and Harrison (2010) in breaking down the landscape in this way using a colour notation of red, amber or green ('RAG' system) adapted from other disciplines. Here 'red' can be used to identify areas of high probability, 'amber' for areas of average probability and 'green' for areas that are of lower importance but nevertheless require searching. This colour coded system can then be integrated with the various stages of search. For example, areas denoted as 'green' could be subjected to Stages 1 and 2 only (subject to findings) and then eliminated; 'amber' areas could then be searched at Stage 3 (e.g. by geophysics and focused dogs) with any responses forming the essence of 'red' areas for invasive action (Figure 4.5).

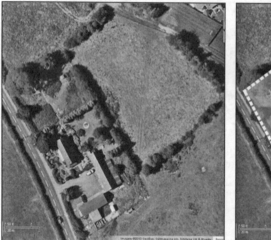 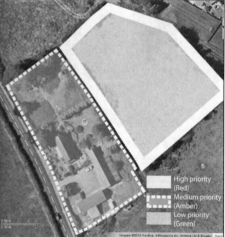

Figure 4.5 Hypothetical example of use of 'RAG' analysis of landscape. The image on the left represents a straightforward aerial photograph of a suspect area. The image on the right shows the same area divided into priority zones on the basis of access points, slope, geology cover or intelligence. Aerial image by permission of Getmapping plc.

On the basis of the prioritisation formed in Stage 1, decisions may then be made to enter Stage 2 by targeting those areas of greatest likelihood on the ground, for example by using a combination of close line field examination and free roaming cadaver dogs. If areas of disturbed ground are identified, or if the dogs respond in a particular location, then the investigation can move directly into Stage 4 and an excavation strategy can be implemented. On the other hand, if there are no obvious pointers to a burial at Stage 2 then the search process may need to be reviewed. If, in the SIO's opinion, the likelihood of the body being in the area is very low, and there are other locations that might bear investigation, the search can be shut down at this point. S/he has undertaken a level of investigation that s/he considers to be reasonable on the basis of the evidence available. In other words, the level of 'thoroughness' was appropriate under the particular circumstances of the case. The domains and target areas together with the methodology will have been logged and can always be returned to for future investigation. Conversely, if levels of confidence are high, Stage 3 can be implemented in those areas already searched by field examination and free roaming dogs.

Stage 3 may introduce methods of geophysical survey, but this may be restricted according to terrain and method and is unlikely to be applied consistently across a full targeted area unless the targeted area is relatively small. The same may apply to the focused use of cadaver dogs, which requires systematic venting of the ground. Because of constraints posed by scale, land use and vegetation, there is often a narrowing of the area addressed at Stage 3. This is not an issue of increased confidence in sharpening the focus of search, but an effect of the constraints presented by the terrain and the methods available. Searching areas simply because they are 'searchable' at this stage not only begins to dislocate the methodology from the objectives, but also introduces undesirable inconsistency at points of perceived focal interest. However, if targets are identified excavation will be required. If the search findings are still negative, the SIO will need to decide whether or not to move into Stage 4 at all, while bearing in mind that not all the target area was consistently examined. Excavation or machine clearance will only serve to sample the area in question further and leave greater areas unattended. It may indeed be possible for the whole area to be examined in this way, for example in a rear garden, but not in larger terrains. In other words the search area has been narrowed down by factors that are outside the control of the SIO; these factors have created patterns of inconsistency and hence the extent to which the search can be deemed 'thorough'. There may indeed be specific areas, perhaps as a result of witness information, that the SIO would wish to strip, but these may be small in relation to the whole area targeted.

But what alternative is there? The only redeeming element here is that the same constraints encountered by the search may also have been experienced by the offender in burying the victim in the first place – hard sub-soils, limited accessibility, intense undergrowth, tree roots, steep contours and so on. In current enquiries where the interval between disposal and search is short (i.e. days), this is less of a problem: disturbed ground is more likely to be evident, levels of vegetation penetrability and density of woodland will be similar and water tables consistent. There are good odds that the landscape available for burial and the landscape amenable for search will match fairly closely. However, in longer term enquiries (i.e. months) or in cold cases (i.e. years) there may be significant changes to all of these factors (see Chapter 5), for example bramble and scrub cover can increase remarkably quickly in the space of a few seasons, and leaf fall will conceal or level out disturbances or tell-tale topographical change. Levels of confidence in search thoroughness and thus in eliminating areas can only be as high as the landscape allows. At the end of day the degree of thoroughness of search is a direct measure of several factors: the size of the search area in question; the impact of the landscape on search methodology; and the stages at which the SIO chooses to enter and exit the search process. These are illustrated in Case Studies 4.7 and 4.8.

Case Study 4.7

In 1976 a lady and her young son went missing in north-east Scotland, her car being discovered a short distance from a sand/gravel quarry which had been used for a trunk road upgrade scheme. Despite an intensive police search the two were never found, but the quarry, which was infilled shortly after the disappearance, was never searched at the time. The decommissioning of the quarry involved using the empty quarry space to dump building material and commercial waste, the upper edges were pushed in to obscure the steep sides but the original terraces and base in which the bodies may have been hidden were undisturbed although the original dimensions and contours of the quarry were completely obscured. A year later the local police force dug a machine trench through part of the quarry (unrecorded), but was unsuccessful in its search. The whole area was then topsoiled and planted with conifers to match the surroundings.

A review of the case almost three decades later led to the quarry being excavated and searched. This was in many ways a response to local rumour and speculation, and important for elimination purposes. Although the location of the quarry was known, the SIO initiated a search at Stage 1 as the quarry had been mostly levelled and its precise edges obscured. Earlier aerial photographs and maps were used to identify the original edges and the area was cleared of vegetation and trees (Stage 2). The idea of using GPR or cadaver dogs was considered at this point (Stage 3) but the depth and nature of the quarry sides and infill was unknown at this stage and their effectiveness considered unlikely. Consequently the search moved directly into Stage 4 using two mechanical excavators under an archaeological watching brief to remove the infill (Figure 4.6). This was undertaken stratigraphically over a period of some five weeks during which time the infilled police trench of 1977 was identified and emptied. A total of over 37,000 tonnes of material was removed. Carried out carefully, this process was able to return the quarry to its original state before infilling in 1976, measuring some 110 m across to a maximum depth of c. 35 m leaving terraces and scree exposed. It also identified the location of the search trench dug in 1977 (Figure 4.6). The sides were then stripped back by machine in order to identify any disturbances or concealment. None were found and the quarry was eliminated from the enquiry with a high degree of confidence. In conclusion, the search area was consistent in its character and the search strategy was able to provide an equally consistent approach, one which was comprehensive and which enabled satisfactory elimination to be made.

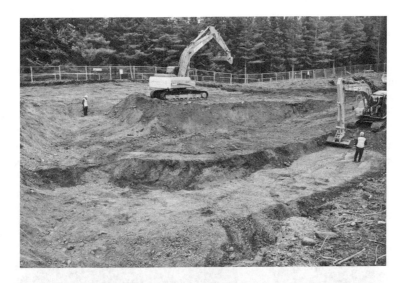

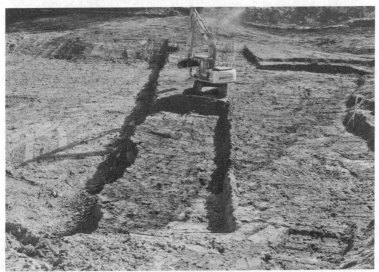

Figure 4.6 Excavation of quarry showing (top) stratigraphic removal of fill using heavy machinery and (bottom) the exposure of an earlier search trench which appears as a darker rectangle.

Case Study 4.8

A small area of overgrown land (some 40×20 m) was identified as being significant in a particular enquiry, partly on the basis of evidence that the body of a victim may have been burnt and subsequently buried there. This was a cold case, the area was partially fenced and the boundaries clear. Search commenced at Stage 2 by physical assessment of the area on the ground. However, this proved impossible, given the thickness of the vegetation. As a result the undergrowth was removed by task force officers taking care to disturb the ground surface and any possible markers as little as possible. Once cleared the surface was inspected and a small number of obvious points of interest identified. Geophysical survey was not used owing to the likely extent of tree roots and other features.

Cadaver dogs were then allowed to free roam but made no responses. Search then moved into Stage 3 mode, the ground being systematically vented to include the points of interest (Figure 4.7). The dogs were re-introduced with some positive response. On the basis of this and the points of interest recorded, small scale excavation took place

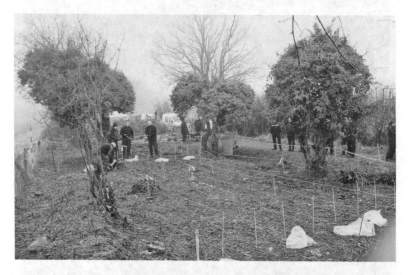

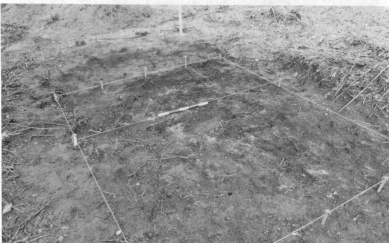

Figure 4.7 Investigation of a defined area of land showing (top) systematic venting for dogs (Stage 3) and (bottom) careful excavation and sampling of area of burning (Stage 4).

in selected areas (Stage 4). These were eliminated with one exception – a spread of burning. This was carefully exposed to its full extent, photographed, recorded, sampled and excavated (Figure 4.7). In order to ensure complete elimination of the rest of the scene, a small mechanical excavator was introduced to strip away the remaining vegetation and topsoil down to undisturbed deposits. This was carried out systematically at a consistent depth under an archaeological watching brief. No further evidence was forthcoming. In conclusion, it had been possible to take a logical, staged approach to the search and to implement a consistent strategy throughout. This was mostly due to the relatively small nature of the search area. The use of a mechanical excavator as a final tool ensured complete elimination of the rest of the site.

4.3 Balancing probabilities

The balance between objective and subjective search is an interesting one. Any prioritisation of the search area is inevitably biased by factors that are believed to influence choice of deposition site (proximity, distance, slope, access, etc.) and these also form the basis of the 'RAG' system (Section 4.2). In the absence of defined starting points these present realistic foci. However, they inevitably assume that the disposal is undertaken according to principles that are logical in the eyes of the investigator, that generally conform to recorded statistical data (Section 2.1) and that are generally in keeping with principles of least effort on behalf of the offender, or that match a perceived profile. The model is theoretical and makes a number of assumptions. It tends to assume, for example, that the offender may have a basic knowledge of the landscape and its soils, an awareness of optimum places that lie out of sight where disposal can take place, or the best route from A to B in the dark through woodland. It assumes that cadavers are unlikely to be carried very far up steep hills, over fences, through bogs and rivers or into impenetrable thickets. The initial assumption, for most search purposes, is that the basis of the deposition is essentially a logical one.

In the authors' experience there are many cases that serve to demonstrate the extent to which the locations of disposal diverge widely from theoretical doctrine, or indeed from common sense. There are some good examples: in one case the authors excavated a victim from below the water table in a heavy clay soil in a relatively open location. From a search point of view the location of disposal ticked none of the likely search boxes other than being a short distance from a vehicle access point at the end of a track. In another, the offender clearly had no knowledge of the local geology and his first attempt at digging was thwarted by a tree root and a bedding outcrop. He was obliged to give up and bury the body elsewhere but left spade marks and characteristic flakes of paint from the spade behind (Case Study 6.3). In a further case all the intelligence pointed to a disposal point that would have required the offender(s) to have carried the body over 100 m up hill and bury it in a hard stony landscape instead of in softer soil in an equally secluded location lower down the slope. Intensive police search and excavation of a wide area demonstrated the impossibility of digging through the compacted stones. A fine example of improbability is demonstrated by Ruffell and McKinley who illustrate an alleged burial site defined by a tarmac patch in the middle of a garage forecourt (2008, 290 and figure 9.11e).

From an offender's perspective, even the best laid plans can be thwarted by a host of different situations: the need for a hurried disposal; fear of being observed; unexpected turns of weather; loss of orientation during darkness; having to review a planned disposal at short notice in view of encountering potential witnesses out for walks; gates being locked, or discovering unexpected new buildings, or changes to access. Case studies suggest that luck seems to play as much a part of an effective disposal as it might in a successful discovery subsequently.

Disposal activities can also vary by homicide type according to whether the offence is serial, premeditated or non-premeditated, and there is a wide literature on criminal and geographical profiling (e.g. Canter 2000; Canter 2004; Rossmo 2006). Serial murderers tend to follow a prescribed pattern that is repetitive and hence ostensibly predictable, but this does not mean that the disposal patterning is necessarily carefully predetermined. Robert Black, for example, in his abduction and murder of young girls, disposed of their bodies in a largely circumspect manner, dumping them in secluded areas at or near lay-bys on main roads where the assaults had taken place or elsewhere on his established commercial routes. He was eventually caught because of his need to keep petrol receipts in order to claim back his fuel expenditure. These showed dates and times of fuelling and, by inference, routes taken. They also flagged up geographical areas of activity, the so-called 'Midlands triangle' within which his criminal activity was greatest (Farren 2004). By contrast, Ian Brady the so-called 'Moors murderer' carefully formulated strategies for the destruction of forensic evidence and disposed of the bodies by burial, usually in locations bearing tell-tale markers that he recorded photographically. Both men followed their own *modus operandi*, and each took satisfaction from their crimes in characteristic ways. But the two could not be more different. Black was probably little aware of the landscape of disposal other than it was immediate and usually concealed from public view. His satisfaction was in the crime, the disposal of the body was secondary – the principle of least effort. Brady was more landscape aware. He was very familiar with the locations of disposal, and he was also obsessed with succeeding with 'the perfect murder'. To him the disposal was part of the satisfaction of the crime. This emphasises not only the dangers of using a 'by-the-book' approach, but also the importance of introducing psychological parameters (criminal profiling) into the overall disposal equation. Both men were predators, in both cases their victims were casually encountered in that they were not specifically earmarked for assault as named individuals. In their own way both men were prowlers: Black took the opportunity to seize children on their own in isolated locations on his routes and bundle them into his van, whereas Brady used quiet suburban streets to lure children away. Their abductions were mostly serendipitous, the victims just happened to be in the wrong place at the wrong time. In serial killings, knowledge of the potential offender and the geography of activity can often be drivers in understanding the likely landscape of disposal.

The general issue of criminal mapping is explored in some detail by Hirschfield and Bowers (2001) whose work tends to focus on sociological and demographic evidence that may have predictive qualities for policing purposes. This examines, for example, types and concentrations of particular crimes in certain socio-economic areas, or crimes committed in certain places in relation to population movement and activity. Moreover, some of the data on which the studies are based demonstrate that a criminal's familiarity with places for disposing of a body is often as important as familiarity with places for committing the crime in the first place. GIS lends itself well to crime mapping (e.g. Laukkanen *et al.* 2008); further case studies illustrating the value of geographical analysis are well documented by Canter (2003).

Ruffell and McKinley use Northern Ireland sectarian examples to illustrate the importance of geography in understanding abduction and disposal patterns; they apply the term 'influence of locality' showing how these patterns can be used predictively (2008, 134). Whilst not being 'serial' killings as such, these gang murders feature many of the signatures that might be recognised in serial killings. Analysis of the geographical patterning showed that Republican victims were generally abducted in a number of specific places where they were vulnerable and where surveillance was poor. Disposals tended to occur either nearby in those same places, or some distance away in the relative safety of loyalist housing estates. The bodies were normally dumped rather than concealed. GIS analysis showed an interesting correlation between sectarian territorial centres, concentrations of gang activity, and communication and public transport routes (*ibid.*, 136). Using a wider data set, trawled from Lane and Gregg's *Encyclopaedia of Serial Killers* (1995) – a useful, if popular, volume that collates general information in a fairly consistent way – the importance of 'influence of locality' is reinforced. However, what is perhaps interesting is that some of the randomly selected data points took on a much more pronounced locational significance in both the place of initial encounter and in the place of the crime than in the eventual place of body deposition (Ruffell and McKinley 2008, 134, table 5.1).

Single premeditated murders can present a completely different set of themes. Premeditation normally assumes that the victim is known to the offender, as (ex-)spouse, business partner, lover/mistress, fellow criminal, etc. The dispute that leads to the murder can embrace a range of potential contexts, but notably divorce/matrimonial issues and drugs activities. In most cases the timing of the crime, including the disposal, has been anticipated and organised, any necessary equipment purchased, and a suitable time frame set out. The location of disposal will have been planned, a potential alibi system set up, and preparations made that will enable the disposal to take place effectively.

In the experience of the authors, offenders who premeditate murder (or who are believed to have premeditated murder) usually manage to engineer a suitable time window between the death and the reporting of the person going missing. This might be planned around times when the potential victim is normally not seen in public or visiting friends, and during which time the movements of both victim and offender are only partially traceable. In due course alarm bells may be set ringing by relatives or friends, or even by the offender him/herself in the case of domestic arrangements. Either way, there is a dedicated period in which assault, murder, disposal and cleaning up can be achieved according to a pre-established scheme. This may even extend to removing superfluous spoil (i.e. soils that can no longer be put back in the grave as the body has taken up the space) off the site to a different location. Where time has allowed, offenders have used various devious methods to conceal the burial site, for example, by the careful replacing of layers (Case Studies 6.1 and 6.2), planting shrubs across the disturbed area, introducing compost to encourage quicker growth of natural vegetation, constructing buildings or terraces over the site (Case Study 4.9), or piling rubbish across the disturbed ground (Case Study 4.10).

The advantage of premeditation is that it presents an adequate time frame to ensure that the disposal is arranged rationally and that the location is as secure as possible. In establishing this location, the offender may need to undertake reconnaissance visits to various sites in order to ensure a place of appropriate access and optimum concealment. Disposal statistics suggest that burial is unlikely to take place in some random area of countryside unknown to the offender. Time taken to identify the 'right' location is probably not an issue, but there is a balance between time spent and the potential risk of being witnessed. There have been some instances where archaeological evidence has been able to demonstrate that the grave has been dug in advance, on the basis of the edges slumping inwards or through silt and organic accumulations in the bottom. The longer a grave is left open, or only partially concealed, the greater the risk of it being discovered. The further off the beaten track the grave lies, the less likely it is to be noticed, but the further and more laborious it will be to carry the body, and thus the greater the risk of being witnessed and the longer the empty time frame to be explained. Moreover, if the location is to be revisited in the dark, or twilight, then the offender will need to be either very familiar with the terrain, or rely heavily on well defined landmarks ('winthrop' points) that will lead him or her to the burial site. Management statistics have these variables reasonably well identified and most search strategies will be appropriately prepared. However, problems may arise when the offender is highly familiar with the landscape in question through activities such as childhood recreation, fishing/hunting, jogging or innocent dog walking, which may present a more intimate knowledge of landscapes and terrain features than mere reference to a map. Anyone who has driven from A to B by car on a regular basis and then walked the same route will recognise how much more detail about landscape features (both urban or rural) and slope can be experienced with the latter. In knowing a landscape, the offender puts him/herself at an advantage by virtue of greater knowledge of quiet places, secluded areas, workings, drains, ditches, vegetation characteristics and soils (Case Study 4.11). In disposals that appear to be premeditated, search strategies will need to assume the detailed knowledge of landscapes as well as the exposition of carefully laid plans, and respond accordingly.

The third and final category of murders are those that are not premeditated and that occur on the spur of the moment, for example, when one party is pushed down the stairs during a struggle, a partner throttled or struck on the head during a heated argument, or where teaching someone a lesson goes too far. Television soap operas provide a reasonable selection of examples and an equally reasonable selection of irrational disposals. In theory these should be the easiest graves to locate as they reflect panic and hurried preparations – the use of rugs or sheets to wrap the body, unusual vehicle activity or soiled clothes, and nearby disposal points that have not been evaluated fully. They have a tendency to involve immediate concealment as opposed to long-term security, and search foci can be directly accordingly. Speed of disposal is probably the critical element, especially if the relationship between victim and offender is not a close one (i.e. in instances where association between the two parties is indirect or not one in which suspicion might readily fall on the perpetrator) and this can be factored into any search design in order to identify priority domains. There are a number of case studies that illustrate this, in which the victim is buried in a secluded area a short distance from a lay-by, or at the end of a track, or even in the back garden. In theory, an unprepared, hurried deposition offers a lower risk of being witnessed simply because the elapsed time during which the event takes place is minimised, but there is a higher risk of the body being found since the event has not been planned and implemented with a view to longer-term concealment.

There will be some non-premeditated murders which do not conform to this general pattern. These are instances where the assault has occurred and the body concealed temporarily while the offender is forced to plan a more appropriate disposal strategy. This 'thinking time' is inevitably constrained by the concealment of the body (and possibly the smell) in a specific place, by the expected daily movements of the offender – such as going to work, keeping appointments, etc. – as well as the expected movements of the victim. But it does offer some breathing space in which a more secure disposal method can be thought out. It may not be as carefully planned as a fully premeditated disposal, but in many senses it will require the same degree of search preparation. Distance, areas of concealment known to the offender, vehicle accessibility and time available for disposal will become much more important in the enquiry.

Case Study 4.9

In another matrimonial case a husband had killed his wife and buried her in the back garden. His hobby was ornamental fish and he was often seen creating or modifying ponds. Here the pre-planning was in creating what was ostensibly a formal pond measuring approximately 1.5 × 1.5 m to a depth of about 1 m. It had clean, straight sides and a flat base. His wife was deposited in the bottom and covered over until the grave was about half-filled. He then laid a compacted layer of slates over the top and used the open upper part, suitably lined, as a fish pond. After a suitable period of time this was emptied, infilled with soil and then compacted as the base for a concrete terrace. The pre-planning here was in the construction of the grave/pond and in the sealing of the body with the layer of slates rather than in the choice of location *per se*. The assumption seems to have been that anyone excavating the disturbance caused by digging the pond would reach the layer of slates, assume them to be the bottom of the pond and investigate no further. The concealment lasted for many years until it was discovered during a police search of the garden that involved using geophysics (resistivity). The grave was too deep to be excavated from the ground surface and required a platform to be excavated out on one side in order to facilitate access (see Chapter 6.1).

Case Study 4.10

A young female had gone missing and her male relatives were suspected of her disappearance and murder. As a result of police enquiries the back garden of a house in a row of terraced houses was identified as a potential burial site. The circumstances of the garden were not conducive to a geophysical survey, so non-intrusive systematic visual search was undertaken by the forensic archaeologist. There was little evidence of disturbance in the garden. Only a small area of ground, close to rear of house, had been dug over leaving indications of lighter soils scattered on its surface. There was however, a single paving slab, lent against the privet hedge near to rear of the house, which had a small amount of soil on its surface indicating that it had recently been laid flat on the ground. Beneath the privet hedge was a small amount of loose thrown soil.

The visual examination now turned to the garden paths that comprised similar paving slabs, but none appeared to have been disturbed. There was a communal pathway, no longer used by the residents, immediately adjacent to rear of the row of terrace houses. This pathway was covered by household rubbish comprising three distinct piles covering the width of the pathway: an old bed; an armchair with a TV set on it; and next to that a table top, on top of which was an old fridge freezer laid length ways, with other miscellaneous items on top. Against this household rubbish were a few black plastic rubbish bags. However, between the gaps in this rubbish pile there were indications of bare soil where the edge of pathway should be.

Each of the objects placed on top of this pathway was photographed and recorded as layers that were potentially part of the stratigraphy of the suspected burial, and examined for trace evidence. Their removal revealed that the flagged pathway had been disturbed, and there were tool marks on the edges of those paving slabs that had been removed. The reason for the paving slab left against the hedge appeared to have been that when the slabs were re-laid they were replaced in the wrong alignment, hence there was no room for this slab. Excavation then commenced by half-sectioning the disturbed ground (see Chapter 6). Beneath the pathway the service pipes for the water supply and waste water from the house both exhibited tool marks. Ground disturbance is inevitable when repair works occur, but the disturbance continued below the level of the pipes and was clearly for a different reason. The depth necessitated the creation of working platform. A burial was exposed approximately 50 cm below the level of the service pipes. Anyone without archaeological skills checking the disturbance might stop at this level thinking that the disturbance was connected with the repair of the pipe (see also Case Study 4.9).

This case emphasises the importance of visual crime scene assessment and analysis, and the fact that the stratigraphy of the grave is not only subterranean but often above the surface. Furthermore, this often provides evidence of the *mens rea* (the state of mind) of the perpetrator(s); in this case it provided evidence that this was a determined effort at concealing the burial, below the service pipes, as opposed to an unplanned and hurried burial.

Case Study 4.11

After a turbulent marital relationship the wife left her partner and went to live on her own. The spouse, as a form of retaliation, chose to threaten not only his estranged wife but also the extended family of the wife, including her younger brother who still lived with their mother. The acrimony reached such an extent that he chose to take revenge on the brother as a way of hitting back at his former partner. He waylaid him, killed him and buried him, then confessed to the killing but deliberately refused to say where the burial was located as a way of taunting and upsetting the family further. By trade he was a building site worker and an expert at digging foundation trenches and drains by hand. The crime had been pre-planned to the extent that he had already prepared a grave of exceptional depth. This had almost sheer vertical sides and had been professionally executed. The location was in a relatively secluded landscape, which was familiar to him and a short distance from where the family lived. However, before the murder took place he decided that the location was insufficiently secure and dug another grave, equally deep and formal, in another location, having filled the first grave in. The first grave was subsequently found by police officers during a search. However, the second grave in which the body lay was only discovered some months later after the man's eventual confession. It was found in the rear overgrown garden of a substantial detached residence in local suburbs. As a builder he had been working in the adjacent house and had used the garden next door as a regular place for relieving himself, thus becoming familiar with its features, seclusion and access. The grave itself had been marked by items of rubble which would have allowed him to return at later dates to maintain peace of mind (Figure 4.8).

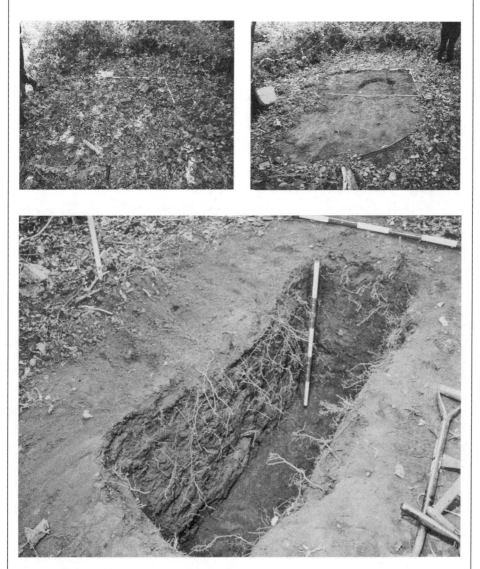

Figure 4.8 Illustration showing grave marked with bricks (top left), identification of grave cut (top right) and fully excavated grave (bottom).

Both burial locations were known to the offender and pre-planning was evident in the construction of both graves, although this did not appear to include using the opportunity to conceal either burial very effectively. The offender may have mistakenly assumed that depth alone would somehow ensured long term concealment. The first grave was so deep (over 2 metres) that officers needed a ladder to gain entry and exit. The second grave was only slightly shallower and the recovery necessitated digging out a platform to a parallel depth in order to extract the body (see Section 6.1).

5   Longer-term 'no body' cases

5.1   Introduction

Although search processes have become more rigorous, organised and interdisciplinary, there are still areas of relative neglect, some of which have yet to be explored in formal literature. This chapter begins to consider one of these: the search processes relevant in longer-term enquiries where landscapes may have changed as a result of both natural and cultural forces – 'landscapes' here being taken in their broadest context to embrace anything from tracts of moorland or an urban centre to the back garden of a small terraced house. Natural processes of change tend to be gradual and unperceivable – increased vegetation growth, woodland expansion or eroding hillsides – whereas cultural processes tend to be more easily defined and observable, most obviously through building activity and construction, but less overtly through agricultural change and land use. As a result of these changes, longer-term enquiries may find that the use of conventional applied 'desk-top' and field methods as outlined in Chapter 2 require some rethinking. There is, however, a diversity of data available, loosely described as 'historical', which is relevant and which this chapter attempts to address.

The number of instances in homicide cases where a conviction has been made without the victim's body ever being recovered continues to grow. This has been particularly in response to the development of DNA profiling, and courts have been increasingly comfortable with convicting under such circumstances. While a conviction effectively completes the criminal justice loop and provides formal resolution of a case in legal terms – that is the offender has been found and guilt proven (Rossmo 2006, 537f) – the lack of a body remains an open issue in personal terms for relatives and friends of the victim. Much has been written on the importance of 'closure' (Beder 2002; Williams and Crews 2003), but while police forces remain sympathetic and helpful they have no statutory obligation to pursue enquiries any further other than under the 'duty of care' element of Human Rights legislation. This might, for example, occur if new evidence comes to light or a new search location is identified. There are also (rarer) instances where renewed investigation has resulted from public or media demand, a notable example being the excavation of a quarry almost 30 years after persons were reported missing, partly as a result of additional evidence, but also as a result of increased community pressure (see Case Study 4.7).

Moreover, and on a practical front, there would normally need to be strong justification to deploy further police resources when the crime is already solved. This is quite distinctive from 'cold case' reviews where the crime remains unsolved (and the body may also be missing), and where regular reviews of the existing evidence take place with a view to considering the potential of new technological developments and techniques. Cold cases could be argued as those where 'perhaps, there were no leads . . . where evidence was lost, or went unnoticed; where for whatever reason, witnesses would not come forward' (Greig 2006, 6). Both types can come under the category of 'no body' murders, the difference being that cold cases are likely to have resources while the resolved crimes are not. 'No body' cases are complicated further depending on whether the victim is considered the victim of a homicide or whether they are simply considered missing, an issue that will be influenced by factors such as age, vulnerability and the circumstances surrounding their disappearance (for further discussion see Section 2.1; Gibb and Woolnough 2007). It is often difficult, without a body, to prove that the subject has been the victim of a crime and even more difficult to prove that the person has been buried or concealed (Preuss *et al.* 2006, 55). 'No body' search scenarios can be summarised as follows:

- *Cold Cases.* An offender, although he/she may be under suspicion, has yet to be convicted and the victim may not have been found. These are reviewed regularly by police (Nichol *et al.* 2004).

- *Resolved Cases.* An offender has been convicted, thus from a criminal justice perspective the case has been resolved. Further searching for the victim will require additional evidence and/or pressure being brought about by the victim's family or the public.

In addition to these two main types we should also consider *allegation cases* – instances where the police are approached with claims that human remains were buried in a very specific location many years earlier, perhaps by witnesses free from earlier restrictions. No missing person may be on record and the identity of a possible victim or suspect may not be known. These differ from the other two types in that no criminal investigation has hitherto taken place; this is discussed in more detail in Case Studies 4.2, 4.3 and 4.4. However, the common factor with all three is the time elapsed between (alleged) burial and a current investigation; all three share potential issues of landscape change.

5.2   History of cold case investigation

Cold case reviews are now undertaken by individual police forces as part of routine operations, often leading to new specialists being bought into the investigation, as initially suggested by the Byford Report in 1981 (Nichol *et al.* 2004, 4). Increasingly, special cold case units have been set up to relieve the pressure that such investigations place upon day-to-day policing. However, these units tend to target specific types of case (below) rather than cold cases in general, and no such part of the police infrastructure exists for cases where the primary aim is the search for the victim's body. It seems unlikely that any such units would be created given that burials probably constitute less than 5% of all murder cases a year according to CATCHEM data (Tony Osborne pers. comm.) For example, *Operation Enigma*, which began in 1996, examined over 200 unsolved murders of women dating back to 1986 and found 72 of them needed 'further analysis'. It was concerned with common factors where the victim was female; this marked the start of a wider trend to create such units as part of the Operational Policing Policy (Home Office 2005). The Metropolitan Police Force quickly followed with the establishment of the Homicide Support role in 'examining old cases for new investigative opportunities, particularly taking into account advances in forensic science', and *Operation Advance* which, although concerned with sexual assaults, serves as an example to demonstrate the increased interest in cold cases in recent years and the belief that, in certain instances, the passage of time can be used to the advantage of the investigator (Metropolitan Police 2006; FSS 2006a).

This interest has been shared in academic circles also. The symposium 'Unlocking Old Cases with a Scientific Key' was held in 2004 and explored 154 cold cases which could benefit from the advances in technology that had occurred since the crimes were committed (FSS 2006b). Although there has been a recent upsurge in literature concerning cold cases, particularly in the USA, there is little attention paid to exploring situations where the victim may be buried or concealed. For example, publications by Grieg (2006) and Walton (2006) are specifically dedicated to cold case reviews, particularly the ways in which modern advances can be used to solve old cases. They comment on a wide range of specialisms, ranging from forensic anthropology to DNA to fibre analysis, but search issues and developing search techniques are barely explored. This is mirrored in Hinkes' *Cold Case Homicides* that gives minimal attention (one and a half pages) to the search and recovery of a buried corpse (2006, 370f) hidden within other more mainstream forensic initiatives. It has been left to the examination of case studies in more specialist areas of literature to flag up appropriate developments (e.g. Hunter and Cox 2005; Ruffell and McKinley 2008), but these seem not always to have been fully recognised as offering new possibilities when cold cases are reviewed.

Part of this apparent neglect is undoubtedly a result of the relative rarity of these cases and the fairly recent sophistication of search techniques themselves (Cox 2001a, 145–57). Ironically, however, this sits in sharp contrast to the immense UK public and media obsession that such searches generate, as seen for example in the longstanding public interest in the disappearance of the estate agent Suzy Lamplugh, and the missing Moors Murders victim Keith Bennett, whose case continues to attract tabloid headlines half a century after the event.

The passage of time carries with it many factors: memories become vaguer; anecdotal evidence and ideas sometimes become established as 'fact'; and the nature of the physical evidence that might connect places with people and people with crimes can alter. This is not just a matter of broad landscape change: over time, the trace evidence that might link an offender to a crime may become eroded or destroyed during burial, deteriorate (see Section 7.3), become hopelessly contaminated, or vanish completely in an open environment. Any renewed investigation will need to understand change at both macro- and micro-levels; it will need to assess the impact of cultural and natural events and the implications of those events above and below the present ground surface. This may present some starting point that enables the critical linkage between offender, victim, crime scene and place of disposal to be established. Without this starting point, or without new positive evidence, a police force is unable to justify the resources needed to commence further investigation; nor can it logically argue a case for further exploration or activity which might otherwise appear random. The following sections begin to explore some of the issues involved and the resources available in identifying new starting points.

5.3   Cultural changes to rural landscapes

Cultural landscape change takes place every day in the form of construction, demolition, farming or the acquisition of the earth's resources. Even after a short period of time, such changes can rapidly alter topography and, in longer-term 'no body' enquiries, these changes may occur to the extent that the landscape becomes unrecognisable from the time when the crime was committed and an original search took place (Wilson *et al.* 2007; see Case Studies 5.1, 5.2, 5.3). In rural environments (those seemingly most commonly selected for burial) areas may have undergone cyclic or continuous processes of change, usually based on agricultural regimes, or have been subject to resource exploitation (extraction, quarrying or mining). Even simple events, such as the removal of hedges, altered access or ditch cleaning and widening, can be disorientating to a perpetrator revisiting a place several years later, especially if the disposal was originally undertaken hurriedly or in half-light.

Case Study 5.1

A relevant case in point involved the disappearance of a woman from Merseyside in 1988. Despite the conviction of her killer a year after her disappearance, the search for her remains has become a 'no body' investigation (McGann 2002). As part of a review undertaken around 2000, the evidence retained from the original investigation was re-examined using new techniques. Pollen analysis on the spade with which the grave is believed to have been dug revealed that it had been used near a hedgerow in a particular habitat. This, coupled with a re-examination of the locations where associated evidence had been found, including the perpetrator's and victim's clothing, made it possible to focus on a likely region for burial. This lay adjacent to an area of brick clay exploitation which had sporadically continued since her disappearance but which had also undergone considerable change: old workings had been waterfilled; new trackways had been formed and old ones overgrown, and both foot and vehicle access points had changed. Even personnel who had been involved in the original search found it difficult to orientate themselves in the changed environment. The appropriate hedgerow was found, but the landscape around it had changed substantially. Areas were targeted and vented for cadaver dogs but no responses were forthcoming. In this instance the passage of time presented both advantages (the development of palynology) and disadvantages (significant landscape change).

Case Study 5.2

In a published case, the victim had been missing 12 years before the offender directed police to where she was buried (Nobes 2000, 715–21). Despite this information, significant natural and cultural landscape change hindered the search. A combination of alterations to the road system and tree felling meant that areas offering concealment at the time of burial were no longer apparent. Developed geophysical survey techniques were employed, notably ground penetrating radar (GPR), resistivity and electro-magnetic survey. A small search area was initially defined but the anomalies discovered in this area were found to be tree roots and areas of industrial activity; above all they demonstrated how the geophysical signatures of tree cavities presented a remarkable similarity to those of burials. The victim's remains were eventually found when the search area was expanded, but the investigator involved admitted that the discovery was serendipitous and that a combination of landscape and geophysical complexities had served to confuse the issue.

Case Study 5.3

A middle-aged couple went missing in 1987 in the Channel Islands where they were resident. Some suspicion over their disappearance lay with family members, but no bodies were found and the investigation eventually went cold. In 1993, the case was re-examined and three areas along the south coast of Jersey were identified as being significant based on police information. Forensic archaeologists were brought in to assist, basing their search strategy on information that the bodies were buried and wrapped, devising their search accordingly in areas of relative concealment in the three areas. The remains of the victims were eventually recovered in a different part of the island altogether as the result of a confession. It transpired that the bodies had indeed been wrapped and buried but that the location of burial had, by chance, been heavily landscaped by the local council as a result of storm and tree damage. Earth had been piled up over the grave site as part of a landscaping process and any indications of vegetation or topographic change, or potential for geophysical survey, had been nullified in the process (Sullivan 2006) (Figure 5.1).

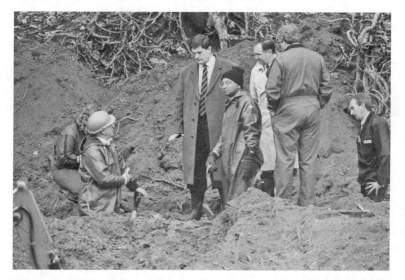

Figure 5.1 Police and a pathologist recovering the remains of buried victims in Jersey. The grave had been inadvertently concealed by landscaping (PA 806390 – Neil Munns/PA Archive/Press Association Images).

In Case Study 5.1 both quarries and landfill sites are known to have been, and indeed still are, active in the area where the victim's body is believed to have been deposited, yet it is unclear from the elapsed time the extent to which the dates of activity coincide. This case falls into the 'resolved' category (i.e. a person has been convicted) and hence researching the relevant information does not become a police priority. Similarly, in Case Study 5.2 the alterations to the road layout caused, 'some confusion about the location of the body' (Nobes 2000, 715) which resulted in the search being carried out in the wrong place. In Case Study 5.3, landscaping of the area around the grave led to the burial being concealed further. It would probably never have been found without the confession. In the first two cases there was always the chance that earlier maps and aerial photographs (Sections 2.2 and 2.3 respectively) might contribute to the investigations, but only if the scale was appropriate. Large scale OS mapping was available for the exploitation site in Case Study 5.1; this was published much earlier than the date of disappearance but depicted the surrounding fields and field boundaries accurately. It showed the historical area of quarrying, rather than the area of quarrying open at the time of the incident. But as such it provided a snapshot of quarrying extent at a known point in time, and allowed plotting of the hedgerow species to be compared to the pollen samples taken from the spade. It is not clear whether maps or earlier photographs would have been available to monitor alterations to the road layout in Case Study 5.2 as the incident is from New Zealand, but it is surprising that this oversight occurred when planning records undoubtedly existed.

There is a further issue that surfaces here, namely the question as to how much background research can be conducted without raising suspicion, whether on site, from the air or in archives, if an operation is required to be covert. In these circumstances police are often reluctant to visit potential scenes other than casually, or conduct aerial surveillance more than once. Moreover, cultural changes involving construction work require comprehensive records to be maintained in the public domain (discussed in greater detail in Section 5.5), access to which may arouse unwanted interest. This poses an awkward dichotomy given that comprehensive researching of landscape history can have a significant bearing as to where and how a search might be conducted. Not researching adequately (for whatever the justifiable reason) presents a risk and poses significant implications. The SIO will need to balance on the one hand the need to retain secrecy and, on the other, the risks of incurring unnecessary expense or not finding the body simply because the techniques were inappropriate or the search undertaken in the wrong place. One such example is outlined in Case Study 5.4 below.

Case Study 5.4

This occurred in a small village where information had been received that a murder had been committed almost half a century earlier and the victim thrown down an old shaft, which had since been sealed. The location was alleged to be within the grounds of an adjacent property but was otherwise not specific. The property had been used commercially and had been concreted over both internally and externally; it had latterly been used as a car sales area. Little background information had been gathered in order to keep the operation as covert as possible. Ground penetrating radar (GPR) was deployed over the concrete and provided several substantial responses. Time-consuming excavation of each response uncovered a mass of metal debris buried below the concrete. It was subsequently established that the site had formerly been used as a scrap metal yard, and before that a place where iron working had taken place. This history rendered the GPR wholly inappropriate, but was only discovered several days into the work. Historic maps were then consulted; these indicated the position of several shafts which enabled the search area to be better focused. As part of this focusing an elderly local resident came forward, he remembered where the shafts had been located and the shaft in question was subsequently found and opened without further difficulty. This occurred a week after the exercise had started. The case demonstrates the difficulties that can be encountered when operations are conducted covertly.

Even a history of relatively minor cultural actions can have a significant impact on burial survival and recovery over the longer term. For example, the effects of ploughing on archaeological evidence are well known, and a much needed study by Haglund *et al.* has identified how primary and secondary tillage, cultivators and fertiliser applicators all impact upon the location of buried remains in a variety of different ways (2002) (see also Section 7.3). In many respects this requires the enquiry to gain some reasonable awareness of farming methods. Additionally, bone may be crushed and its level of exposure to fertilisers and chemical change increased (*ibid.*, 134–46). Remains may be moved from their original position by machinery, exposed and subsequently scavenged by animals, thus removing evidence connected to the deposition site. Continuous ploughing, even over a short period of time, will also disguise the depression left by a grave; conversely, of course, ploughing can also lead to the serendipitous discovery of remains and provide a starting point for search.

In rural areas, land managers (farmers, gamekeepers, woodland managers, park rangers and green keepers on golf courses, etc.) can constitute a useful human resource. These are occupations that require a high degree of personal familiarity with the landscape, in the case of some farmers, a familiarity that goes back generations. These individuals may, through documented record or memory, recall changes that occurred 10 or 20 years earlier that are relevant to a renewed search. This is especially pertinent in instances where different locations are flagged up on the basis of new information and where there are no records in an existing crime file. There are various key areas here that the authors have experienced, for example with respect to cultivation: as to whether a particular field was under crop, stubble, ploughed or 'set-aside' at a particular time in a certain year (this will be significant for the feasibility of burying); or recollections of when deep or chisel ploughing was undertaken, which may have implications as to when remains are more likely to have been disturbed. Other examples might include whether a vehicular track (now overgrown) was passable at a particular time in the past, or when certain large trees blew down leaving open tree cavities that were subsequently levelled off. In another case it was necessary to establish when the dumping of farm rubbish occurred creating a concealed area for disposal, and on one golf course it was important to establish when the 17th hole was redesigned as it had the effect of marginalising a small piece of woodland away from active golfers. Few of these events are likely to have formally documented records in the same way as required by building development (below), but all may have significant implications for earlier body disposal. However, some rural work will require local authority sanction (such as certain levels of a/deforestation) and there will be formal records. If major agricultural changes were externally funded then there will be dated documentation for grant-aided work from DEFRA (Department for Rural Affairs) or its predecessor MAAF (Ministry for Agriculture, Fisheries and Food) as well as from European funding agencies. In short, there is a resource, albeit limited and not always easy to access, which can be drawn upon to track even relatively minor cultural changes to the landscape. It is a matter of knowing what to look for, or who to ask.

5.4   Natural changes to rural landscapes

Perhaps more difficult to detect are changes to the landscape that are largely free from human involvement: trees grow, brambles spread and coastlines erode or collapse. These occur throughout time according to environment and climate and there is no linear timeline by which changes can be measured. Specialist botanical input may provide some level of guidance, but only for the very recent past and not for the period of time that many older cases cover. Botanists have developed methods for counting plant species and stands of species within defined sample areas (typically one square metre) and have a broad understanding of colonisation rates, although this is habitat dependent. Appropriate techniques for assessing the abundance and population dynamics of plants and other sessile organisms or those with low capacity of movement are now well recognised (e.g. Krebs 1999). Forensic botany *per se* tends to be more concerned with plant biology and identification (e.g. Coyle 2004). More recently, the counting of species has been used experimentally in assessing the extent to which disturbed ground caused by burial can become re-colonised (Caccianiga *et al.* 2012), but the corollary has not yet been investigated. Plant colonisation is not the type of micro-data identifiable cartographically: published maps only define certain types of land form (e.g. bog, moorland, woodland, etc.), not always with clearly defined boundaries, and rarely at the desirable scale. Nor is examining sequences of map editions likely to helpful unless the time span covered between maps is very great or the landscape changes of some magnitude. A useful example pertains to the search for Moors Murder victims (see also Case Study 5.5 below) where one of Ian Brady's photographs taken in the 1960s can be compared to the modern day landscape (Figure 5.2). The rock formation in the background is recognisable in both, but the extent of the current vegetation coverage (which now also conceals surface rocks exposed in the 1960s) is significant over the intervening period of time.

'Historical' aerial photographs tend to suffer from similar issues of scale according to altitude of flight unless the changes are of observable size. However, one useful avenue of investigation has been the monitoring of peat exposure on sloping moorland landscapes. On the Lancashire/Yorkshire moors this has occurred at a sufficient scale to be identifiable from runs of aerial photographs taken since the war and has been used in an attempt to locate the grave of Keith Bennett, an unrecovered victim of the so-called Moors Murders in the 1960s (Case Study 5.5).

Landscape erosion of this type is fairly well confined to certain types of moorland terrain, but erosion in general tends to be more prevalent along coastlines, particularly with regard to the presence of sand. The geomorphology of many coastal zones is the result of the continual shifting of dune systems caused by gradual deposition and erosion. This occurs according to natural forces of wind and sea and is only partly predictable. Even

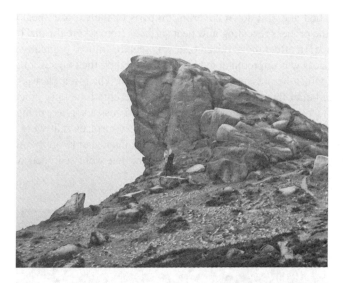

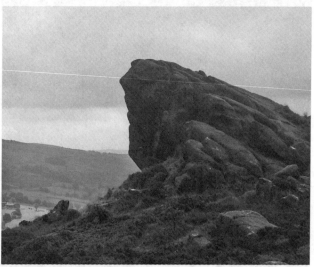

Figure 5.2 Comparison of photograph taken in the 1960s (top) and in 2012 (bottom), courtesy of Duncan Staff. The earlier photograph shows a barren scree landscape which is now heather covered. Only the very obvious rock reference points are still identifiable.

Case Study 5.5

Keith Bennett, aged 10, was murdered and allegedly buried on Saddleworth Moor in 1964. Despite intensive efforts in the late 1980s and in 2008 his body has never been recovered. As one part of the search, images from aerial photographs taken in 1964 and in 1968 available in the public domain were compared to the modern landscape. Comparison showed how the open peat scars had 'moved' as eroding turf surfaces became detached and slid down covering up parts of the exposed peat on the lower slope, but in the process revealing new peat surfaces from where the turf had shifted on the upper slope. In effect the exposed peat was seen to 'move' gradually up the valley sides; the process was unpredictable but was captured by the two sets of aerial images and plotted against the present landscape (Figure 5.3). The research was carried out in the justifiable belief that exposed surface peat represented the only practical location for burial of a body in the moorland, the turf and tussock grass being too hard to dig into. The key point, however, was that the peat surfaces that were exposed and appropriate for deposition in the 1960s were no longer visible on the ground during subsequent searches. As a result those peat scars that were searched were likely to have been incorrectly targeted.

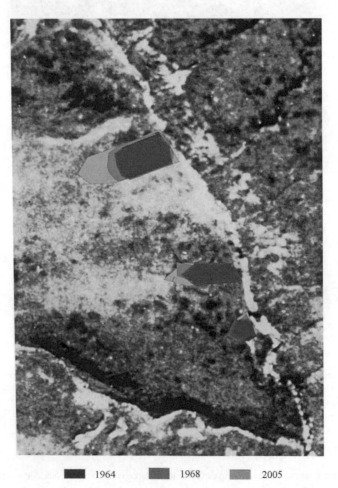

███ 1964   ███ 1968   ███ 2005

Figure 5.3 Changes in the erosion patterns of moorland peat exposure. Shadings represent different areas of exposure over time recorded on aerial imagery. (*For colour details please see colour plate section.*)

with specific information as to where a body might be buried, locating the victim becomes increasingly difficult as time passes, not only because the sand contours alter in character, but also because there are often few reliable static reference points by which the location can be identified. An ancient burial in sand may remain concealed for centuries but may be serendipitously uncovered during storms, and more recent depositions run a similar risk. The process of exposure can be both random and unpredictable. The following two cases, Case Studies 5.6 and 5.7, both 'archaeological' in their own way, illustrate these points.

Case Study 5.6

A walker on a cliff side footpath in South Wales noticed a bone projecting from underneath the pathway which ran just above the shoreline. The bone was later identified as human and an excavation was undertaken in order to clarify the nature of any burial. Figure 5.4 shows the results of the excavation that uncovered the partial skeleton of a supine male. Part of the grave had been eroded by the sea and the right arm was missing. The grave cut was evident on the landward side and the grave itself had (fortuitously) been sealed underneath a compacted pathway that had been used by the local community for as long as people could remember. The burial was not deemed to be of forensic interest on that basis alone. It was assumed that the individual was a victim of the sea in earlier times, and was buried where he was washed up. By coincidence the location later became part of a route from the beach to the top of the cliff. Eventually, processes of erosion brought the sea closer to both the path and the grave until the grave itself was breached and spilled on to the shore.

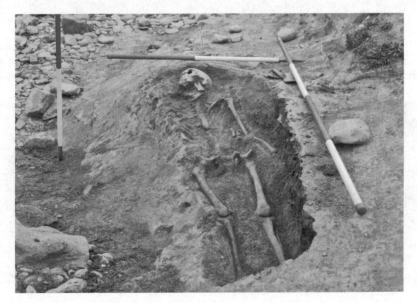

Figure 5.4 Human remains discovered as a result of coastal erosion. They constituted an articulated burial and lay beneath a well used footpath.

Case Study 5.7

Police were alerted to the presence of bones projecting from a sand dune in a remote part of western England at a considerable distance from the nearest vehicle access point or footpath (Figure 5.5). They were identified as human and their position in the vertical stratigraphy showed that they had been deposited on the surface of an exposed dune and later sealed by the formation of topsoil. They lay at the interface of the two

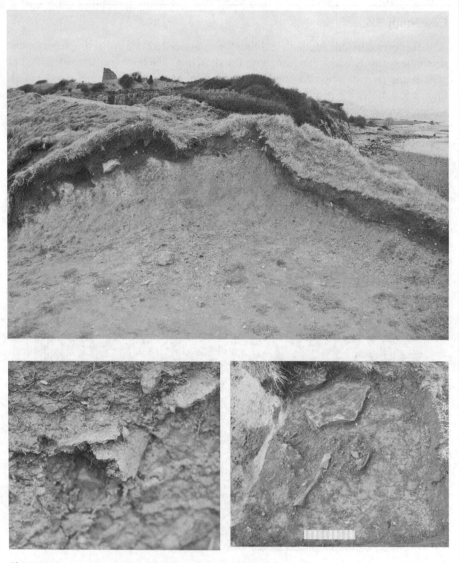

Figure 5.5 Human remains discovered as a result of coastal erosion of sand dune (top), lying at the interface of the sand and the topsoil (bottom left). Excavation (bottom right) demonstrated them to be both incomplete and out of anatomical order.

layers and there was no evidence of a grave cut. Excavation revealed what was essentially a dump of human bones – an incomplete skeleton of a single individual deposited in non-anatomical order. The only viable interpretation was that the remains had been dug up elsewhere, taken to a remote spot and dumped on a sand dune where they eventually became sealed by natural formation, became exposed through erosion, and then noticed. Where the bones originated will probably never be known, but the most obvious explanation is that they were uncovered during building work or gardening and hastily taken to a remote place in order to avoid building delay or issues with the police. This would explain why the skeleton was both incomplete and jumbled. The remains could have been modern, illegal and requiring forensic investigation; conversely they may have been archaeological and irrelevant in any forensic sense. Samples were taken and radiocarbon dating placed the remains around 3500 BC. The case demonstrates the complexities that can arise from even relatively simple erosion situations.

There are other equally unpredictable natural phenomena, albeit on a smaller scale, such as flooding, cattle trample, or the localised movement of soils by burrowing animals, especially badgers. Some changes might be viewed as 'catastrophic', for example the presence of sheep on hitherto marginal land can have an immense impact on how the vegetation of a landscape can change and is well illustrated in parts of rural Scotland where sheep have destroyed local vegetation. Anyone revisiting the general area of a scene where animals had been active at this level would be hard pushed either to become easily orientated or recognise reference points.

Seasonality can have similar disorientating effects (Case Studies 5.8 and 5.9). A deposition site used in spring during a time of thick vegetation, or in autumn with heavy leaf fall, may be difficult to re-identify in a different season. Equally, a deposition carried out in winter utilising evergreen cover may not be as obvious in the summer. Water tables change according to both natural seasonal and cultural events, trees fall down and, lately, some species have become diseased and died. In short, there are a host of natural factors that can come into play in attempting to reconstruct a former landscape. This has particular implications when witnesses are brought to an area after many years – a situation well illustrated when Myra Hindley and Ian Brady were taken to the moors some 25 years after burying bodies there. Both were seemingly disorientated, partly because the ground was snow-covered and featureless – very different from how they remembered it – and partly because they were taken via an unfamiliar route (Staff 2008). With the best will in the world even well-meaning witnesses can find themselves disorientated or confused when returning to a site to pinpoint a spot after a period of elapsed time. Two further case studies illustrate this.

Case Study 5.8

An informant had agreed to take police to the location where drugs had been stashed in a buried container for distribution. The location was in a woodland and it was assumed (although not indicated by the informant) that the location would somehow be marked. The police were led into a clearing with dense woodland on one side and a steep

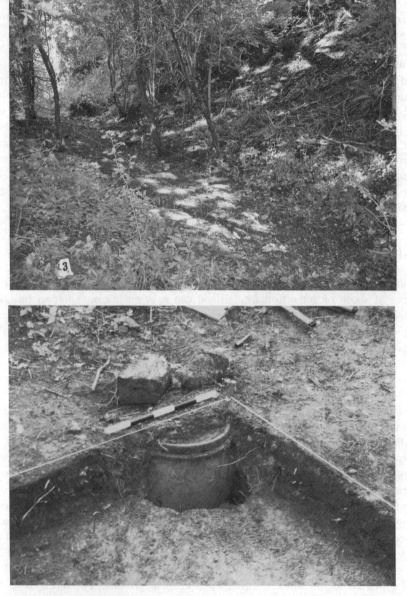

Figure 5.6 A woodland search showing (top) area of interest and (bottom) location of buried container. Note the marker stones over the container.

wooded bank on the other (Figure 5.6). A path ran along the top of the bank and was sporadically visible from down in the clearing. The informant attempted to position himself where he could stand in the clearing and see a gap in the trees through to the path. After a period of walking around and looking he expressed some confusion, being unable to position himself with any accuracy. His difficulty, he explained, was that the trees and path 'looked different' from how he remembered them, even although this had only been a few years earlier. A number of trees had fallen, and there had been some collapse of the banking leading up to the path. Eventually he indicated a general area some four metres long within the clearing. This was subsequently searched and excavated, nothing being found. The area was then extended, the surface stripped and the buried container was discovered approximately 10 m further away.

Case Study 5.9

A shooting had taken place and the body allegedly buried in a different part of the countryside. Several locations were targeted and assessed without success until an informant agreed to take the police to a field in a semi-rural area in Yorkshire. The place lay at the end of a rough track and was in dead ground away from a farmhouse and hidden from the playing fields of a local school. The part of the field in question (*c.* 75 × 75 m) had been used as storage for agricultural purposes – manure, a turnip heap and other deposited material – and these mounds constituted the informant's reference points in relation to the field gate from eight years earlier (Figure 5.7). The character of the dumping was clearly different from how the informant remembered it (albeit in half-light), and the seasonal level of the water table creating boggy ground was clearly confusing to him. As a result, his pinpointing of the deposition transpired to be flawed; it was only when machine stripping of the whole site took place as part of a process of elimination that the body was eventually found.

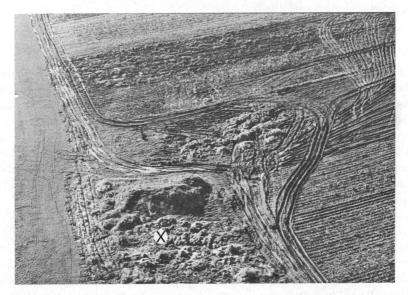

Figure 5.7 Aerial photograph of field containing manure heap. The informant used this as a reference point, but the location of farm dumping had changed over time. The cross identifies the approximate location of burial when eventually found.

In longer-term 'no body' searches it now seems accepted practice for an enquiry to pay serious attention to what the landscape might have looked like at the time of deposition. But this requires much more than uninformed subjective observation if an inquiry is to have any credence. It would, for example, be a mistake to assume landscape vegetation merely grows and flourishes evenly as a natural course of events. Some species grow and dominate, others become repressed or diseased, and cultural activities, including those based on agriculture practice, can create significant change not only to visual character, but also to the prominence of those landmarks and features likely to have been paramount in defining the precise location at the time of deposition. At the micro-level, the survival of features that can characterise disturbed ground above a grave – topographical expressions and vegetation anomalies (see Sections 2.3 and 7.3) – can also become obscured by time according to environment. Hidden within the grave itself there will also be changes over time brought about by taphonomics, bioturbation and other natural agencies. There are many factors to take into account, and there is no easy solution as to how best to reconstruct a rural landscape from 10, 20 or 30 years ago. Archaeologists have attempted to visualise ancient landscapes using GIS, for example by creating virtual landscapes according to hypothetical values of vegetation (e.g. Vitale *et al.* 2011; Ch'ng *et al.* 2005) in order to ascertain visibility from one place to another. This has only a broad relevance in forensic cases, but GIS can also be used to create DTMs from early edition maps, allowing the superimposition of relevant 'historic' aerial images, or previous access points. It can at least provide a platform on which cultural activity, witness observations and recorded changes can be added, interrogated and tested. With or without GIS, any inquiry needs more than just a passing knowledge of the various ways changes can occur; it requires an awareness of the equally varied sources by which the chronology of those changes can be evidenced.

5.5   Planning controls and building controls

Many longer-term enquiries are faced with large scale urban changes – new buildings, demolition sites, roads and so on, the construction of which may have occurred around the time of an individual's disappearance many years ago and which may have presented convenient opportunities for body deposition. Structured information regarding the nature, extent, time frame and technology of a particular development may be available; it may be complex and not always easy to track down. However, this is a desirable research avenue if an enquiry is to identify those potential deposition sites available to an offender when the construction was taking place. Simply knowing the stages of a development at any given time could include or eliminate a building, or part of a building, accordingly.

Questions may need to be asked as to the feasibility of disposal during the development process, the time frame of construction, the depth of ground works or the materials used. Fortunately, in the UK, urban development in its many forms is constrained by legislation and directives that require specific routines to be undertaken and specific records to be maintained. These laws and directives have been amended or changed over time and enquiries will need to consult those relevant at the time of the incident in question. They relate principally to planning and construction processes, local authority inspections undertaken during certain stages of these processes, 'green' and 'brown' field land use, as well as the progress of landfill and waste disposal facilities. Moreover, there are also specific processes which pertain to the repair, alteration or demolition of listed buildings, not to mention those which deal with ecclesiastical buildings in use, as well as graveyards and burial grounds. Together, these constitute an essential documentary resource that allows a non-invasive search framework to be constructed and an opportunity to focus more closely on some potential deposition sites and eliminate others. These records can be of great value; Case Study 5.10 provides a simple example.

Case Study 5.10

The importance of records research can be highlighted by a recent 'cold case' forensic search in the north of England concerning the re-investigation of the disappearance of a missing 6-year old child from 1944. The investigation was concentrated on a domestic rear garden and the initial expert advice to the SIO, in the non-intrusive phase, concentrated on the technological non-intrusive methods available, such as geophysical survey. The advice was that the target of the search was too small to be detected by geophysical survey and therefore that total excavation was necessary.

After five days of searching by excavating the whole garden to a depth of around one metre, the police abandoned the search having found nothing. Towards the end of the search, local newspaper reporters discovered that 10 years previously the rear gardens where the police search was concentrated had, for up to two thirds of their length, been heavily excavated by plant machinery. Mechanical excavators had been brought in to excavate a 3×1.5 m trench to hold a new sewer pipe. The enquiry had hitherto concentrated almost entirely on witness credibility and on technological feasibility. It had proceeded without the benefit of researching planning documentation relating to the site – something which the local media reporters managed to research with little difficulty. It is easy to be critical with hindsight, but the case highlights the value of a thorough search of existing records in advance of a field operation in order to achieve the most effective and efficient use of money and resources.

Planning and building controls are evolutionary, and it is useful here to outline their general development before any discussion of their practical application. Planning as such has its roots in the thinking that saw the creation of 19th century 'model' townscapes, such as those at Welwyn Garden City (Hertfordshire), Port Sunlight (Cheshire), Bourneville (Birmingham) and Saltaire (Bradford). These planned environments embodied the concept of land use for living, working, social and recreational purposes as envisaged by enlightened industrialists of the time. Their underlying philosophy went some way to underpin the Town Planning Act 1909 (TPA 1909) and subsequently the Town and Country Planning Act 1947 (HMSO 1947a; 1947b), which established the major rebuilding programme in England after World War II.

This 1947 Act made local authorities responsible not only for dealing with planning applications, but also for preparing local plans for future planning developments. This still forms the basic structure of the current planning system today (Telling *et al.* 1993). Local government reorganisations in 1972 delegated planning responsibilities; these were further revised by the Town and Country Planning Act 1990 (HMSO 1990a) and amended by the

Planning and Compulsory Purchase Act (HMSO 2004c), the latter providing a strategic framework within which the planning process could operate. In summary, the legislation now provides for detailed planning reporting at both local and regional level together with an increased depth of information being available locally. Much of this is necessarily in the public domain, for example, the construction of new buildings requires permission from local planning authorities (LPAs) and involves a process of public notice and consultation. Moreover, much planning information, together with local planning history, is now available electronically and is readily accessible. Definitive details of boundaries and ownership of properties are held by H.M. Land Registry, a body which has acted as the sole agency for the holding, transfer and archiving of titles since 1862.

Building controls (as opposed to planning controls) essentially have their roots in the Rebuilding Act of 1667 (subsequent to the Great Fire of London), followed by numerous other Acts, notably the Public Health Act of 1875 and its revisions which all sought to introduce controls (e.g. Fraser 1978; Noy 1998). Most significant was the 1961 revision of the Public Health Act which led to the introduction of the first independent set of national building standards, the Building Regulations. These came into effect in 1966 (Cullingworth and Nadin 2002, 14–15) whence it became mandatory for local authorities to maintain records certifying that all construction work (essentially pertaining to building materials and structural integrity) complied with their provisions. Building legislation was formally separated from public health policy in 1984 with the passing of the Building Act (HMSO 1984b). Subsequent revisions to regulations have been brought about by changes in construction technology or by major disaster (e.g. the collapse of the flats at Ronan Point, East London). Current regulations are the Building Regulations 2010, (HMSO 2010a) and the Building (Approved Inspectors etc.) Regulations 2010 (HMSO 2010b) which came into force on 15 July 2011, and include provision for the supervision and certification of building work by 'approved inspectors' who were first introduced into the process in 2000 (HMSO 2000a).

5.6 Current planning arrangements

Although planning is delegated to local authorities, the 1990s witnessed increasing involvement by central government in planning matters with the publication of Planning Policy Guidance notes (PPGs) covering a wide range of issues. These Guidance notes were not laws as such, but they had a strong influence on planning matters and brought with them a string of records as to what is required (for example in groundworks) in order to satisfy the interests of the local authority. These interests might be historical, cultural or of amenity value and reflect what is perceived as being of local significance. As a result guidance might stipulate the position of a proposed building's footprint, the need for trial trenching or the required extent of an excavation. Some of the original PPGs were updated and replaced by Planning Policy Statements (PPSs). Both the PPG notes, and their replacements, the PPSs were prepared by the government (after public consultation) in order to explain statutory provisions and to provide guidance to local authorities and others on planning policy and the operation of the planning system. Since 2012, however, these Statements have been effectively superseded by the National Planning Policy Framework (NPPF) (DCLG, 2012), which drew all the previous separate acts and guidances under a single 'legislative umbrella', but in essence required the same information to be placed on record in the future.

Any search requiring data from *before* the implementation of the NPPF in 2012 (i.e. those longer-term cases that are the subject of this chapter) will need to rely on the processes and records operating at the time of interest. These are detailed below. Searches for persons missing *since* 2012 will require a slightly different strategy according to the wording of the NPPF which presents a number of amendments. These are not pursued further here.

Local authorities were required to take the content of all these documents into account in preparing plans. The guidance was also relevant to decisions on individual planning applications and appeals. In total there were 25 PPGs/PPSs many of which required the keeping of records and have implications in researching an urban area, or indeed a rural area, for potential deposition sites. Many of the original PPGs from the 1990s, with revisions, remain in force within the NPPF. However, the early years of the 21st century saw several PPGs superseded by PPSs issued initially under the authority of the Office of the Deputy Prime Minister (OPDM) as planning legislation and planning strategies changed. This oversight of the planning process is now under the authority of the Department for Communities and Local Government (DCLG 2011a). One of the more significant documents, PPG 16: Archaeology and Planning (HMSO 1990b) was replaced by PPS 5: Planning for the Historic Environment (DCLG 2010); this could involve significant ground intervention and is discussed further below.

The underlying purpose of these PPGs/PPSs (now vested in the NPPF) was to promulgate government policy in an attempt to create a balanced and sustainable planning policy to protect the built environment while still allowing growth and development. However, in terms of criminal investigation, the positive effect of the planning legislation was to increase further the levels of process and records available. Planning strategies demanded the establishment of an evidential base by LPAs to underpin and justify the phasing in of new Local Development Frameworks (LDFs) under the requirements of PPS 12 – Local Spatial Planning (DCLG 2008) and the Planning and Compulsory Purchase Act 2004 (HMSO 2004c). Their implementation specifically advocated the incorporation of relevant information from existing and previous plans and surveys, together with records obtained from other stakeholders, for example, English Heritage, English Nature, the Environment Agency and the British Geological Survey. This process ensured the retention and local availability of many detailed maps, both current and historical, together with a great deal of information about current and past land use within the LDFs. All these agencies kept records.

Moreover, local authorities increasingly came to use their own digital mapping and Geographic Information Systems (GIS), or employed outside consultants to record and display current land use and developments, in order that plans were capable of constant update. Consequently the use of GIS and digital mapping systems provide an enquiry with the opportunity to explore layers of recorded information in order to identify townscape and landscape characteristics at moments of time in the past – an especially useful facility in dealing with 'cold' or historical cases. This can be supplemented by 'historical' aerial photographs, taken at various intervals in time, for military or land use purposes since the 1950s. The location of archives for these are noted in Section 2.3.

A survey undertaken by the Royal Town Planning Institute (RTPI), in 2000, into the use of information technology by LPAs, illustrates the type of data capture undertaken even at that time (RTPI 2000). An illustration of the depth of information currently available from local authority databases (and which also relates to prime potential deposition sites within an urban area) is the local authority research in respect of 'brown field' sites. 'Brown field' sites are those that are derelict, disused or abandoned, often classified as 'contaminated land' due to their previous industrial usage. Part of the national planning strategy under Planning Policy Statement 3: Housing (DCLG 2011b) was the use of such brown field sites for future urban development to avoid further encroachment on to green belt land.

An LPA, when researching brown field sites for re-development, is still required to consider the physical and environmental constraints in the development of such land, for example, the levels of contamination, stability or the flood risk. This also provides an example of how previous and existing plans are capable of incorporation in support of the new LDF, as well as their value to the enquiry. Under the provisions of Pollution Prevention and Control Act 1999 (HMSO 1999), all local authorities had to inspect land within its area to identify contaminated land, and to publish a Contaminated Land Inspection Strategy. Relevant guidance is also contained within Planning Policy Statement 23: Planning and Pollution Control (DCLG 2004). For practical purposes, in the Contaminated Land Inspection process, the local authority officers are likely to have undertaken desk-top research involving: current and historical land use maps, aerial imagery and photographs, together with many other documentary records. A Geographical Information System (GIS) stores all the relevant information, documentation, photographs, maps and possibly also site visits, and the information is available to the public through the appropriate local authority department. In addition to the mapping, photographs, documentary records and site inspection visits, information may also be held regarding closed landfill sites, waste disposal sites, scrap yards, sites involving regulated industrial processes, information in respect of geological, hydrological and topographical issues and planning records as far back as 1984. The inspection also uses and maintains within its database relevant information from other sources, for example from: English Heritage; English Nature; British Waterways; the Environmental Agency and the Geological Survey. It stands as a unique source of detailed current and historical information for any enquiry to use at the assessment stage of an investigation. Being continually updated it is also dynamic and can provide a useful timeline of events.

5.7 Planning records

At the micro-level of planning there are further detailed sets of documentary record available. These arise from applications made for planning permission and from those made under the building regulations (see below). Planning permission and building regulation requirements are often confused. In simple terms, planning permission is the authority required to erect a new building or alter an existing building to more than 10% of its current footprint, while the building regulations lay down the physical construction requirements for new building(s). Both lie under the direct control of the LPA and both require the submission and retention of separate and detailed records under separate legislation. The local authority is the depository for both sets of records generated by the process.

The current legislation and regulations in relation to the registration and validation of planning applications are vested in various Town and Country Planning legislation (HMSO 1988; HMSO 1990a; HMSO 2004d). Although they also deal with a plethora of planning types, including listed buildings and waste and mineral applications (below), they deal predominantly with outline planning permission (permission in principle for a construction, but subject to detailed plans) and full planning applications where such detailed plans are approved. Outline planning permission automatically lapses after three years if no full planning application is made. Equally, full planning permission lapses after a similar period of time if no construction has taken place. This has important search implications in that it potentially presents a three-year disposal window between full permission and a new build. In other words, a missing person enquiry that wishes to determine the date of a house extension needs to consider the date of planning permission as a *terminus post quem* only, rather than as an absolute point in time.

The documentation required for full planning applications is set out by the Department of Communities and Local Government (DCLG 2007). It includes a defined location plan based on Ordnance Survey 1:1,250 or 1:2,500 scales, a site plan at 1:500 or 1:200, floor plan drawings, elevations and sections, including any changes in ground levels. The level of detail required is considerable and the information is subsequently archived by the LPA. There may be instances where this detailed information may potentially be extended by further 'additional matters' required by the LPA depending on the nature and type of application (*ibid.*). Some of this may be of little value in search terms (e.g. the design of buildings, affordable housing statements, regeneration issues, noise impact assessment, etc.), but other factors, such as the inclusion of information on landscaping, the creation of car parking or access roads, historical or archaeological information, tree or arboricultural statements, or methods to deal with the disposal of foul sewage, may prove relevant in identifying potential disposal sites.

Figures maintained by the UK Statistics Authority for the Department of Communities and Local Government show how many planning applications are made. Taking a random selection, in the period January to March 2011 local authorities undertaking district level planning received around 119,400 applications (DCLG 2011c). This gives some idea of the size of the database available. Full planning applications provide essential information on what existed *before* the development outlined in the planning application, and what was proposed to be built in its place; they represent an important primary resource. That said, however, planning permission merely authorises the building. The actual construction process generates a further documentary record in relation to the site through building regulations.

5.8 Building records

Once planning permission is granted the next set of documentary records that the process produces are those required under building regulations. The main function of these is to control the design and construction of buildings and the provision of services, fittings and equipment (HMSO 1984b; HMSO 2010a; HMSO 2010b). As in the case of full planning applications, submission of detailed plans relating to proposed construction work is required, but with the addition of further information on drainage, structural design and calculations (HMSO 2010a). This supplements the plans and records submitted with full planning applications. Moreover, the importance of building regulations is that they provide a further set of potentially useful documentation through the system of inspections required during the various construction phases. The Building Act 1984 also introduced a system of building control to enforce those standards. Building control involves the checking of plans for approval by the local authority, and making visits to inspect the work on site for compliance with the technical requirements of the building regulations.

Visits are undertaken either by Inspectors from the LPA or by private sector 'Approved Inspectors' (HMSO 2010b), both working to common national guidelines. In this way, the building regulations establish a detailed system of on-site inspections to ensure compliance with the national building standards. The inspection timetable is set out (HMSO 2010a, Reg. 16) and formal notice must be given to the local authority by the builder to ensure that inspections take place at certain intervals during the construction process. From an investigation point of view key visits by inspectors may occur and reports made the day *before* the following events:

- when excavations are covered

- when foundations are covered

- when damp courses are covered

- when site concrete or any other material is laid over a site

- when any drain or sewer is covered.

Visits and reports are also likely to be made five days *after* drains are completed and when the work is completed and/or before occupation of the building. Failure to comply with any of these regulations can result in the building being pulled down. The advantage to an investigation is that the prioritised inspections occur at the most significant periods during the construction process for a potential body deposition to have taken place; they provide dates as to when potential locations for a deposition were either open or closed. Basic records of inspections (locations, times, dates, etc.) are maintained in a public register, and some LPAs also include additional material (notes, plans, etc.) as good practice.

The construction site records will also contain valuable information that may be useful in respect of the sub-surface construction, and this is of particular interest in identifying feasibility of disposal. The geology of the site is a key factor in calculating the required depth and design type of foundation structure to be used, for example: traditional strip foundation; deep strip or trench fill; solid slab raft; beam and slab raft, isolated pad or combined pad or the use of reinforced concrete in the foundation (Chudley and Greeno 2004, 185–226; Chudley and Greeno 2005, 45–86). This sub-surface information record will be available to assist in briefing for a geophysical survey or assessing and planning any proposed excavation. The information is not a substitute for cadaver dogs, geophysical survey or aerial imagery; it is simply a method of enhancing information sources to enable better targeting of these methods. The searching of internal completed buildings is well documented elsewhere (ACPO 2006, Appendix 4) and is not pursued further here.

However, not all development requires planning permission, and not all building construction work is subject to the building regulations, for example: patios, hard standing, sheds, greenhouses, accommodation for pets and domestic animals, swimming pools, ponds, sauna cabins and even enclosures such as tennis courts. The process is complicated: some cases require neither; some requiring planning permission but not the buildings regulations, and other cases *vice versa*. These minor developments are usually either moveable or can be investigated non-invasively, for example by ground penetrating radar if required.

Overall, the practical value for a forensic enquiry is the increasing local authority-driven research and database creation, employing GIS and digital mapping systems. This provides a detailed and authoritative source of both current and historical information on the local landscape. The legal requirements to continually update the information makes these records 'databases in action' enhancing their continued value as a search tool. Additionally, this procedure is supervised by an independent inspection process, which produces further records, to ensure compliance with the relevant legislation. The following flow chart (Figure 5.8) offers a simplified outline of approach for any enquiry where this type of documentation may be of relevance.

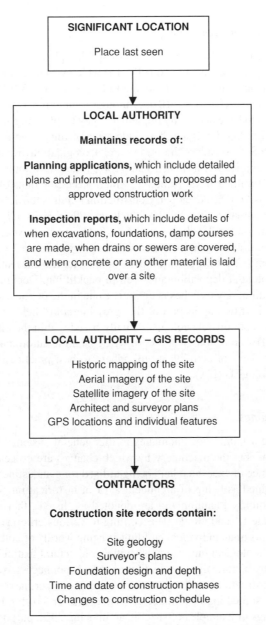

Figure 5.8 Flow chart for searching locally based planning and building documentation.

5.9   Special circumstances

The planning world appears to be full of anomalies or special circumstances. Three of these with potential relevance for clandestine disposal are outlined here: the possible requirement for developers to undertake *archaeological investigation* in advance of construction; the issues presented by *listed buildings*; and the special cases posed by *ecclesiastical buildings* and *burial grounds*.

5.9.1   Archaeological investigation

The buried history of the landscape is a matter of specific planning concern and is flagged up in Planning Policy Guidance Note 16 (PPG 16) which was first issued in 1990 (HMSO 1990b) (and was replaced in 2010 by Planning Policy Statement 5 (PPS 5) – Planning for the Historic Environment (DCLG 2010)). Although a directive as opposed to a piece of legislation, it appears to have been fully implemented by all planning authorities since 1990 in the UK (NPPG 5 in Scotland) and has made a major impact on the planning process. In short, PPG 16/PPS 5 considers the buried archaeological environment in those areas for which planning application has been made for building development, even at a small scale. It reflects the 'polluter pays' principle, which places the onus of the archaeological investigation (and cost) on the developer. Construction requires the developer to satisfy any local archaeological demands as defined by the local authority (usually through the county archaeologist) that might involve desk-top survey, field survey or excavation. Specification for any work will be drawn up by the county archaeologist and put out to tender. It may require anything from test-pitting to 'full-blown' archaeological excavation leaving exposed trenches open as potential deposition sites before backfilling. Documentation relating to the location and detail of any trenches is unlikely to lie in the public domain, but the detail will be recorded and written up as part of the 'grey literature' held by the archaeological contractors used, the county archaeologist (usually based within the planning department) and the developer. The archaeological record will contain location maps, details of depth and size, as well as dates of activity; it will adhere to best practice as laid down by the Institute for Archaeologists (IfA).

5.9.2   Listed buildings

Inevitably, there are a number of anomalies in this general system of building controls. These are exceptions, but the machinery by which changes are processed is important to note, even if the chance of excavated land being utilised for clandestine purposes is remote. Many buildings defined as being of architectural or of historical interest under the terms of the Town and Country Planning Act are denoted as 'listed', that is, they are given a grade (Grade I, Grade II* and Grade II) according to various criteria. The listing process identifies key elements of an individual building as being worthy of note. These can include period qualities, technological innovation, specific architectural features, or even buildings formerly inhabited by historically famous figures. Age is not necessarily a factor and even relatively recent constructions (railway stations, cinemas, supermarkets, etc.) can qualify providing they have something of intrinsic or local character to offer. However, most tend to be period dwellings or examples of specific architecture. The purpose is not to fossilise an individual structure but to ensure that its specific merits are taken into account when any changes are undertaken, and that any change is sustainable. The built environment was the focus of a separate planning policy guidance note PPG 15 (DOE and DNH 1994) but this has been superseded by PPS 5 (above) in an attempt to unify various heritage directives.

The listing process is monitored at local authority level and any owner wishing to alter a building of listed status is required to obtain formal listed building consent (LBC) in order to do so. The process requires a more rigorous procedure if substantial building work is to be undertaken, and consent usually requires specific conditions. Details of the application will receive a wider scrutiny and, if an application for demolition is requested, consultation with external bodies. LBC may require more specific conditions regarding materials, construction technique and design than for non-listed buildings, as well as the usual planning requirements.

It is important to note the issue of curtilege; for example, some listed buildings may also include land within the title boundary as part of the listed area. This is likely if the gardens have been formally landscaped, or if the house and grounds are considered to be a combined period entity. In these cases details of excavations or small developments within the gardens will also require LBC, and the data will be recorded and archived accordingly. This is quite different from work undertaken in gardens of non-listed buildings, which can be adapted or excavated privately without prior public notification. Again, the chance of excavation within or around listed buildings being used for clandestine purposes is remote, but the detailed documented information available may be of use, if only for elimination purposes in historical cases.

5.9.3   Ecclesiastical buildings

Churches, or more precisely, ecclesiastical buildings in use, are exempted from listed building controls and have been since 1913 (Bianco and Monckton 2006). Their exemption has been argued on the basis of their specific liturgical function as opposed to more general or variable secular use. Changes within an ecclesiastical building, including the graveyard and irrespective of whether the building is listed or not, are monitored by internal church processes. This applies to ecclesiastical buildings of all denominations. By far the most significant here is the Anglican Church, which owns the greater majority of all listed buildings in England (and the Churches of Wales and Scotland in other parts of the UK).

The procedures used by the Anglican Church are very formalised, but those used by other denominations less so. The Anglican Church requires any change to be approved by the Diocese Chancellor (a legal appointee) who relies upon his Diocese Advisory Committee (DAC) for comment and recommendation regarding individual applications from parishes. This position remains in force despite revisions, the most recent being in 2010. These applications can range from minor changes, such as repainting or movement of objects within the building, to lavish re-ordering schemes or to the construction of meeting rooms or church extensions. The DAC acts as a filter to ensure that the effects of any change will not be detrimental to the historic character or fabric of the building, and that any change will be for long-term benefit rather than short-term gain. Minor changes can be dealt with locally through the offices of an Archdeacon's Certificate, larger changes by means of a Faculty issued by the Chancellor. In both instances plans and full meeting minutes, decisions, conditions and dated documentation of any construction are maintained within the diocese records, usually filed under the name of the parish concerned. This means than any historical investigation will be able to draw upon appropriate documentation and plans detailing when the event took place, the materials and duration of construction, and the points at which excavated trenches might have been exposed.

Ironically, cathedral churches lie outwith this process but, since the Care of Cathedrals Measure 1990, they too are now bound by a formal set of constraints. These are vested in the Fabric Advisory Committees of individual cathedrals, themselves bound by the Cathedrals Fabric Commission for England (in the case of England). As with parish churches, appropriate records for any construction are archived, but within the cathedral offices as opposed to diocese offices. It might be remembered too that the curtilege of the cathedral has, from medieval times, also included the cathedral precinct and all the buildings and dwellings which are contained within the precinct. Development or excavation anywhere within this area requires similar levels of detailed documentation. In the cases of either parish church or cathedral, it can be argued that the formal planning framework is somewhat more rigorous than those functioning in the secular world.

5.9.4   Burial grounds

The clandestine burial of victims within legitimate graveyards, or the search for such, is not uncommon and merits some discussion. As in the case of building construction and waste management, there are formal regulations, processes and records for legitimate burials; these are useful starting points for any investigation that requires a burial ground to be searched. The relevant legislation that supports these processes has its origins in the 19th century and, with amendments, still forms the basis of the current legislation relating to the formal burial of human remains. The historical background is worth summarising and essentially involves two major 19th century events: changes in the burial practices from the overcrowded churchyards to large new cemeteries or burial grounds, and changes to recording of death from the church to the state.

The major milestone was the Burial Act 1853, which enabled parishes and boroughs to establish and administer their own new cemeteries under local burial boards. Many of the new cemeteries created in this period are of historic interest but are still actively used today (English Heritage 2011). In 1894, district and parish councils were allowed to adopt the powers of their local burial boards if they so resolved. These burial boards were set up to supplement rather than replace local churchyards; additionally, many private cemeteries established themselves as limited companies. There are no fewer than 15 specific Burial Acts passed by Parliament between 1852 and 1906; additionally many other Acts concerning local government and churches also impinge on burial law, notably the Registration of Burials Act 1864 (HMSO 1864) which required details of burial to be recorded and maintained in registers by all cemetery authorities.

The country was divided into registration districts, each district lying under the control of a Superintendent Registrar who was responsible for the issuing of birth certificates and death certificates that occurred in that district. They also produced records of the births and deaths that occurred and sent them on a quarterly basis to the Registrar General. These records were originally archived at Somerset House, Central London, but since the end of World War II the records have been held at the Registrar General's Office in Southport.

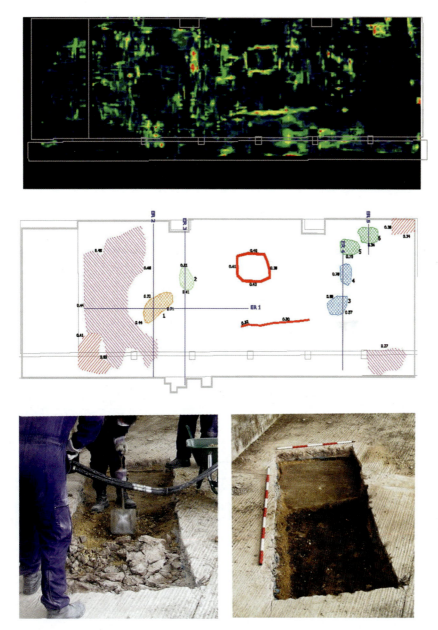

Plate 2.1 Excavation of the concrete floor of a barn marked out on a common grid resulting from GPR responses. The top image shows a horizontal radar slice at an estimated 0.5 m depth; the middle image shows the overall interpretation of radar responses at different depths, and the bottom images show the excavation of one of the potential targets. Geophysics images courtesy of Stratascan Ltd.

Forensic Approaches to Buried Remains, First Edition. John Hunter, Barrie Simpson and Caroline Sturdy Colls.
© 2013 John Wiley & Sons, Ltd. Published 2013 by John Wiley & Sons, Ltd.

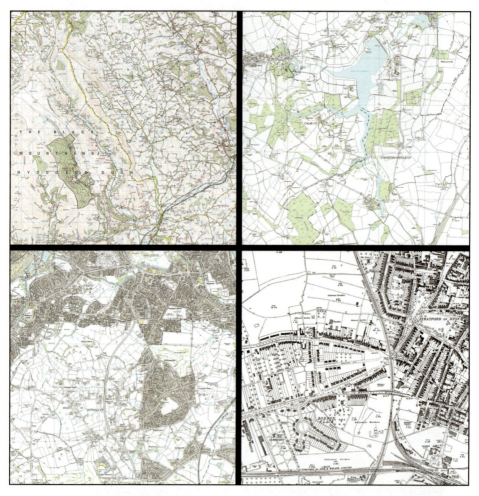

Plate 2.5 Examples of different scaled maps illustrating differences in detail: top left scale 1:50,000; top right scale 1:25,000; bottom left scale 1:10,000; bottom right scale 1:5,000. © Crown copyright 2013 Ordnance Survey.

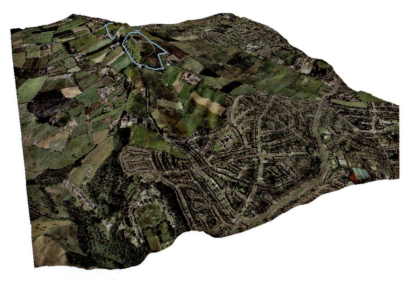

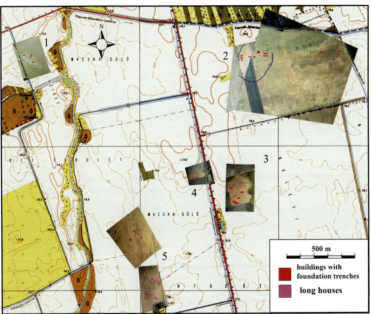

Plate 2.7 Superimposition of aerial photographs: top, full coverage over a DTM at Barr Beacon Image by courtesy of K. Colls and P. Breeze on behalf of Birmingham Archaeology; bottom, partial coverage over a simple contoured map of a Hungarian landscape. Image by courtesy of Zoltán Czajlik.

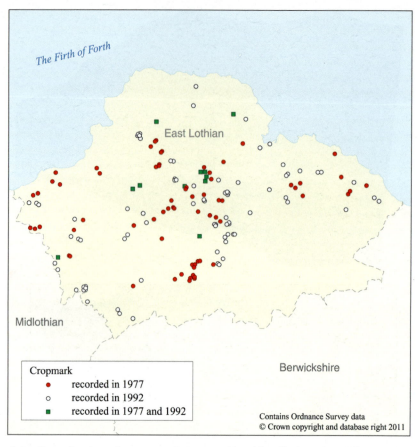

Plate 2.8 Plan showing discrepancy between sites identified under different conditions (Image courtesy of RCAHMS. © Crown copyright: RCAHMS. Licensor www.rcahms.gov.uk).

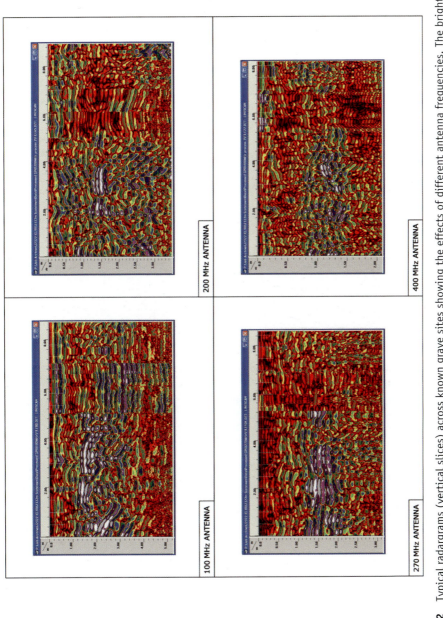

100 MHz ANTENNA

200 MHz ANTENNA

270 MHz ANTENNA

400 MHz ANTENNA

Plate 3.2 Typical radargrams (vertical slices) across known grave sites showing the effects of different antenna frequencies. The brightest responses at approximately 1.5 m depth indicate the presence of graves. Images by courtesy of Stratascan Ltd.

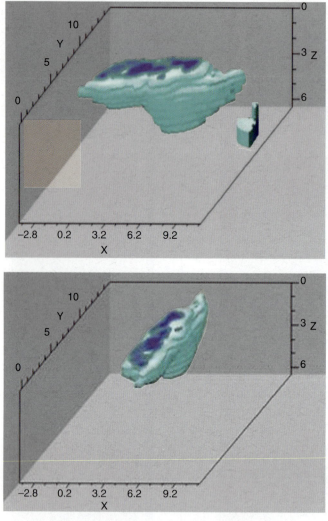

Plate 3.4 Three-dimensional view of mass grave generated using electrical resistance tomography. Image by courtesy of the International Commission on Missing Persons.

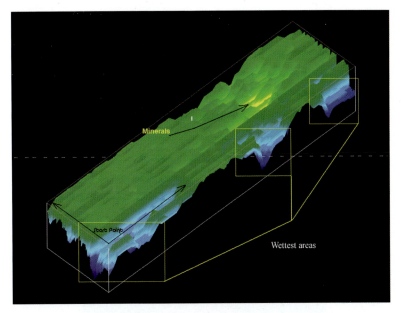

Plate 3.7   Three-dimensional model of moorland landscape from a ground penetrating radar survey showing wettest areas and underground water-coursing. Area covered is approximately 12 × 3 m and depth 2 m. Image by courtesy of Malcolm Weale.

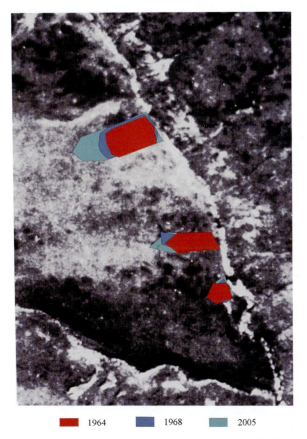

1964   1968   2005

Plate 5.3   Changes in the erosion patterns of moorland peat exposure. Shadings represent different areas of exposure over time recorded on aerial imagery.

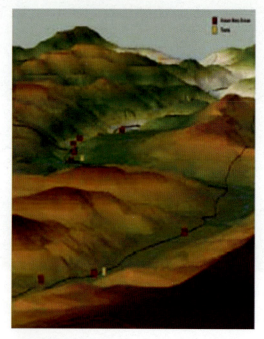

Plate 8.3 A digital terrain model (DTM) showing the location of mass graves in Bosnia. Image by courtesy of the International Commission on Missing Persons.

The registration process for births and deaths became compulsory from 1874; the onus for registration of a birth was passed to the parents, or the occupier of the house where a birth took place, and this has some implications in searching for the remains of neonates or small children (see Section 4.2). In respect of deaths, a relative of the deceased now became responsible for registering a death with the Registrar. This registration had to be supported by a death certificate issued by a doctor and the death had to be registered within five days.

In 1926, to further prevent the irregular disposal of bodies, the Births and Deaths Registration Act introduced the requirement for a Registrar's Certificate or Coroner's Order to be produced before a burial or cremation could take place (HMSO 1926). Importantly from a forensic point of view, this Act introduced the registration of the deaths of stillborn children. It also required cemeteries to maintain records and plans of all graves, the details of the individual(s) within a specific grave, and the dates of interments or re-interments; this constitutes prime data in any graveyard investigation. To summarise, in the UK there is a long established data bank of information on births and deaths, including the precise location of a grave in which the remains are finally buried.

Formal legitimate burials are now subject to additional requirements under terms contained in a Statutory Instrument, the Local Authorities' Cemeteries Order 1977 and Burial England and Wales (HMSO 1977), issued under the Local Government Act 1972 (HMSO 1972). It is worth citing parts of the latter verbatim (Schedule 2, Part 1: Exercise of Rights) as it has direct relevance to any graveyard enquiry, as well as to any formal exhumation (see also Section 6.1.3). Items 1–4 deal specifically with graves, and items 5–6 with vaults.

(1) No burial shall take place, no cremated human remains shall be scattered and no tombstone or other memorial shall be placed in a cemetery, and no additional inscription shall be made on a tombstone or other memorial, without the permission of the officer appointed for that purpose by the burial authority.

(2) No body shall be buried in a grave in such a manner that any part of the coffin is less than three feet below the level of any ground adjoining the grave, provided that the burial authority may, where they consider the soil to be of suitable character, permit a coffin made of perishable materials to be placed not less than two feet below the level of any ground adjoining the grave.

(3) No body shall be buried in a grave unless the coffin is effectively separated from any coffin interred in the grave on a previous occasion by means of a layer of earth not less than six inches thick.

(4) When any grave is reopened for the purpose of making another burial therein, no person shall disturb any human remains interred therein or remove therefrom any soil which is offensive.

(5) Every walled grave or vault shall be properly constructed of suitable materials.

(6) Within 24 hours of any burial in a walled grave or vault, the coffin shall be – (a) embedded in concrete, and covered with a layer of concrete not less than six inches

thick; or (b) enclosed in a separate cell or compartment of brick, slate, stone flagging or precast concrete slabs of a 1:2:4 mix, in any case not less than two inches thick, in such a manner as to prevent, as far as may be practicable, the escape of any noxious gas from the interior of the cell or compartment.

(7) Any person to whose order a body is buried in a grave in respect of which an exclusive right of burial has been granted shall, as soon as conveniently may be after the subsidence of the earth has been completed, cause the surface of the grave to be covered with any tombstone or other memorial in respect of which a right has been granted by the burial authority or any predecessor of theirs, or with fresh turf, or, where the burial authority permit, with such flowering or other plants, or in such other manner, as may be permitted.

(8) Where the burial authority permit uncoffined burials, any reference in this Part to a coffin includes a reference to the wrappings of an uncoffined body.

It is interesting to note that there is no requirement to bury to the apocryphal depth of 'six feet under'. The specified depth may only be three feet to the top of the coffin, or even two feet if the coffin is deemed perishable (presumably cardboard, wicker, or similar) and the soil of a 'suitable character'. The phrase 'suitable character' has been defined in a Memorandum of the then Ministry of Health to accompany the Local Authorities' Cemeteries Order 1977 thus:

The soil of a burial ground should be preferably of an open porous nature, with numerous close interstices, through which air and moisture may pass in a finely divided state freely in every direction. In such a soil decay proceeds rapidly, and the products of decomposition are absorbed or oxidised. The soil should be easily worked, yet not so loose as to render the work of excavation dangerous through the liability to falls of earth. It should be free from water or hard rock to a depth of not less than 4 feet 3 inches if only one interment is to be made in each grave. This would allow 1 foot 3 inches for depth of coffin and 3 feet for cover of earth above the coffin. If more than one interment in a grave is contemplated the soil should be free from water or hard rock to a proportionately greater depth, allowance being made for a layer of earth not less than 6 inches in thickness between any two coffins. If the soil is not naturally free from water, it may be found necessary to drain the site to the required depth, and hence the site should be sufficiently elevated above the drainage level of the locality, either naturally, or, by filling it up to the required level with suitable earth.

A dense clay is laborious to work and difficult to drain; by excluding moisture and air it retards decay, and it retains, in a concentrated state, the products of decomposition, sometimes to be discharged into graves in the vicinity, or sometimes to escape through cracks in the ground to the surface. A loose stony soil, on the other hand, may allow the passage of effluvia, and of imperfectly purified drainage water.

(ICCM 2004, Appendix 1)

An interesting observation from an investigative point of view is the requirement to seal vaults, or concrete over coffins within 24 hours of interment (item 6); if adhered to, this gives a precise and well-defined disposal window.

In addition to the regulations under the Local Authorities' Cemeteries Order 1977 (HMSO 1977), if the grave that is the subject of an enquiry or investigation falls within a part of a cemetery that has been consecrated for burials according to rites of the Church of England, then it falls within ecclesiastical law. Such areas are subject to the jurisdiction of the Diocesan Bishop, which means that no work may be carried out without authority granted by way of a Faculty from the Diocesan Chancellor via the Diocese Advisory Committee. Here the committee's deliberations, decisions and the time frame of events are well documented (see Section 5.9.3 above).

The cemetery records are obliged to identify the grave on a plan, the specific grave number, the type of grave (earth dug, walled or vault), details of the individual(s) within the grave (referred to as the 'lair' in Scotland), the date of burial, and any subsequent actions relating to the grave. Often the records have useful details about the burial itself, for example a record of the depth of burial, or the depth of soil between the top of the coffin and the surface. These details are maintained by the cemetery in case in the future there may be a need to disturb the grave for any reason, i.e. a second burial within the same grave, or the need to bury cremated remains, or if there are retained organs and body parts that will require burial some years after the original burial under the various human tissue acts involving a Coroner (England, Wales or Northern Ireland) or Procurator Fiscal (Scotland), or if there is need for police investigation.

A slightly more complex situation for forensic search has now arisen with the emergence of 'natural burial sites', defined by the Ministry of Justice as places 'where the burial area creates habitat for wildlife or preserves existing habitats (woodland, species rich meadows, orchards, etc.), sustainably managed farmland, *in-situ* or adjacent aquatic habitats or improves and creates new habitats which are rich in wildlife (flora and fauna) (MOJ 2007, 1). These 'natural burials sites' sometimes termed 'woodland' or 'green' burials were first introduced into the UK in 1993 in Carlisle in an unused woodland area within an existing local authority cemetery. Other local authority cemeteries followed by creating similar areas for 'green burial' within the existing cemeteries; they were thus covered by existing burial legislation.

As these 'green burials' gathered popularity among the environmentally minded, private burial sites were developed and, by 2009, when the Ministry of Justice produced its Natural Burial Grounds – Guidance for Operators (MOJ 2009) there were an estimated 220 natural burial grounds operating in the UK. It was the first time since the 19th century that large scale development of cemeteries had taken place nationally within the UK. In 1994, the Natural Death Centre, a Registered Charity, set up the Association of Natural Burial Grounds (ANBG) to promote the 'natural burial' movement in both the public and private sectors. This organisation has produced a professional code of practice (ANBG 2011) based on the Ministry of Justice's Guidance and provides advice and support to ANBG members. It does not act as an inspectorate or monitoring body; nor is it an archive-holding authority.

These private natural sites lie outside of the majority of ecclesiastical and state legislation, which pertains to 'ordinary' local authority cemeteries and the older established 19th century private cemeteries – many of which had Acts of Parliament specific to individual cemeteries, or had passed from private ownership to local authority, or had simply 'closed'. The Ministry of Justice Guidance includes references to: UK burial law; ecclesiastical law; authority for burial; health and safety; contract and employment; planning regulations and environmental and wildlife law. However within this Guidance the Ministry of Justice makes the point that 'privately owned natural burial grounds are not covered by the *Local Authorities' Cemeteries Order* provisions and are largely unregulated' (MOJ 2009), although aspects of the burial itself in terms of depth and spacing tend to be followed. Part of the ethos, it seems, is that natural burial sites tend to avoid coming under any regulatory controls, either ecclesiastical or state, and hence any of the constraints associated with them. Basic requirements, however, must be met and these include: a certificate from the Registrar that records the death; a register of the burial by the burial ground owner or burial authority, and notification of the physical act of burial to the burial ground owner or burial authority no less than 96 hours after it has taken place. Natural burial sites, however, appear to fall outside the 1926 Act which requires burial grounds to maintain appropriate ground plans; as a result of this the Guidance offers suggestions as to how the position of the grave might be recorded. Many of the natural burial sites, by their very nature, fail to conform to the Victorian easy plan 'grid system' with their main drive and cross-drives; instead they often lie within woods or a meadow, on a wooded hillside with a view over a valley, or next to a simple bare earth pathway where people have selected their favourite place to be buried, often with a grave marker in the form of a tree, a bush, or some wild flowers. The Guidance suggests that operators consider various options: surveying each plot and recording the coordinates and locations on a digital plan; using electronic tags with each burial, or using fixed markers from which individual graves can be located by triangulation. These may sound unnecessary, but they ensure that graves can be located in the future for remembrance, or if additional family members need to be buried, or even for post-mortem exhumations. From a forensic investigative point of view, it allows burials to be identified as being legitimate or not.

Finally, it may come as a surprise to learn that it is also legal to bury a person outside a formal burial ground, or even at home, subject to certain conditions. There is nothing in law that prevents the burial of a deceased person in a place other than a cemetery. The only exception to this is where a proposed burial on private ground might constitute a public health risk. The Quaker movement, which used to practice 'home burials', is often quoted as an example. Wealthy families with large estates have, for centuries, built a mausoleum or burial chambers and vaults on their land for the burial of a family member; more recently families are keen to have 'green' or alternative burials, and the number of burials which have taken place on private land (i.e. farmland or within gardens) has significantly increased. Some local authorities take a very open position on 'garden burials' and address the subject on their websites, with all pro and cons. Home burial does not require planning permission, nor does it appear to need approval from the local Environmental Health Department (unless the deceased died of an infectious disease), but it does require the Department of the Environment to be reassured in terms of the proximity of the burials to boreholes, wells, ditches or water coursing, and to the natural drainage of local soils. This itself constitutes a source of information in any forensic enquiry. That apart, the main requirements are permission from the land owner, and record of the burial in the deeds of the land or property under the terms of the Registration of Burials Act 1864. This record also requires a location map confirming the position of the grave and details of the name of the deceased, age, date and place of death to be recorded. This reduces the potential complication of the police being called if human remains are discovered during future garden maintenance or building work, or in the case of a missing family member (see Case Study 5.11). A certificate for burial issued by the Coroner or Registrar of Birth and Deaths (called the 'Green Disposal') will have to be obtained and any other procedural matters of the Registrar satisfied. The detachable section of this certificate needs to be completed and returned to the Registrar by the person who is arranging the burial. The Registrar does not record the place or location of the burial and this is why it is necessary to consult the property deeds to ensure legitimacy.

Case Study 5.11

An elderly man and his son lived a secluded life together in a suburban town until neighbours noticed that the father had not been seen for some time. The son, who had learning difficulties, refused to comment on the whereabouts of his father and the police became suspicious over his role in the man's disappearance. As a result of this, the house was searched and the garden became the subject of an archaeological investigation. The secluded areas of the garden were searched first, notably those out of view from any neighbour or public gaze, as well as areas below sheds and flagging. The body was eventually found in a shallow grave towards the centre of the garden beneath a paved area that facilitated its concealment. The son's story was that his father had died and had requested that he should be buried in his own garden. The post-mortem could find no suspicious cause of death but the police and the Crown Prosecution Service progressed with a case of murder, fraud and unlawful concealment of remains. Following two trials, successive juries failed to convict the male, and with some reluctance the body was handed back to the son who promptly buried it in the garden again, this time having been made aware of the necessary protocols.

5.10   Landfill sites and waste disposal

Society continually creates and changes the landscape by the erection of new buildings and the alteration of existing buildings; it creates large quantities of unwanted waste in the process. In December 2002, the EU Waste Statistics Regulation (EC 2150/2002) was published in the *Official Journal of the European Communities* (EU 2002). The Regulation requires Member States to provide the Commission with information on the generation, recovery and disposal of waste every two years. As an example, the total waste produced in the UK from industrial, commercial and domestic sources in 2006 was 307,053 thousand tonnes of waste of which 7,629 thousand tonnes was hazardous, and 299,424 thousand tonnes was non-hazardous (DEFRA 2008). The majority of this is conveyed away through regular local authority refuse collection or in builders' skips. Skips of various sizes are regularly seen on construction sites, at the rear of commercial premises, on the highway, or on the front driveways of houses currently undergoing repair, renovation or development. These skips, together with other assemblages of bagged waste awaiting collection, have the potential to become the means of a clandestine disposal of 'least effort', albeit on a temporary basis. Fortunately, however, legislation requires each individual skip to be tracked by a documentary record in respect of its location, load and ultimate destination, from its source to final disposal site. Similarly, the removal of large piles of rubble or rubbish by lorry from building or demolition sites for disposal, generates the same records. In both cases, the normal final disposal place in the UK is within a landfill site or recycling centre.

Current UK legislation and regulations relating to UK waste legislation are numerous, based on European Union Directives and require the specific maintenance and retention of records. Only those Acts and regulations with forensic search relevance are included here; an awareness of these can provide an enquiry with a clear avenue of approach. Under the terms of the Control of Pollution (Amendment) Act, 1989 (HMSO 1989) the required documentation makes it possible to trace all firms involved in the transport of controlled waste within the area surrounding a search location, and to ascertain the location and destination of their skips or lorries on any specified date. Section 1 makes it compulsory for all firms involved in the transport of controlled waste to be registered as a Carrier of Controlled Waste with the Environment Agency. The details of these registered carriers are maintained in a register at the local area offices of the Environment Agency, as required under the Controlled Waste (Registration of Carriers and Seizure of Vehicles) Regulations, 1991 (as amended) (HMSO 1991, Reg. 3).

Once registered, the Registered Carriers must follow a Code of Practice regarding the 'duty of care' in respect of any waste transported in order to prevent illegal disposal; important here is the requirement for the transference of waste to be accompanied by a full written description which needs to be sufficient for each person in the disposal chain to understand what they are disposing (DEFRA 1996, 39). The Registered Carrier must maintain a written record of all waste received and transported, and make those records available to the Environment Agency. Each party to the transfer process (the waste producer, the transporter and the receiver) must keep a copy of this record at the disposal point. 'Model' forms for this are made available in the Code of Practice (DEFRA 1996). Documentation requires, *inter alia*, a description of the waste, but this description needs only to be generic and is of little value in a forensic investigation – it simply directs the carrier to undertake 'a quick visual inspection to see that it appears to match the description, but he need not analyse the waste unless there is reason to suspect an anomaly' (DEFRA 1996, 50). Moreover, multiple consignments of a consistent nature, such as weekly or daily collections of waste from shops or commercial premises, can be undertaken on a 'season ticket' basis for a maximum of 12 months covered by only a general description. The onus of the description is placed on the waste producer unless the person producing the waste is a householder producing domestic waste, in which case the responsibility for the description passes to the person first taking waste from the householder, i.e. the weekly council refuse collection – 'the bin-men'. More useful, however, is the requirement to record the time and date of transfer and the names and addresses of the parties involved. Additionally, all parties are required to keep the records for a minimum of two years – a period useful for recent enquiries, but less helpful over the longer term.

It is easily possible for a skip, loaded with 'innocent waste' consisting of rubble or domestic or commercial waste, often consisting of a large quantity of non-descript black plastic bags, to become a deposition opportunity of 'least effort'. The statistical odds of any clandestine addition being immediately noticed are low, as the checking requirements are essentially visual and do not require the total contents of the skip or lorry load to be checked by the waste carrier, particularly if it is part of a 'season ticket' arrangement. There is, however, a recommendation in the Code of Practice to place the onus for checking on the waste managers receiving the waste for disposal, to increase the level of scrutiny at this final stage. Waste managers are viewed by the Code of Practice as being, 'in a stronger position to notice discrepancies between the description and the waste and therefore bear a greater responsibility for checking descriptions of waste they receive' (DEFRA 1996, 51). However, any sampling is only a visual random test at best, and the majority of loads will normally progress on to the landfill for final deposition without more than the required visual check.

The management of landfill sites is covered by further legislation, and the actual land-filling operation is stringent and highly technical (HMSO 2000b; DEFRA 2010), but the controls present considerable benefits for search purposes. Much of this legislation reflects the environmental and pollution impacts of waste disposal generally, and landfill sites in particular in terms of surface water, groundwater, soil, air, traffic, noise, odour, pest control and human health. Landfill sites are also subject to planning permission and strict licensing controls through the Landfill Regulations; these demand engineering skills in the design, construction, maintenance and completion phases. Landfill sites cannot be simply regarded as large disorganised rubbish tips, and there is within the Regulations key legislation of significance for a forensic enquiry. The relevant regulations (HMSO 2000b) require land-fill managers to visually inspect and randomly sample the material, register the quantity submitted (usually by weight), record the origin, delivery date and identity of the producer, operate records at the site in question and, in the case of hazardous waste, record its precise location on the site. Also available from the documentary records maintained at landfill sites are detailed scale maps of the site. Prior to the Environment Agency issuing a licence, landfill operators must provide an accurate scaled map, based on the Ordnance Survey, of the whole site, indicating its external boundaries and internal boundaries of each proposed phase of disposal. Due to the engineering demands and the monitoring of emissions of water and gases, operators regularly survey or GPS the site in order to produce updated site maps. In this way it is also possible to ascertain the approximate depth that any particular load may be located.

Overall, it can be seen that the documentary record maintained within the various aspects of the waste process, as with those from the planning and building process, represent an important source of ready, and often neglected information which is available to be consulted for the non-invasive search and locate phase of an enquiry (see Case Study 5.12). It can provide a continuity record for individual skips or lorry loads from their source, through all those who handle it, to its final destination, and even to the final approximate three-dimensional location within a large landfill site. A suggested approach relevant to an enquiry that can be adapted to need is shown in Figure 5.9.

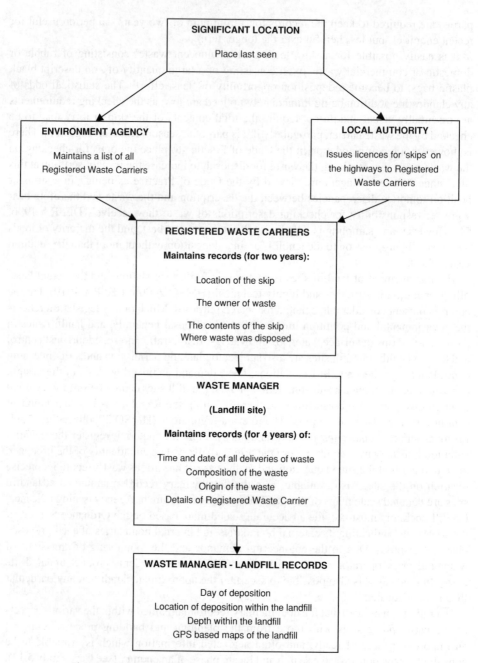

Figure 5.9   Flow chart for searching potential landfill disposal sites.

Case Study 5.12

In November 2004, a murder occurred in the Midlands. The offenders dismembered the victim's body and passed the soft tissue through a domestic mincer, then used bin liners to secure the human remains using two 25-gallon plastic oil drums for their transport. The remains were later carried by vehicle to East Anglia where the bin liners were dumped in a builders' skip where they merged with similar looking bin liners. The skip was situated on the approach driveway to a building site at the rear of shops that were subject to building work. It was subsequently collected by a waste carrier and taken back to the waste carrier's premises where the load was visually examined and mixed with similar building waste before it was deposited on a nearby licensed landfill site.

The bin liners containing the body parts passed though the waste process undetected and, as the victim was a transient person, with no connections in the Midlands except through the offenders, the crime and deposition passed completely undiscovered. The potential for the 'perfect crime' ended when the offenders walked into a local police station in Norfolk to confess the crime. By that stage, the skip concerned was no longer *in situ*, but the documentary records relating to that skip were available and contained the essential information to locate the whereabouts of the body. The waste producer and the licensed waste carrier were located and both were in possession of copies of the required waste transfer record, based on 'the model' format under the Code of Practice (DEFRA 1996).

The information from the waste record enabled the investigation to obtain continuity information in respect of the time and date of the depositing and removal of the skip, the identities of the individual drivers involved in the process and also the time date and location of the final deposition of the waste on a local landfill site. Enquiries at the landfill located the third copy of the waste record, furthering the continuity of the skip and its load. The operating records maintained at the landfill site identified which phase of the landfill was operating on that date, the specific working face and the landfill cell where waste on that date was being deposited and compressed. In this particular case, mapping was available in respect of the infill phase, working face and cell and recorded the depth of the waste layer before it was capped as being 1.5 m. The search was successful and the body parts (as well as the domestic mincer) were recovered.

6 Recovery, stratigraphy and destruction

The crime scene is the place where the main elements of a crime interact with each other – the place, the victim(s) and the offender(s), and is rightly considered the paramount aspect of the investigation. In the case of burials, this is most likely the body recovery scene. While the recovery of the victim is obviously an important facet of the investigation, it is not the sole purpose. Equally important is the recovery of evidence to prove what occurred, as well as identifying evidential links to other scenes, and links to other persons who may not even have been at the scene. The implications are much wider than the burial itself. The forensic archaeologist is not simply exhuming a body, but is reconstructing events by identifying them in the reverse order in which they occurred, and presenting the investigation with an accurate and archaeologically supported reconstruction of the actions that took place there. Rudyard Kipling's lines from the 'Just So' stories are worth bearing in mind:

> *I keep six honest serving-men*
> *(They taught me all I knew);*
> *Their names are What and Why and When*
> *And How and Where and Who.*

This reflects the basic matrix deployed in an investigative approach used by SIOs and Crime Scene Examiners today (Cook and Tattersall 2008). Recovery is about interrogation. Each piece of evidence recovered poses a question: 'How does it inform the investigation?'; 'What more does the investigation now need know?' and 'Where or how does the investigation find this?'. Like the concentric circles of a stone thrown into a pond, the investigation works from the primary crime scene based on evidence recovered, and the questions asked of it, to link it to other places and individuals. This brings in another major consideration: while an archaeologist may be an expert in understanding burial environments, this particular knowledge coupled with experience also entails an appreciation of other sciences that are capable of recovering evidence within and around the burial. In the UK, forensic archaeology has long advocated a multidisciplinary crime scene approach (Hunter *et al.* 1996; Hunter and Cox 2005), for example, the use of additional expertise, as appropriate, in anthropology, palynology, entomology or soil science. Either the appropriate scientist visits the crime scene, which is the preferred option, or a relevant sampling strategy is devised and included within the investigation of the burial.

Forensic Approaches to Buried Remains, First Edition. John Hunter, Barrie Simpson and Caroline Sturdy Colls.
© 2013 John Wiley & Sons, Ltd. Published 2013 by John Wiley & Sons, Ltd.

The methodology of excavating graves is well recorded elsewhere (e.g. Hunter and Cox 2005; Blau and Ubelaker 2009) and this chapter takes 'as read' knowledge of basic archaeological excavation processes. All forensic excavations differ according to context, environment and the nature of the questions posed by each particular police enquiry; approaches may differ, but there are consistent underlying principles that guide those approaches. This chapter explores certain areas of concept, as well as some practical difficulties that the forensic context poses and which are distinctive from those encountered in a conventional archaeological setting.

To be of any archaeological value (forensic or otherwise) the recovery of human remains from the ground has to recognise two key factors: the principles of stratigraphy, and an acknowledgement that the process of recovery *per se* is wholly destructive. Each of these needs amplification with regards to forensic contexts as the implications are significant. Furthermore, associated buried materials (including trace evidence) tend to be dissimilar to those encountered in conventional archaeology and can require different techniques of recovery. The same applies to sampling design, particularly with regard to environmental (ecological) evidence. As emphasised throughout, the forensic excavation process is modelled according to the questions asked: these questions underlie the design, the methodology and the recovery processes.

6.1 Stratigraphy

6.1.1 *Layers and contamination*

The importance of stratigraphy has been outlined in Section 1.2; it has a specific forensic relevance that has been introduced by Hanson (2004), and a number of relevant forensic case studies have been presented by Hochrein (2002, 47–51). The principles of stratigraphy follow empirical laws that demonstrate the relationships between individual layers in the ground; they have a geological pedigree and are fundamental to conventional archaeology where they provide a controlled and systematic approach to the removal of buried remains and the reconstruction of events (see Harris 1979). Reconstructing sequences of events is key to forensic recovery; finding the body is often an achievement in its own right, but being able to recover evidence and interpret what happened is of equal or greater importance. Stratigraphy recognises the ways in which one layer may overlie, seal, cut into or underlie another layer. This is straightforward, it enables a temporal relationship between the individual component layers, and hence a relative chronology. An absolute chronology (i.e. a fixed point in time) is another matter altogether and is discussed in Section 7.5. Stratigraphy also requires the boundaries of each layer to be defined physically. This is important because each layer is likely to have its own evidential value according to its position in an overall matrix of layers. To merge, confuse or ignore differences between layers will result in contamination. Fortunately, most forensic burials have an uncomplicated matrix containing, at a minimum, only a few layers. At the most simple level there may just be two: the mixed fill of the grave itself and a single layer of ground into which the grave has been dug. It is more likely, however, that the surrounding ground will contain a number of layers (especially in residential or urban areas) and that the top of the grave may have become sealed by topsoil formation or by deliberate addition of other layers undertaken to disguise it (imported topsoil, hardcore, paving, etc. (see for example,

Case Study 4.10)). Additional stratigraphic complications may occur innocently through subsequent landscaping, building work or animal burrowing. But they are all important.

If the ground into which a grave is dug contains several layers, then the infill of the grave will consist of a mixture of those layers. It may not be a completely homogeneous admix, but all the layers will be represented within it. If the fill of the grave does *not* contain evidence of the ground substrates, or only some of them, then something unusual, possibly sinister has occurred and needs to be explored further. For example, it may be that the soils have been 'imported' from a different place to fill in or disguise the grave, or that some material (e.g. large stones or brightly coloured bedrock such as chalk) has been deliberately removed to prevent the disturbance from being obvious on the ground surface. This may have significant implications in Court, for example in demonstrating that the offender was not acting hastily nor could justifiably argue a case for diminished responsibility by evidencing the *mens rea* (state of mind) and the *actus reus* (the physical act) of the perpetrator. There are good case studies to illustrate this (see Case Studies 6.1 and 6.2) and this is one reason why the recording of soil types (below) is so important. Under most circumstances, however, the fill of the grave will represent a mixture of the layers already in the ground, typically topsoil and different coloured substrates (Figure 6.1). In more complex cases the grave may have silting layers at the bottom if, for example, it has been left open, there may be re-cuts into the grave fill if items or parts have been added to or removed from the grave, and there may be layers of additional material dumped in it from elsewhere in order to provide further concealment. Interpreted correctly, each layer has its own statement to give: together they provide an interpretation for the overall grave digging, body disposal and infilling of the grave.

However, the definition of individual layers is not always simple, especially if the grave is very old. This is because there is normally interaction between the surfaces of individual layers. As a result their boundaries can sometimes become difficult to distinguish. Over time this phenomenon can become exacerbated, *inter alia*, by water action, roots, faunal perturbation, the fluids released during the human decay process and the gradual biochemical breakdown of the soils themselves. As a result, instead of clear-cut boundaries between layers there may be a series of interfaces where adjacent layers have merged and where it is difficult to distinguish one layer from another. The grave sides are a case in point: a newly created burial is likely to have a very clear distinction between the edges of the grave and the soil infill, in fact when excavated the soil will often fall away easily from the grave sides leaving a sharp edge where the grave has been cut, possibly with tool marks still being visible. There is good evidence to show that impressions and tool marks from digging implements and machine bucket teeth, especially in plastic soils such as clay, can survive well (e.g. Hochrein 1997). Techniques need to be applied to ensure their identification and preservation (for a good example see Hanson 2004, 43). However, over time and depending on the character of the local soils and layers, this distinction may become harder to make. Even an experienced archaeologist may have difficulty in following the edge despite differences in colour and texture. Hochrein (2002, 64) suggests creating a 'small rectangular window' in the centre of the disturbance, and then widening it out until the sides of the grave are properly recognised.

Some environments can be particularly difficult, for example where a grave is dug into peat or sand and then infilled with the same material. A recent murder in Scotland, where a body was excavated from a sand dune approximately one week after burial, posed this

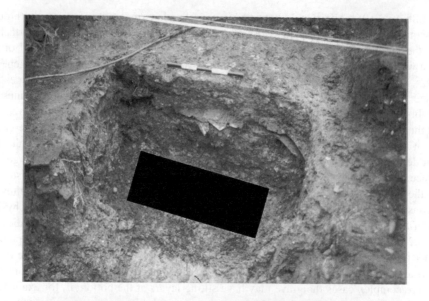

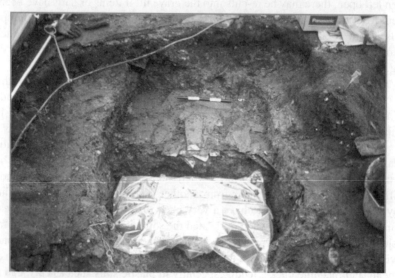

Figure 6.1 Half-section of grave stratigraphy showing (top) cleaned vertical section containing layer of slates, and (bottom) excavation to expose the layer of slates.

specific problem, but the archaeologist was eventually able to identify the grave edges and recover the body and associated evidence appropriately (Cecily Cropper pers. comm.). Given that it is the fill of the grave that contains any physical evidence that may link the digging of the grave to an offender (see below), it is essential to make this distinction correctly in order to avoid accusations of contamination (Figure 6.2). In training exercises for Crime Scene Investigators (CSIs) the authors regularly press small copper coins into the

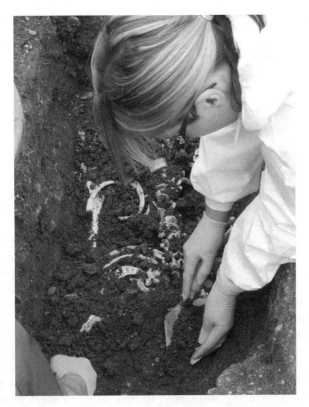

Figure 6.2 A CSI being trained to recognise the grave edges.

grave wall of training graves. The coins do not belong to the grave fill and are, therefore, not of evidential value. If they are recovered by the CSIs during excavation (as often happens, and with some misguided excitement) they indicate that the grave wall has been overcut and the evidence contaminated.

There is a good argument to recognise the grave and its contents as a mini crime scene in its own right. Within the boundaries of the floor, walls and surface of the grave is contained all the evidence that pertains to the victim, the grave construction, associated materials and linkage to the offender. The only evidence types likely to permeate beyond these boundaries are toxins and volatile fatty acids which may infiltrate the grave sides and base, or projectiles which may have entered the surrounding substrates if the victim was shot in the grave. That said, it is as well to remember too that if the surrounding ground surface is contemporary with the digging of the grave, both will belong to the same forensic landscape; the crime scene will be wider than the grave itself and evidence in the form of impressions, trampled vegetation, footprints or, in the case of some mass graves, cartridge casings, may be associated. This is not only important in very recent graves, but also in older burials where, despite erosion caused by climatic and cultural factors, there is always the possibility of some evidence surviving. Irrespective of age of burial, it should be standard crime scene protocol to explore and record the surface around the grave before the grave itself is tackled.

Case Study 6.1

A young woman had been murdered in the south of England. The offender was a building worker who had transported the body to a construction site where he was working. At the rear of the site, concealed from the road, foundations were being prepared for a garage. This consisted of concrete footings for the walls and an infill of compressed gravel as bedding for a concrete floor. He dug a relatively shallow grave into the gravel bedding and was able to conceal the body with the gravel infill. He then compressed the surface as well he could to make it indistinguishable from the surrounding bedding, and left the scene. Unfortunately for him the gravel over the grave was not compacted enough and was observable, especially after a rain shower when differential drying out occurred. The building site was high on the list of locations indicated through a CATCHEM analysis (see Section 2.1) and the disturbance was subsequently vented for a cadaver dog. The dog's response was positive.

Archaeologists were brought in and half-sectioned the disturbance, noting a consistent grave fill of gravel above and around the body (Figure 6.3). This was excavated and recorded in a series of numbered spits and retained for any further work. However, it was also noted that the grave had been dug through not only gravel, but also into compacted hardcore consisting of heavy rubble and stones. It must have taken considerable effort to achieve this as the offender was obliged to use a mattock in order to hack his way through the rubble, leaving tell-tale mattock marks embedded in the grave sides. What was of particular interest, however, was the fact that none of the hardcore or rubble that he had struggled to remove appeared back in the infill of burial. In other words the offender had removed substantial parts of the spoil from the grave off-site and introduced new material (gravel from a builder's gravel heap nearby) to cover the body and level the surface. Had the same mix of rubble and gravel that had been removed from the grave been put back in again, then the presence of rubble indicating a disturbance would have been very visible on the surface. The prosecution barrister could use this information in order to illustrate that the offender's actions were calculated and logical, and that there were no grounds for diminished responsibility, i.e. the *mens rea* (the state of mind) that accompanied the *actus reus* (the physical act).

This particular burial also had another interesting aspect. The offender had collected all other incriminating evidence that would link him to the murdered woman and secured them inside a supermarket plastic bag. After dumping the body in the grave the bag was placed on the body and the grave filled in with gravel. As such the plastic bag was not part of the gravel infill, but represented an interface layer between the body itself and the subsequent gravel layer. On this occasion the time interval between the three events – deposition of body, placing of plastic bag and infilling – is likely to have been minimal. After infilling the grave then became a sealed unit and the presence of the plastic bag directly over the body was incontrovertible proof of the offender's link to the grave and the body.

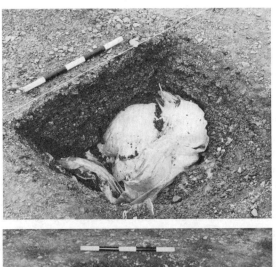

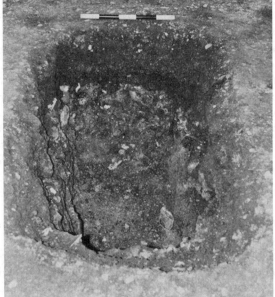

Figure 6.3 Half-section of grave showing (top) infill of gravel and (bottom) how full excavation demonstrated how both gravel and builder's hardcore had been dug out to create the grave.

Case Study 6.2

A wealthy estranged couple had argued over a divorce settlement. In an ensuing event the husband killed his wife and deposited the body in a large plastic garden storage unit which was buried in woodland. Inside the container was the associated death material including the murder weapon. The burial location was found as the result of a confession, and the storage unit was excavated and recovered archaeologically.

The case presented a number of interesting aspects. Given the distance into woodland (approximately 300 m) and the absence of vehicle access, the storage unit, which measured some $1.2 \times 0.7 \times 0.8$ m, would seem likely to have been carried manually, presumably flat-packed, to its chosen destination. The hole in the clay ground into which it had been sunk was so regular and tight fitting that it was probable that the base of the container was used as a template for digging. The body was transported and placed in the container some time later, the interval in question subsequently being a particular matter of interest to the Court.

On clearing the ground surface of leaves and twigs, the disturbance appeared to be broadly rectangular with irregular edges and a darker fill than the surrounding undisturbed ground. In fact, on excavation, it transpired to be of a black, greasy consistency and more like heavy garden soil than the lighter, sandier soil in the woodland round about. Removal of this black soil showed a much more regular rectangular shape to the disturbance with well-defined edges; it exposed a dense brown/yellow clay which was sufficiently hard and compacted to give the impression of natural clay. The upper surface of the clay lay at the same height as the upper surface of the natural clay in the surrounding ground, presumably to give the impression that no further digging had occurred in this place. It was a clever ruse in an attempt to conceal the container underneath. Closer examination showed the clay to be re-deposited, it contained a number of leaves, and it acted as a seal to the container (Figure 6.4). On excavation it peeled away very easily from the sides of the hole. During this process it was immediately apparent that the upper edges of the hole had slumped inwards, effectively sealing the top edges of the container, but still allowing the lid to be opened. The slumping of the sides of an excavated area is well attested on most archaeological sites that are left open. It can occur especially with clays when pressure from the undisturbed strata force the excavated sides of a trench to lean inwards slightly at the top. The question that was posed was how long must the hole have been open for this level of slumping to have occurred?

The prosecution were arguing that the murder had been premeditated, that the hole had been dug and the empty container buried well in advance of the crime. The defendant argued that he had only buried the container after having killed his wife, approximately one week before it was recovered by police and archaeologists. The question asked was whether this level of slumping could have occurred within the space of a week? Archaeological opinion, based on analogy and experience, was that it could not, but equally that it was not possible to say how long other than perhaps an interval of weeks or months. Assessment of slumping is not an exact science, but the Court was interested in gaining professional archaeological opinion.

The defence subsequently changed tack and admitted that indeed the hole had been dug well in advance of the murder, in fact almost 18 months earlier. The defendant's argument was that he had used the container to conceal important documents. However, absence of any roots growing into the excavated hole suggested that this time interval might be contested too. Botanical opinion was sought but the argument progressed little further. The defendant was convicted of manslaughter and was sentenced to imprisonment for 26 years. The case was fascinating from an archaeological point of view in that it sought archaeological opinion not only in a number of predictable areas, namely the way the grave was dug, the question of the 'importation' of the

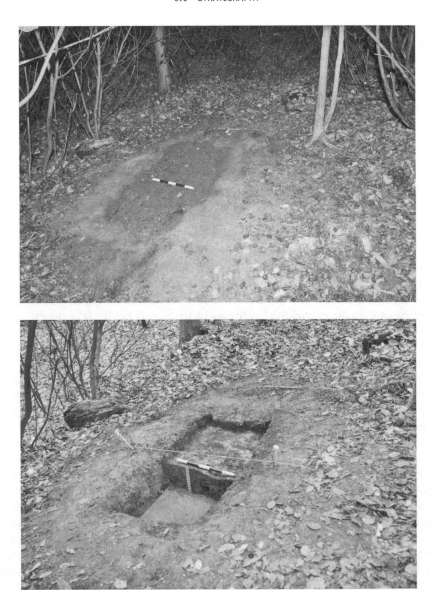

Figure 6.4 Grave in woodland showing (top) evidence of disturbance on surface and (bottom) the half-section illustrating the clever use of re-deposited clay in concealing a container. Image courtesy of Cecily Cropper.

topsoil, and the significance of the re-deposition of the clay over the container, but also in less predictable ones, notably the time interval between burying the container and interring the victim inside the container. Moreover, it became clear too that the Court was concerned with the dynamics of the burial process and the archaeologist was asked to give evidence regarding the volume of excavated material involved. In burying the container the defendant had been required to dig out approximately 0.6 cubic metres of hard natural clay, but only approximately 0.2 cubic metres of clay was used to seal the container. This required the defendant to dispose of clay weighing somewhere between 500–700 kg according to water content. The Court wished to know how and where this might have been carried out. The archaeologist involved was in the witness stand for the prosecution for approximately 45 minutes, and almost twice that time under cross-examination by the defence.

An undisturbed grave is effectively a sealed unit and the role of the archaeologist is to recover not only the victim but also the trace evidence potentially representing other persons or objects at the scene, or links to other places. Discussion of trace evidence invariably reverts to Edmund Locard's 'Exchange Principle', usually expressed as 'every contact leaves a trace'– a statement not actually made by Locard himself, whose early researches on the exchange principle were initially concerned with the presence of dust particles in criminal investigations (Locard 1920). This principle of trace exchange encompasses a wide array of potential transferable materials. These are more commonly associated with surface crime scenes, such as visible bloodstains from the victim, fingerprints, footprints or mud stains from the ground. Alternatively, the traces may be 'latent' in nature, i.e. not obvious and invisible to the naked eye, and require collection and observation by a variety of enhancement techniques, for example, by chemical analysis or electron microscopic examination off-scene at a laboratory by the scientific community (e.g. Houck 2001 and 2003; Blackledge 2007; Coyle 2010). Both types of trace evidence can occur in either surface or buried contexts, but they may differ in terms of visibility and preservation according to environment. Some may survive better buried, or *vice versa*. Any worthwhile encyclopaedia of forensic science demonstrates the range of potential evidence types available.

The behaviour of various trace evidence types in buried conditions has been the focus of growing research (e.g. Janaway 2002, 2008; Wilson 2008). However, to be of value the trace evidence transfer has to be *primary* to the incident in reflecting linkage of one person to another person, one object to another object, an object to a person, or potential suspects to crime scenes. This type of evidence does not necessarily equate to proof that a particular person committed the crime, but it can corroborate or contradict a statement given to an investigation, or provide another avenue of enquiry. Although effectively 'circumstantial' trace evidence is of value as it allows the court to make informed inferences (English and Card 1999). The recovery of trace evidence from a burial, even if it is invisible, should be viewed as part of a standard collection strategy even if it is not considered relevant at the time.

The practical difficulty, especially in a buried environment, is avoiding *secondary* transfer, that is when trace evidence is passed on to a third party, for example through contamination at the crime scene. In excavating a grave there are standard protocols against bringing trace evidence into the crime scene (normally by wearing protective clothing), but it is harder to devise a strategy that avoids contaminating trace evidence that may not be visible (see sieving, Section 7.1 below), or which may not even be there in there first place. To put it bluntly, the archaeologist needs to know what *might* be there in any given circumstance and adapt a recovery methodology accordingly. Furthermore, the significance of identified trace evidence may not be recognised until much later, or it may lead to a re-direction

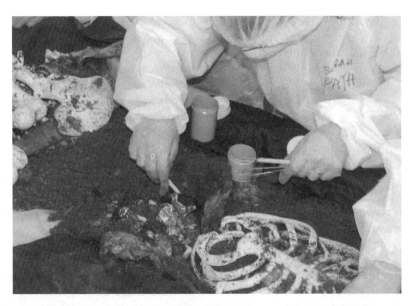

Figure 6.5   The use of small implements to recover trace evidence.

of interest (see Case Study 6.3). In the small volume of material contained in a grave fill (as opposed to larger volumes of material in conventional archaeology) sampling for trace evidence is not an option – the entire volume requires examination. This can be done carefully by hand trowel or other small implement *in situ* during the recovery process itself (Figure 6.5), by bulk transfer of material in numbered units to a more controlled indoor environment for careful investigation, or by a combination of both. Experience suggests that in most enquiries, locating and recovering the victim's body takes priority as this allows the investigation to progress rapidly. The painstaking grain by grain, clod by clod analysis of a grave *in situ* does not always sit well with pressure on crime scene time, natural light and the need to answer fundamental questions, for example, whether the disturbance contains a body or not. There are some practical levels of compromise, for example the application of A4 size taping sheets across the exposed grave fill at arbitrary depths during excavation in an attempt to recover fibres or hair. This may be random in its collection, but it lacks the rigor of a comprehensive examination and is arguably tantamount to sampling anyway.

   Recovery of trace evidence in more controlled environments is not a complete answer as it may fail to reflect the issues posed by the interfaces between one layer and the next. These can only be addressed *in situ*. Interfaces are curious beasts and often cause archaeologists difficulties in interpretation. If, for example, a layer is left exposed and a coin eventually becomes dropped on it, and then in time another layer is deposited (or forms) over the top of the original layer, to which layer does the coin belong? The answer is that it belongs to neither, although an unskilled excavator would invariably associate the coin as belonging to one layer or the other. In fact the coin belongs to an interface layer that is physically invisible and that can be defined only in terms of a time dimension. What we do not know, of course, is the extent of the time interval involved between the three events – the creation of the first layer, the dropping of the coin and the superimposition of the second layer. It might have been only a matter of seconds between each, or it might have been several years. Alternatively one of the intervals may have been very short and the other very long. It is prudent to remember that depth of layers is not a linear measure of elapsed time. Some layers can be created very quickly, others very slowly; some very ancient layers can lie very close to the surface. We can only see the layers that are tangible, not the intervals of time that separate them. What is important is that the exposed layer on which the coin was dropped might constitute a *surface*, in the same way that a grave floor constitutes a surface. In conventional archaeology, it is standard practice to define and clean buried surfaces thoroughly for recording and photographic purposes; in forensic work where surfaces may retain impressions such as tyre or track marks, footprints, fabric impressions (Hochrein 2002, 62), or even exhibits caught at the interface, the evidential requirements are different and the approaches need to be adapted accordingly. It is worth noting that implement marks have even been observed on a clod of earth found within the grave itself (Clarke 2011).

The importance of surfaces and interfaces brings into question how deeper (or mass) graves may need to be approached, given that some may require a platform to be dug out at one side of the grave in order to facilitate access for careful excavation. A relatively shallow grave can normally be excavated safely and carefully from the adjacent ground surface, but only up to a depth of 0.5–0.6 m. Beyond that it becomes necessary to adopt a different approach. Physically entering the grave itself has the potential to create catastrophic forensic disturbance, not to mention damage to the body lying buried below the soil. One solution widely used, especially in mass graves, has been to excavate around the circumference of the grave and then excavate the core or pedestal from the sides (Figure 6.6). This is widely, but not universally, denounced as the method serves not only to break the forensic sealing element that the grave sides provide, but also destroys any marks or other evidence impressed into the grave walling or at the interface (Hanson 2004, 44; see also Wright *et al.* 2005, 148–49 for a discussion on the relative merits). A better solution is to excavate from the ground surface in the normal way until such time as difficulties are encountered and/or the quality of forensic recovery is compromised. At that point, and providing the grave wall has been planned and recorded, the side can be dug out and excavated down to, but not beyond, the level that the excavation has reached inside the grave. The process can continue in stages as the grave becomes deeper; it allows full access to the grave itself on one side, greater ease of movement for the archaeologist and pathologist, and has the added bonus of allowing in more light. The method has been effective on a number of occasions (see Case Studies 4.9 and 4.10), but impossible in some others (Case Study 6.4).

Interfaces are less of an issue in the excavation of burials, but much more common on sites where the time interval tends to be greater and the stratigraphy more complex. Nevertheless, the issues and the implications need to be borne in mind. There is the general assumption that the grave is dug, the body put in and the grave then filled in again as components of one continuous rapid process, and that there is little in the way of a definable interval between the three elements. This makes sense if the process is a hurried one and the grave is a stand-alone event, but the issue becomes more important, for example, if human remains are discovered within the context of building work where the surrounding layers create a greater stratigraphic environment and a broader chronological dimension. If this lies within

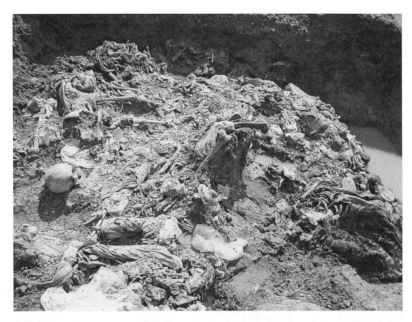

Figure 6.6 Excavation using a pedestal method, in this case necessitated by the presence of a high water table. Image by courtesy of Cecily Cropper.

building history it may be possible to utilise building and planning records (see Chapter 5) to identify the duration of exposure of individual construction elements, i.e. the time intervals between building 'layers'. Construction work is essentially upstanding stratigraphy and the same principles apply. Equally in the excavation of mass graves, there may be identifiable time intervals between individual depositions (for example if a secondary grave is used to conceal victims from different primary graves). Hanson cites a striking example where it was possible to identify how individual machine dumps of victims were separately covered by earth before being pushed to one end of the grave. The next deposit of victims sealed and preserved the machine tracks of the previous deposit (2004, 41). The simple fact of being able to identify that intervals occurred, even if those intervals are not necessarily measurable, can have a significant bearing on interpreting grave construction and infilling and is evidence in its own right (see Case Study 6.2).

It would be wrong to assume that existing layers into which the grave is cut are sterile, although in most rural areas they will be. In urban or brown field sites the layers are more likely to be cultural (as opposed to natural) and will represent activities such as demolition or made ground. These deposits may contain material drawn in from elsewhere or from activities during their formation, mostly detritus. A good (if unlikely) example of the difficulties of this would be the presence of a small rusty kitchen knife that had managed to find its way into one of the layers as part of sporadic rubbish deposition. A clandestine grave is dug in the same spot, the knife is dug out unnoticed in a soil mass as part of the extraction process and then thrown back in as part of the grave infill process over the body.

When the forensic investigation takes place, the knife will be seized (no doubt with great excitement) and taken away for examination. It will of course have no bearing whatsoever on the murder: the fingerprints on the handle will not be the offender's, and any blood on the blade will not match the victim's blood – in fact the knife will be a complete red herring. The same might apply to other potential evidence types, notably part-pages from newspapers or magazines (with dates), items of clothing, or fragments of glass or metal. The archaeologist's job is to interpret the layers in a wider context than just the grave itself and draw conclusions accordingly. He/she will not be able to *prove* that the knife was or was not part of the murder scenario, but will be able to demonstrate from other material within the grave fill and the associated layers into which the grave was cut, that doubt exists as to the value of the object to the investigation. This may, of course, necessitate a wider excavation of those layers into which the grave was cut.

Case Study 6.3

A young female teenager had gone missing and her step-father was suspected of her disappearance and murder. Having first denied any involvement he eventually confessed to having buried her body behind a specific lay-by some miles from his house. The lay-by was identified alongside a mountain road and a search was instigated in an area of unmanaged woodland in waterlogged ground, adjacent to a small stream fed by a spring.

The first search was a visual assessment which revealed no sign of obvious activity, except for a shallow disturbance close to the lay-by; this was left for later examination. However, the visual assessment identified an unexplained area of surface stones that exhibited moss facing different directions and an area of overlying dead branches. These stones appeared to have been taken from a nearby drystone wall and the branches were not beneath any trees from which they could have fallen naturally. It was assessed that they were potentially being used to conceal an area of disturbance underneath.

The stones and branches were all recorded and recovered for later examination for trace evidence (fibres or hairs), followed by excavation. It was an interesting excavation in that the grave was difficult to define in the boggy ground – the spring, the stream and recent heavy rainfall that month, all worked against the investigation. However, the grave cut was identified and the archaeologist was able to identify curved tool marks in the grave sides (it was known that suspect had purchased a shovel around the time the girl disappeared). Despite the conditions the archaeologist was able to safely recover and seal the various soil spits from the excavation and have them securely retained against any future needs.

After the body had been removed, the smaller disturbance was excavated by the same archaeologist but using a different scene suit and a different set of tools to prevent cross-contamination between the two excavations. The new disturbance transpired to be both smaller and shallower than the girl's grave and contained a very stony base and a large tree root which bore marks indicative of scooping action of the digging instrument (Figure 6.7). It was interpreted as being an initial attempt at digging the

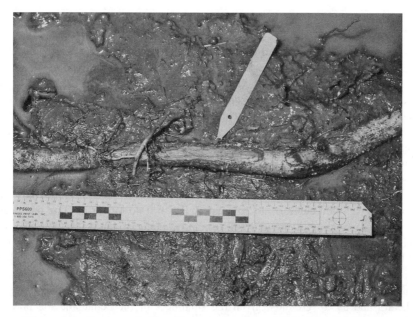

Figure 6.7 Spade marks identified on a root from the digging of the grave.

grave that was thwarted by hard bedrock and root. The root bearing the tool mark was cut and recovered together with some stones that appeared to show a tiny speck of green paint. Subsequent laboratory examination found the paint on the stone and on the root to be identical to the green paint on the new shovel that the offender had purchased. This discovery led to a re-examination of the fill from the grave proper: the soil was carefully sieved off-site and yielded a further speck of the same green paint on the rock within the fill. This was also found to be identical to the paint on the shovel bought by suspect. The circumstantial evidence provided links to connect the paint used on the type of shovel bought by the suspect to the paint found on the stone in the main grave, and also to the root and the stone from what was interpreted as an 'attempted grave'.

The case demonstrates the importance not only of trace evidence (here the transfer of paint from shovel to rock, soil and root) but also how sometimes trace evidence does not always manifest itself at the time of recovery. Furthermore, it emphasises the importance of being able to return to the fill (in this case two months later) and the scene after the excavation has been concluded. It is also shows the importance of reading the wider scene for potential indicators of the actual burial under difficult circumstances, i.e. the movement of the stones from the drystone wall. Careful use of different excavating equipment for the 'attempted grave' to avoid any cross-contamination maintained the integrity of evidence recovered. The archaeological evidence was more than a simple exhumation of a buried body and in this case it was a major evidential contributor to the finding of a 'guilty' verdict of murder.

Case Study 6.4

A 14-year old girl had been murdered by her step-father and his associate and buried under the flagged floor of a cellar in his terraced house. The cellar was small, approximately 3×3 m. A short line of flags had been lifted to enable the burial to take place, and then re-laid. In order to conceal this further the whole floor had then been crudely concreted over – an action which had the effect of attracting police interest when the girl was later found to have gone missing. After removal of the concrete (a sealing layer in its own right) it was obvious which flags had been disturbed and an excavation was undertaken to see if the disturbance contained a burial. It was initially half-sectioned and was seen to contain a fill of dirty mixed clay and some rubble. This was removed in spits and was also found to contain various items of clothing and various objects. At a depth of approximately 0.6 m it no longer became practicable to continue excavating: it was difficult to remove material, the water table had been reached and the level of care necessary was becoming compromised (Figure 6.8). Not knowing how much deeper the body may have lain (if indeed there was a body there) it was decided *not* to enter the disturbance physically in case post-mortem damage was inflicted. The option of creating a platform on one side was rejected on health and safety grounds, given the smallness of the cellar and the potential weakening of foundations. Furthermore, it was not possible to use a mechanical pump

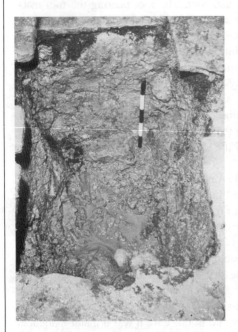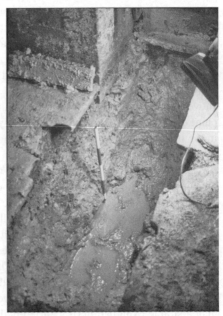

Figure 6.8 Excavation of grave in cellar showing (left) half-section demonstrating the difficulties of access and waterlogging in the recovery process (the victim has yet to be exposed), and (right) the fully excavated grave.

to remove the water because of the danger of fumes in a confined space. After due consideration the only option open was to cut planks of wood, wedge them across the excavated sides of the grave and use them as a platform from which to continue to work (and from which to extract water in a small container). Before this was done, however, the grave outline was recorded and surveyed into the cellar, and the sides were examined carefully and recorded for any impressions and marks. The excavation was a slow but effective process and the girl's body was eventually found, exposed and lifted. The bottom of the grave was over 1 m below the surface of the cellar floor.

6.1.2 Fire scenes

Most fire scenes contain stratigraphic elements, but these lie above as opposed to below ground, and their nature requires a slightly different treatment. Fire investigation is often a complex process requiring knowledge of, *inter alia*, chemistry, material science, structural engineering and combustion, and is the subject of much specialist literature (e.g. Dehaan and Icove 2012). It can also require approaches that are essentially archaeological in character in terms of both search and recovery, an observation first identified by Cooke and Ide who devoted a chapter entitled 'Excavation' in their book *Fire Investigation* (1985, 109). A more recent comparison between fire investigation and archaeological investigation has been made by Harrison (2008) who demonstrates ways by which the respective methodologies might be usefully shared to mutual benefit.

Most fires involve stratigraphy in one form or another, usually brought about by the collapse of a building and the formation of layers which reflect the sequence of that collapse. These sequences depend on many different factors, for example the nature of the combustible materials present (e.g. timber, fabrics, etc.), the way in which the fire spread and the heat generated. Fire scenes present a much more rapid and concentrated sequence of stratigraphic events than those represented in conventional archaeology where formation processes tend to occur over the course of centuries. Nevertheless, the same principles apply: at fire scenes an understanding of the debris stratigraphy allows the process of collapse to be reconstructed with a view to answering specific questions. Typically these might relate to finding the seat of the fire, identifying the use of accelerants, or the focused locating of victims. The investigation needs to be question-orientated because, like any other archaeological intervention, the process is a destructive one and requires record. However, unlike conventional archaeology, it is not often possible to create vertical sections through detritus: sequences may need to be determined in specific locations by the equivalent of 'test-pitting', for example by careful removal of debris in order to assess the sequence of collapse in a given place. The fire investigator will know where best to locate these sondages in order to answer specific questions. Just because the collapse sequences are 'fresh' does not necessarily mean that the individual layers will be easy to distinguish: the same problem of interfacing encountered on archaeological sites may occur as a result of the water used to extinguish the fire. This can cause soft materials such as plaster spalling and ash to become matted and congealed, a problem likely to become exacerbated by any machinery brought in to remove major structural elements. There are also unusual health and safety issues, such as structural instability and the presence of toxic materials.

The interrogation of the debris can be undertaken by targeted investigation rather than by the removal of the entire mass of debris as part of the process. However, there are also instances where total 'excavation' is required because the questions asked require it. A case in point occurred in the aftermath of the fire at Windsor Castle in 1992 where an archaeological team was deployed to undertake the controlled removal of debris with specific objectives in mind (Kerr 2008). These objectives pertained to the proposed reconstruction of the burned out interior: it required knowledge of the original timber joints, and the nature of the plasterwork, panelling and other decorative elements in order to provide the necessary information for restoration. The archaeological response entailed gridding of the individual rooms and sifting through the debris systematically on a grid by grid basis (Brian Kerr pers. comm.). 'Coarse' manual sifting was used in order to recover appropriate items and materials that would aid the reconstruction, and a process of finer sifting was carried out in defined locations in order to recover the remains of specific known items, such as collapsed chandeliers or displayed artefacts (Figure 6.9). The remainder of the debris was taken off-site and manually sifted on a conveyor for any other items that may have been missed. The time necessary for this final sifting was both considerable and labour intensive. The castle rooms were unoccupied at the time of the fire, and in this particular case a strategy for searching for any human remains was not needed. However, in instances where missing persons, or potentially missing persons, might be involved, the process may need refining as illustrated in Case Studies 6.5 and 6.6 below. It is perhaps worth remembering that the human body is extremely difficult to destroy completely by fire, many parts of the skeletal framework being resilient to high temperatures even under modern cremation circumstances. Brickley's review of burned human remains makes clear how advances in anthropological techniques, in many cases developing out of archaeological research (see, for example, McKinley 2000), have enabled even small fragments of burnt bone to contribution to general identification (e.g. Case Study 6.7; Brickley 2007; see also Section 7.3). Burned human bone is still largely recognisable as such, despite potential changes in colour, although it tends to become highly brittle and vulnerable to crush damage under structural collapse. Locating it among similarly charred remains requires careful debris processing, often involving laborious sieving to maximise recovery for identification and cause of death purposes. An unusual case that exemplifies the advances in identification techniques on burned human bone occurred in the central England (Case Study 6.7); it also serves to illustrate the value of stratigraphic recovery.

Case Study 6.5

When the immigration detention centre at Yarls Wood, Cambridgeshire was burnt down by arsonists in 2002 it was unclear as to whether persons had been trapped and had perished within the building. As a result the investigation strategy differed from that at Windsor Castle in that a high degree of sieving was also employed (Corrine Duhig pers. comm.). The building was of a single storey and the rooms were each divided into four grids, each grid being separately numbered, and the debris from each individual quadrant was sieved separately down to a mesh size that would capture the most tiny of human bones (the ossicle). The work was undertaken by archaeologists and police officers under anthropological supervision. No human remains were ever found and, as at Windsor, the work off-site was both lengthy and labour intensive. In this instance the priority issue was deemed to be the search for human remains, not identifying the seat of the fire, which was viewed as a secondary consideration.

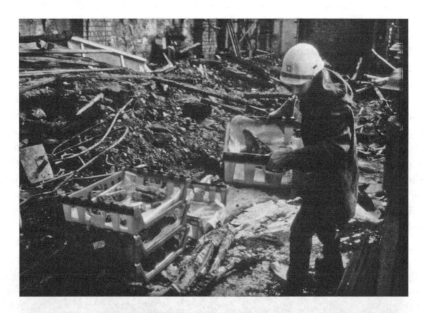

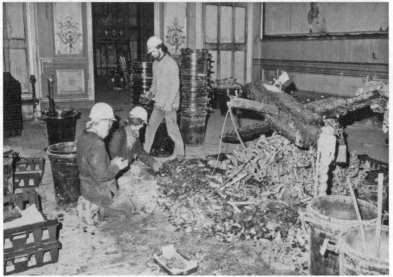

Figure 6.9   Archaeologists excavating in the fire debris at Windsor Castle showing (top) the coarse level recovery of material and (bottom) the specific recovery of a chandelier. © English Heritage.

Case Study 6.6

A scene where victims were known to have been buried under collapse occurred more recently in a fire in a large rural house in the Shropshire countryside. The building was occupied by a family of three (father, mother and teenage daughter) and appears to have been burnt down by the father, seemingly as a result of business/money problems. The key questions here were directed to finding the victims, identifying them and establishing cause of death. The father, it transpired, had shot his wife and daughter before setting fire to the house. His own cause of death is unclear. Here the building was of three storeys with the parent's bedroom being on the first floor and the daughter's bedroom on the second floor. The burning had caused the house to collapse internally providing a straightforward stratigraphic relationship between the ground, first and second floors which could be identified from the structural debris (Julie Roberts pers. comm.) (Figure 6.10). The recovery was undertaken accordingly, the area was gridded and numbered, and the debris removed on a grid by grid basis by CSIs. It was then transferred into labelled containers and sieved through a 4 mm mesh. Both dry and wet sieving methods were employed (see Section 7.1 below). All three bodies were recovered in the house by CSI intervention, but not all were complete. The sieving recovered further remains that enabled cause of death to be established on all three. The sieving process took three weeks, followed by a further three weeks off site.

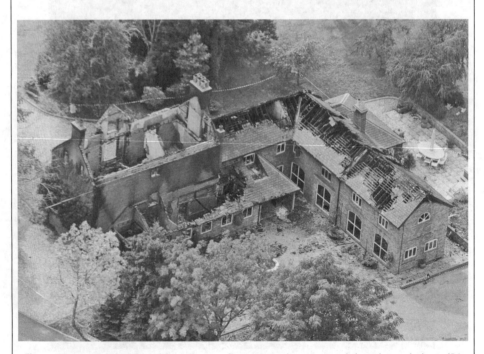

Figure 6.10 The stratigraphic collapse of a country house containing three victims. (PA 6282522 – Rui Viera/PA Archive/Press Association Images.)

Case Study 6.7

A young sex worker went missing in the central England. She had a small child and her disappearance was unprecedented. A police enquiry failed to locate her

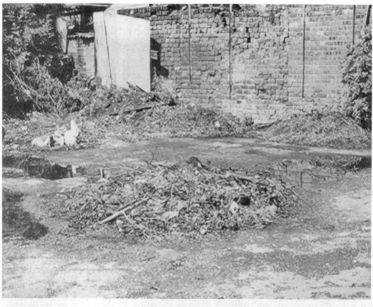

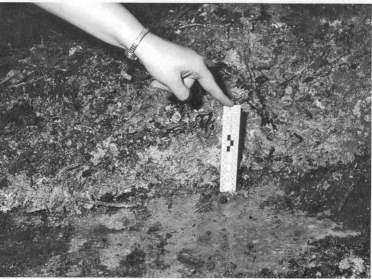

Figure 6.11 The seat of successive bonfires showing (top) the overall context and (bottom) the section through the stratified bonfire deposits. The victim's remains were discovered in the primary ash layer.

but triangulation of her final mobile phone calls was used to define her movements on the night she went missing. The general area identified embraced the residences of a small number of likely suspects with appropriate criminal records. Their houses were searched, one of them being found to contain blood spatter which matched her DNA. The house owner was a frequent user of prostitutes and had a number of favourite haunts where he took them. The search for her likely remains focused on several locations, including a graveyard and various woodland sites. The suspect worked as a garden clearance operative and had a small yard in the city where he stored equipment, tools and rubbish. The day after the girl went missing he was known to have had a large bonfire in this yard, the debris of which had since been subsumed under subsequent bonfires, each creating its own successive layer of ash. The upper levels of this bonfire had been the subject of investigation by CSIs but they had not delved further.

Archaeologists were introduced into the yard two months later and investigated the bonfire remains as one of several potential disposal loci. Their approach was a stratigraphic one and the bonfire ash was excavated in quadrants each of which provided a section (profile) through the ash deposits (Figure 6.11). There were several layers of ash but the primary deposit (i.e. the one resulting from the suspect's bonfire) was found to contain numerous small fragments of bone which were identified as human. Several hundred fragments were recovered through sieving and a number of anthropologists were commissioned to examine them. The consensus was that the remains belonged to a female of the appropriate age and stature of the missing girl; it was also partially possible to reflect her dental record from the few teeth recovered. While this personal level of identification was not conclusive, the presence of the girl's door keys in the same layer of ash provided sufficient evidence for a conviction. In many respects the case was a landmark in anthropological studies regarding fragmented burned bone.

6.1.3 Formal exhumations

The use of archaeologists is becoming more common in the formal exhumation of burials in churchyards and graveyards, although the practice is by no means widespread. Formal exhumations undertaken by the police are typically in order to undertake a post-mortem where death has been suspicious or, more rarely, for identification purposes. Licences from the Ministry of Justice are required for exhumations in non-consecrated land, but not for those in Anglican consecrated ground where Faculty Jurisdiction applies (see Section 5.9.3) and where a Faculty is required from the Chancellor of the diocese. The legislation that permits exhumation reverts to the Burial Act 1857 (with amendments) and has been subjected to review during 2011–12, but no changes have resulted to law affecting exhumation to date. Exhumations are normally required to take place early in the morning (before the general public have access to the cemetery) to maximise privacy, and behind screens.

There are a number of issues worthy of commenting on, not least being the practical issues involved in lifting the coffin. Not all graves are dug to the traditional depth of six feet (see Section 5.9.4); some are less, depending on the nature of the bedrock and whether or not machinery has been used. Also, many older graves are multiple-occupancy with the latest occupant lying relatively close to the surface. The shape of most graves is rectangular with vertical sides and of a proportion that allows the coffin to be accommodated with little room to spare. Some graves are 'coffin-shaped' and may have been created using a template. In either case there is rarely room for manoeuvre between the sides of the grave cut and the coffin itself. Nor should there be, given that the nature of inhumation is such that coffins are buried with the intention of staying buried indefinitely. Moreover, graveyard land is finite and the gaps between graves are often as little as 15 cm (six inches) in order to maximise on burial space. This can cause a number of constraints during excavation, most significantly because of the difficulty of extracting a coffin when there is little working space around it at a depth of some five feet. Creating a working platform to one side is not usually an option if there are graves either side. There is a significant health and safety issue here that is exacerbated by the potential instability of the thin band of soil separating one grave from the next, not to mention the potential collapse of headstones and memorials.

Although exhumation is required to take place in the early morning, working time can be optimised by excavating the grave down to just above the coffin the previous day. This means that the coffin can be exposed and lifted fairly soon the next morning, avoiding unnecessary publicity in the process. Most modern coffins are constructed of solid wood or veneered materials. All decay completely according to burial environment and depth of deposition, although sometimes they can survive as dark stains in the ground. Although coffins are structurally stable at the time of burial, once decay begins to set in they become unable to bear the weight of the grave infill (typically 1.5 tonnes for a normal-sized grave), the coffin lid caves in and the sides splay out. This makes it even harder to extract from the grave cut. Experience has shown that the coffin base tends to retain its stability longest, but that to try and raise it from the ends is likely to be catastrophic. The reason for this appears to be the vacuum effect brought about by the weight of the grave infill pressing the coffin into the grave floor (Figure 6.12). This creates a strong suction effect, particularly if the surface is waterlogged, and it needs to be released gently by allowing air to circulate under the base. This can be achieved by lifting the edge of the base gently all the way around, and then by sliding straps underneath in order to raise the casket in one piece.

The value of an archaeological presence lies in establishing the definition of the grave cut in order to execute the exhumation effectively and safely, and to ensure complete recovery of the remains within the context of the grave cut. It also provides the SIO with some reassurance that the crime scene (for that is effectively what it is once the coffin has been exposed) is not contaminated by material from within the grave sides or below the base, and that this can be achieved according to professional standards that may need to stand up in Court. Moreover, in instances where toxicological sampling is required, this can be carried out and logged according to basic stratigraphic principles, i.e. from defined points in the grave fill and from the side and base of the grave as appropriate. The archaeological involvement is very different from that in a clandestine grave, but the underlying ethos of answering specific questions and resolving practical difficulties remains unchanged.

Many people are surprised to see television or press pictures of gleaming coffins being carried by undertakers from behind exhumation screens. This is not the painstakingly exhumed remnants of the buried coffin, but a new one designed to contain those remains, and therefore larger than the one which has been exhumed. This in itself poses practical problems in that this new (larger) coffin will be buried in the same grave once the

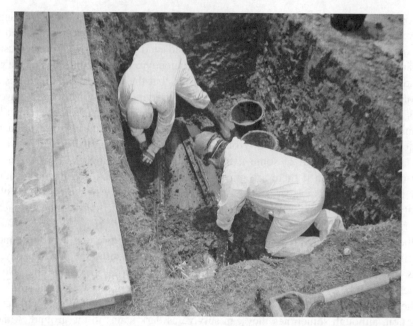

Figure 6.12 The archaeological recovery of a coffin from an established graveyard. On this occasion, and unusually, it was possible to create a platform on one side. The photo shows efforts to release the vacuum effect below the coffin.

post-mortem has been concluded and will necessitate a widening of the existing cut and all the dangers that may incur to accommodate it.

6.2 The destructive process

6.2.1 Documentation

Because archaeology is a destructive process and cannot be replicated, it requires a comprehensive record; this is carried out by documentation, scale plan/drawing and photographing. All of these records are disclosable. From a forensic point of view the documentation element is probably the most important and the most detailed, although also probably the one least understood in Court. It normally consists of context sheets or record cards which describe the character of individual layers, each layer being given a unique number and a separate record. Context sheets such as these are universally used in conventional archaeology and are easily adapted for forensic purpose. However, given the relative simplicity of a forensic matrix these forms tend to be over-comprehensive in the level of information requested. Context sheets have evolved over time to be more user-friendly, often utilising tick-box methods to facilitate speed of completion and for ease of computer input. Neither of these factors are necessarily pertinent at a forensic scene. Using adopted pro formas that are unnecessarily comprehensive is to beg embarrassing questions in Court as to why some boxes are left empty. An example of a possible forensic record sheet is shown in Figure 6.13 and Figure 6.14.

CONTEXT RECORDING FORM

POLICE FORCE	OPERATION REFERENCE:
LOCATION:	OUR REFERENCE:
CONTEXT TYPE:	CONTEXT NUMBER:
AREA:	ASSOCIATED FEATURE:

DESCRIPTION	SHAPE	☐ V. Clear ☐ Clear ☐ Medium ☐ Indistinct
	SIDES	☐ V. Clear ☐ Clear ☐ Medium ☐ Indistinct
	PROFILE	☐ V. Clear ☐ Clear ☐ Medium ☐ Indistinct
	ORIENTATION	
	METHOD	☐ Machine ☐ Pick/Shovel ☐ Trowel ☐ F. Trowel ☐ Lift
	DIMENSIONS	Length: m Width/diameter: m Depth: m
	EXHIBITS RECOVERED FROM CUT:	
	DESCRIPTION:	

STRATIGRAPHY

equivalent – – – – – – equivalent – – – – –

ASSOCIATED RECORDS

PLAN AND SECTION NUMBER(S)	PHOTOGRAPHIC RECORD:
EXCAVATED BY:	DATE:

Figure 6.13   Example of possible forensic record sheet (front).

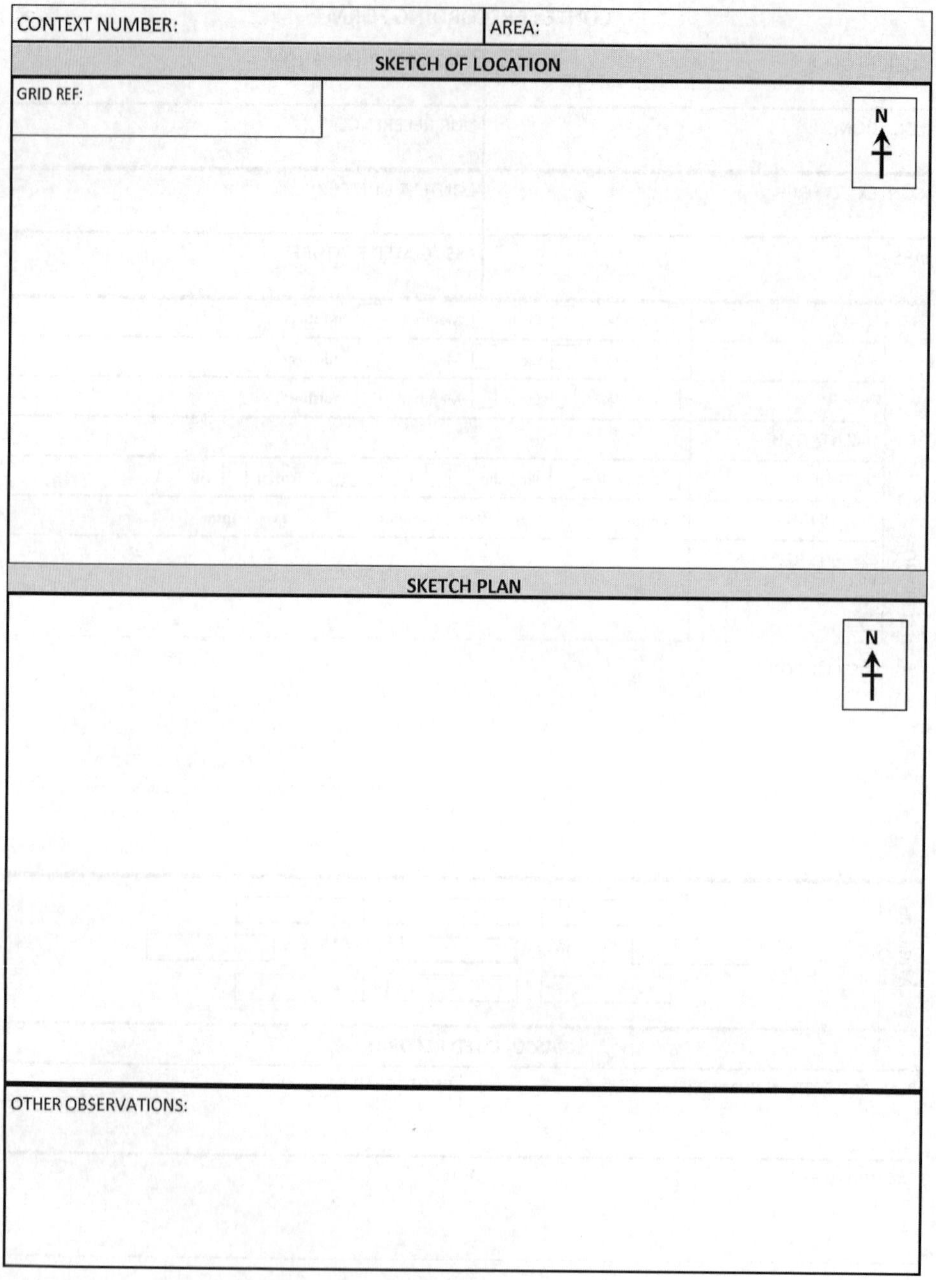

CONTEXT NUMBER:	AREA:

SKETCH OF LOCATION

GRID REF:

N ↑

SKETCH PLAN

N ↑

OTHER OBSERVATIONS:

Figure 6.14   Example of possible forensic record sheet (back).

In view of this the best context sheets for forensic work are those that provide good basic records for a small number of individual layers and their relationships, rather than those that have been created to record complex multi-layered archaeological sites. The main elements required for documentation per layer are those that relate to the nature and character of each layer defined in terms of colour, consistency and physical matrix (e.g. the nature and type of any inclusions, approximate percentage of inclusions, etc.) so that they can be compared to other layers, what artefacts (exhibits) were contained in each particular layer, and the layer's three-dimensional position (usually portrayed in plan and section). There may also need to be a statement regarding the layers' boundaries and their level of distinctiveness, as well as the position of any objects seized in relation to layers and their interfaces. On completion, this constitutes a unique and comprehensive record of each layer. The soil descriptions contain some elements that are more subjective than others, but in general any two experienced archaeologists are likely to differ little in their records. What is also important is a record as to *how* individual layers were excavated (e.g. by trowel or machine) as this may have some implication regarding the nature and extent of material recovered (see Case Study 6.8).

Most clandestine graves contain a single mixed layer which is a composite of the various layers through which it has been cut, for example a dark topsoil (the 'A' horizon), a lighter, browner sub-soil (the 'B' horizon) and a more compacted natural bedrock, such as clay (the 'C' horizon). Put bluntly, components of these will end up in a heap by the side of the grave, their relative distribution being a function of how the offender dug the grave, for example from top to bottom, or from end to end, or a combination of both. They will be further mixed when the grave is filled in again, unless the offender has taken the trouble to separate out certain elements in order to increase concealment or for some other nefarious reason (for example see Case Study 4.10). It is good practice to excavate a small test pit just off-scene to gain some understanding of the layers likely to be represented and their relative depths. When excavation commences, usually by half-section, and there are found to be no obvious layers present, the infill can be removed in 'spits', or arbitrary narrow layers typically about 10 cm or less in depth. Each spit can be recorded in the same way that a layer would be recorded, with a unique context number and description. The description of each spit will also include a record of any exhibits seized in that spit, allowing a coarse three-dimensional reconstruction of spits and exhibits. The use of a total station recording system can produce this graphically but is often thwarted by sight lines and practical difficulties.

Because the fill is inconsistently mixed, the soil descriptions will tend to differ from spit to spit in the percentage ratios of the dark soil, the lighter soil and the clay. Careful recording of these and the relative positions of the various ratios within the grave as a whole may give some coarse insight into the method of backfilling. The planning of several short sections cut across the grave may supplement this, but is time consuming; the production of a single profile resulting from the half-section itself is the best compromise and creates a single record of a part of the backfilling process in the central area of the grave. It is sometimes overlooked that the 'pure' layers exposed in the walls of the grave can also be of potential value. Sampling them for future use provides an uncontaminated sample (as opposed to a contaminated mixed sample from within the grave) that may be of value for soil type, soil micromorphology or pollen that may have become transferred to the offender's clothes or shoes (see Section 7.2.2 below). This entails additional context sheets for those layers

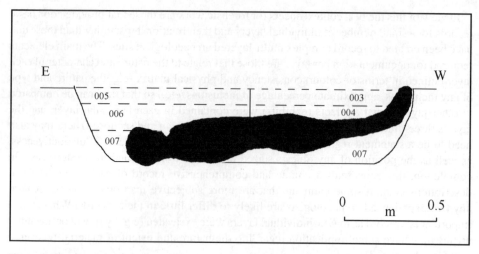

Figure 6.15   Example of measured drawing through grave showing location of individual numbered spits.

exposed in the edges of the grave; it emphasises the desirability of making records beyond the grave itself.

Once the body has been exposed the spits can be better defined spatially in relation to the sides and top of the body. In the same way, the material below the body is normally recorded as a series of separate layers in relation to the body itself, i.e. below the head, or below the legs (Figure 6.15). In many cases this may present no benefit whatsoever, but it may offer unexpected rewards if later sampled for toxins, personal effects, projectiles, or even missing elements of the skeleton (see Case Study 6.9). The more comprehensive the record of individual units of infill (either as defined layers or as spits) the greater the potential for answering questions that may be asked later (Chapter 1.1). The smaller the unit of record the greater the level of interpretation that can be presented, but in practical terms there has to be a compromise between what can be reasonably achieved, the resources available and the outcomes that are essential. One of the skills of an experienced forensic archaeologist is an ability to balance these and produce a workable methodology that fulfils the demands of the investigation and the evidential requirements of other specialist personnel to the satisfaction of the Court.

Case Study 6.8

Whilst conducting a homicide investigation, police were led to an area of farmland where the suspect claimed to have buried a victim several years earlier. The location was fairly exposed, but the suspect was able to point to a particular spot that he remembered. For a number of operational reasons, it was believed that that there was some truth to the story, and the SIO deployed archaeologists to investigate the immediate area of interest. No disturbances were forthcoming and it was agreed to strip a wider area, this time using a mechanical excavator to eliminate the area fully. An 8-tonne 360° tracked excavator with a wide toothless ditching bucket was deployed and this was used to strip a wide area around the alleged burial location under an archaeological watching brief, initially in 10–15 cm spits. During this process human remains were disturbed and partially moved from their original buried position.

At this point work halted and a review of the methodology took place. The grave outline was partly identified as the machine had scooped away the topsoil from the lower half of the grave but left the top half intact. There were also piles of spoil created by the machine, some of these had been scooped from directly above the grave, others had not, but they all constituted topsoil and had the same physical characteristics as the unexcavated soil from the upper half of the grave. Despite their similarity, all these different locations of topsoil were numbered differently for recording purposes: the unexcavated topsoil above the grave was removed by hand trowelling and given one number; the machined topsoil *more* likely to have come from over the grave according to position was given another number, and the machined topsoil *less* likely to have been derived from over the grave according to position was given a third number. When the grave was finally excavated and emptied, and the machine stripped an additional adjacent area in the vicinity, the topsoil removed was allocated a fourth number.

This division of the same topsoil into separate contexts allows the recording system to recognise the manner of excavation and the relative reliability of any material recovered. It also more securely underpins any interpretation of the site and serves to inform any subsequent investigative strategy such as sieving.

Case Study 6.9

A dog walker had stumbled across badly decomposed human remains lying face down in a low-lying waterlogged clearing. The upper part of the back was visible, and presented some residual clothing *in situ*, but the remains were effectively skeletonised. The front of the body, however, because it had been partly sealed in the wet ground had decayed differentially, much of the soft tissue having turned to adipocere. The adipocere had covered the ground surface around the body and had also permeated into the ground. The body was not buried as such, but archaeological techniques were needed in order to recover it together with the associated adipocere. It was not clear whether the death was suspicious or not.

A 3 × 2 m rectangular grid was set up around the body (Figure 6.16). This was then sub-divided into smaller grids; the position of the body was then planned in relation to the grids, the spread of adipocere and to fixed points; each sub-grid was numbered separately. It was not possible to lift the body as a single entity; nor was it possible to remove it in systematic elements in view of the differential preservation and fragmented clothing. Once the main parts of the body had been removed from the scene the recovery of the adipocere was addressed. It was excavated grid by grid in narrow spits and bagged; each spit was approximately 5 cm deep, numbered uniquely and cross-referenced to the individual grid from which it came. At the post-mortem, when individual small elements of the skeleton could not be located, reference was

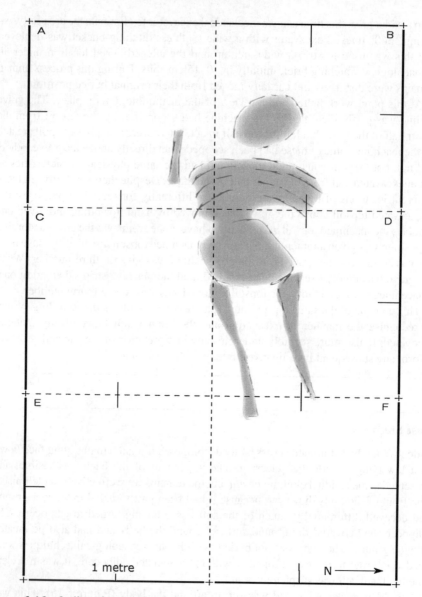

Figure 6.16 Outline of grid and sketch of position of body for recording and examination of surface remains.

made to the plan of the body in relation to the numbered grids. This allowed the likely anatomical position of the missing part to be identified with a particular grid and the appropriately numbered bag of adipocere to be searched accordingly. The method transpired to be particularly effective in locating specific small bones that were found to be missing at the autopsy.

In police work many locations are excavated because they are potentially significant but subsequently transpire not to be. There is a good argument for not entering a detailed level of documentation until such time as a genuine crime scene has been identified. This is not to destroy evidence or lower standards, merely to defer making records. For example, if a suspect disturbance in the ground is being investigated, it can be half-sectioned in spits, each spit being numbered and deposited separately on an adjacent tarpaulin or plastic sheet. If the disturbance proves to be negative a note can be made of the soils and the location and the site eliminated. Conversely, if it transpires to be positive, then full context sheets can be made of each soil spit, and the individual soil heaps can still be bagged and sealed separately for further work. Unlike in conventional archaeology, it is normal to retain individual layers from a grave bagged in sealed containers (usually newly purchased lidded plastic dustbins) where they will constitute exhibits. These may be later used for sieving (see below, Section 7.1) or eventually released and disposed of. A small sample of each is normally retained in case of future enquiries.

In conventional (as opposed to forensic) excavation some layers have greater integrity than others. For example, on a settlement site layers that sit on occupation horizons are likely to reflect specific events over specific timeframes as opposed to layers which have been collected over time, mixed and dumped in pits or wall fills. This is less relevant in a clandestine grave, but there is always doubt over the integrity of the uppermost layer of a grave and the surrounding ground where organic material accumulates and where the surface is most vulnerable to cultural influence and contamination (sometimes referred to as the 'O' horizon). Moreover, as excavation commences, there is always the potential for material to fall from the 'O' horizon into the grave and contaminate individual spits that are otherwise securely sealed (Steyn *et al.* 2000, 237). This can only be controlled by sporadic but thorough cleaning of the ground surface surrounding the grave and by ensuring that the grave walls are fully excavated as each successive spit is removed. As excavation commences, sometimes cleaning is necessary and the resulting residue, which can be composed of in-blown material, residual soils falling down from previous layers or trample (i.e. material introduced by the excavator's footwear), needs to be designated a 'cleaning' layer. This can still have forensic integrity and a unique numbered description, but the likely sources of the material need to be documented and the potential contamination flagged up.

The 'O' horizon itself is often an underestimated source of information, particularly in the discovery of partly buried human remains. These remains may have been buried by a third party and scavenged, or eroded out by natural agencies or animals, in which case they were buried as a result of specific intention; equally they may have originally existed as surface remains that became buried and subsumed wholly or partly by natural soil formation or hill wash (see also Section 7.3). In this case criminal intent may not necessarily be relevant. The distinction can normally be resolved by archaeological means rather than by psychological interpretation. But it does not necessarily mean that the remains are themselves not of forensic interest: while it is possible, for example, that a missing person may have died from natural or quasi-natural causes (e.g. hypothermia), it is equally possible that they may have been murdered and dumped in a quiet location before becoming buried by natural processes (see Case Study 1.1). That particular determination is a medico-legal one, while the archaeologist's role is to present the investigation with a starting point in determining whether the body was buried or not. Older disposals, where the body has been dumped in woodland or remote locations will, in time, result in the body becoming buried by natural processes. The body will also decay and is likely to be scavenged. The distinction that the archaeologist must make is whether the individual was deliberately buried or not, and therefore the extent to which any associated contexts (layers) may contain forensic evidence.

The documentary record provides the basis of the report or witness statement. Whilst it may allude to associated material (exhibits) such as context sheets, plans, illustrations and notes, the report needs to strike a balance between being sufficiently comprehensive to be credible and sufficiently succinct and lacking in jargon to be readable. It is the report that will go to Court and that provides the basis for witness examination. A report that contains too much personal opinion and too much slack invites criticism and unwelcome exploration of detail; one containing too little information and absence of supporting facts might be seen as reflecting lack of competence and professionalism. For simplicity it needs to be couched in a language and style alien to most archaeologists (see Section 1.7) and quite distinct from a typical excavation report. Often it is no more than a clinical account of 'where', 'what' and 'how' couched in simple terms with minimal description of mechanical detail. The basic requirements for this are outlined in the IfA document *Standards and Guidance for Forensic Archaeologists* and are reproduced here in Chapter 6 Appendix (below); also see www.archaeologists.net). Increasingly, archaeologists are being consulted by both sides of the adversarial system and the report will effectively be peer-reviewed and therefore open to archaeological as well as judicial criticism. The same report and the data that underpins it will almost certainly be wheeled out in the event of future work on the same case, or at the same site, possibly with a different archaeologist. The archive of plans, context detail, methods and findings needs to be easily understood and have all data cross-referenced if professional standards are to be maintained. There are no short cuts.

Forensic archaeological practice differs somewhat from its conventional counterpart, and protocols and standards diverge accordingly. Archaeologists might argue over the definition of 'minimum standards', but most archaeologists working in conventional contexts are in healthy positions to implement a 'best practice' drawn up and agreed by peers. The Institute for Archaeologists (IfA) has devised, for example, various *Codes* that relate to watching briefs, evaluations, competitive tendering, etc. (see www.archaeologists.net). However, while these can be benchmarked and monitored in the controlled situations defined by planning directives for the construction industry, they are harder to implement in a crime scene where archaeology is likely to be just one discipline in a complex matrix of other investigative disciplines, all of whose implementations may be constrained by the evidential requirements of others. Additional factors include the need to gather evidence speedily, or the relegation of archaeological evidence to one of minor status according to its perceived relative value in the context of the overall investigation. The archaeologist may simply not be allowed to do what he or she wants to do (a position more frequently encountered overseas in different political and cultural circumstances) or will agree a compromise with other experts in view of the relative value of certain evidence types. Examples of this might be the use of mechanical excavation in a way that allows areas to be eliminated rapidly, even if the upper part of the grave fill is destroyed in the process. Equally, the base of a grave may have to be sacrificed to allow the pathologist to recover the body in a certain way in order to ascertain cause of death.

Most archaeologists are uncomfortable with what might be seen as a lowering of standards from prescribed professional practice, but forensic archaeology tends to be about answering specific questions and problem solving as opposed to the strict adherence to prescribed archaeological methodology. At a crime scene the protocols reflect the *forensic* framework of the work. Within this the archaeology is adapted according to need, not the other way around – it is the servant not the master. Divergence from conventional archaeological work is reflected in the guidance provided by the IfA's 'Expert Panel' (the full set of *Standards and Guidance for Forensic Archaeologists* can be found at www.archaeologists.net/sites/default/files/node-files/forensic2010.pdf; see also Section 3.1) in which a key element is thus:

> Thus the Standard defines a required outcome . . . the attainment of which is covered by non-binding guidance detailing how the profession currently anticipates that the outcome will be reached . . . Any departure from the guidance should be documented, and justification provided as to why the alternative approach is better suited to attaining the required quality Standard.

Key here is recognition of the flexibility required, *provided* that reasons for divergence are recorded. This is important, not only for retention of professional standards, but also for clarification to any defence expert, and for justification in Court under cross-examination. There is, however, a certain standard of excavation that might be considered minimal and which represents a fundamental distillation of more comprehensive codes and guidelines:

- The need to ascertain fixed points for the burial or place of investigation.
- The recognition of grave sides/edges and base.
- The recognition of stratigraphic principles.
- The recognition of the potential for, and implications of, contamination.
- The importance of a written, graphic and archive record.

Lack of justifiable adherence to any of these might be considered non-archaeological and untenable in evidential terms.

6.2.2 Planning and photography

There also needs to be a visual record of the excavation process. In conventional archaeology this is carried out in a series of layered plans that can be superimposed to create a total record of what has been exposed and removed; it enables subsequent interpretation of how sequences of events may have occurred in a given place over time. For example, the first plan might illustrate the rubble collapse of a stone building, the next the foundations and floor of that building, the next the residual traces of a previous building underlying the last building, and so on. Figure 6.17 is a simple illustration of two of the seven structural phases of an Iron Age building that utilised the same outer walling. To achieve this, fixed points are needed in order that the superimposition can be accurate, traditionally by gridding the whole area into 1×1 m squares and using a planning frame strung into at 20×20 cm squares. Features and stones are then planned individually by eye and measurement using the planning frame. There is inevitably slight human error, but the level of this error is contained within each 1×1 m grid and the total result is normally a reasonably accurate portrayal of event sequences. GPS or EDM systems are now more frequently used depending on the size and nature of each site, but the philosophy is the same, namely that the archaeological process is destructive and that the creation of an accurate record is a fundamental part of the excavation process. Planning is normally undertaken at a scale of 1:20 or less depending on the size of the site.

All plans need to be tied into a wider spatial context in order that their precise position on the landscape or on a map can be identified for reference purposes, or so that they can be revisited or re-examined in the future. This is most easily carried out by engaging police vehicle collision investigators, whose job involves frequent total station (EDM) survey work in recording significant landscape features and providing essential mapping data. Total station mapping has the advantage of rapidity. It works well at certain scales, but is less accurate for the more detailed picture. Figure 6.20 illustrates the total station recording of a crime scene at close quarters: the right-hand image provides a coarse but rapid outline of the body, the stones in the vicinity, associated items and breaks in slope (curved lines), and the left-hand image ties in the detail to wider fixed points. If there is no support available 'fixing' can be established by using at least two external fixed reference points (typically a fence or building corners) and two internal reference points from the excavation grid. If a GPS system is being used then only two internal reference points will be needed provided the system is accurate (i.e. <10 cm per point). It is also normal practice to provide a height dimension to each feature or layer recorded, height here being defined as an absolute height above sea level (OD). These heights were traditionally derived from local Ordnance Survey bench marks, but now can be read off automatically using a GPS. Forensic scenes, especially those with burials, are no exception here: those in back yards are easily tied manually to local points (fences, gates, walls, etc.), but those in more remote areas can be more problematic, especially if tree canopies inhibit GPS connections. As a matter of routine grave outlines can be tied into two 'fixed' points established nearby using two pegs set into the ground with a defined separation (typically 5 m), measurements being made either by triangulation or (less accurately, but quicker) by offset. The two pegs can be used as temporary base points that can later be tied in more accurately when time and facilities permit.

Archaeological excavation is a three-dimensional exercise and proper understanding and record of individual archaeological features can often only be made by constructing sections (profiles) across individual features. Plans show sites horizontally, sections show vertical formation. Sections, because they tend to show more detail, are normally planned at a scale of 1:10. Their position is shown on the horizontal plans in order that individual features can be understood in both planes. The sections need to match the horizontal plans: success here is a good measure of accuracy. Comparison of the plan in Figure 6.17 and the section (S76) in Figure 6.18 have to match, albeit at different scales. Like horizontal plans, section drawing is time-consuming and laborious, but is the only way by which a three-dimensional aspect of important parts of the site the site can be portrayed. In the case of a clandestine grave the section needs to be across the grave itself: this will show the grave profile at the point where the long and short axes meet. Recording a section across a grave is the only way that a detailed record of how a grave was filled in can be shown.

If plans and sections are *not* created, there is no measured record of what has been excavated and removed (and effectively destroyed), and no opportunity to re-visit or explain

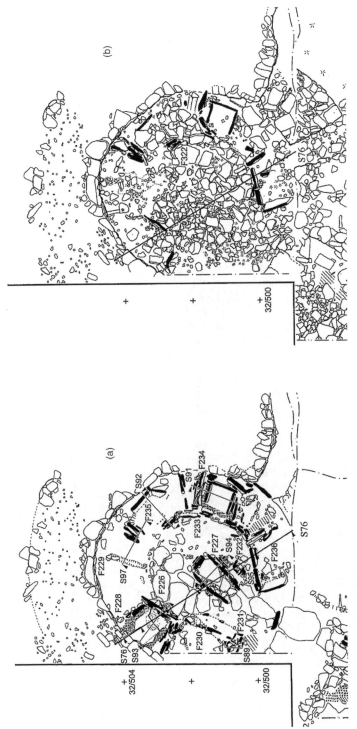

Figure 6.17 A typical stone by stone plan of an archaeological site showing two phases (a and b) of an Iron Age building. Note the position of the vertical section S76. This is illustrated in Figure 6.18 and needs match the features on the ground plans here (blacked-in stones are those which are earthfast, i.e. set into the ground).

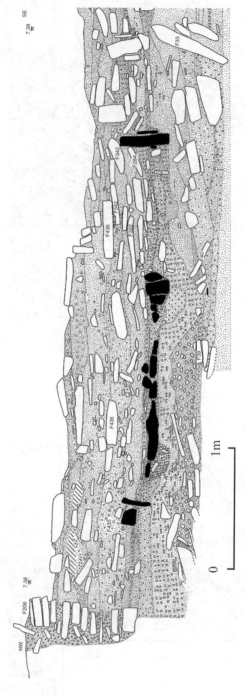

Figure 6.18 S76 is a typical section through an archaeological site. Note its position on the ground plan shown in Figure 6.17 and how it has to match the features illustrated. The phasing of the building is just one of seven phases recorded in this vertical section. For ease of identification, the main stone elements of phase (a) in Figure 6.17 are blacked-in in the section.

what has been found. Plans are a fundamental part of the evidence that allows archaeologists to interpret what they have discovered. Manual planning is slow and can be painstakingly tedious, but is unavoidable because it provides a basic visual record. Manually created plans and sections can be scanned and electronically formalised for publication, thus creating a two-tier system – the raw archive plan produced on site (typically mud-stained, grubby, rubbed out and amended until the planner is satisfied with the result), and the electronically 'tarted up' version that appears in excavation reports and which may embody a degree of selectiveness to it in order to clarify events to a readership. Planning is inevitably a part-subjective process: undertaken manually it depends on the interpretation of the planner as to where the outlines of features or layers lie (especially if they are three-dimensional) – the same issues arise if the points are recorded electronically (i.e. although the record is made electronically, the points which are taken are defined manually, see Figure 6.20).

What are the forensic implications of this? Forensic excavation is normally a relatively simple operation in which planning is usually necessary over a relatively small area. But the same issues still apply, namely that the process contains a subjective element, and that there are likely to be *two* outputs, a raw field plan and a more formalised version of that plan which appears in forensic reports, statements or as an exhibit. Both are disclosable, but it is the former that should matter most to a Court because it is the one that embodies the field interpretation of the evidence as recorded. The latter is normally a simplified version of the former that 'looks nicer', is annotated better and is easier to understand. A general lack of awareness among barristers and Courts that there is such a thing as a primary field record tends to reflect a wider lack of understanding as to how archaeology actually works. Any defence barrister worth his salt should request the raw excavation archives, whether context/record sheets or plans, as these contain the primary evidence that needs to be scrutinised or cross-examined most carefully.

Plans do not satisfy the same requirements as photographs; the two are different recording media with different functions. One is not a substitute for the other. Plans are orthographic representations of what the planner interprets in terms of layer boundaries, edges and the dimensions of individual features. They depict what the planner identifies as significant in a manner that is clinically defined and easy to understand; they effectively communicate how the planner chooses to select visible elements in order to represent the site in hard copy. In other words, plans formalise the interpretations of the person who plans the site. This does not detract from a plan's value, but it is worth remembering that there is always a degree of subjectivity in its production, particularly in the drawing of sections where the boundaries of individual layers do not always lend themselves to the clear-cut definition required by the medium of graphic representation. This issue is exacerbated when the site plan is scanned and transferred into a digital medium for 'cleaning' for formal publication (in conventional archaeology), or for appending to a witness statement or being presented as an exhibit for Court purposes (above). In effect the plan risks becoming further 'simplified' in the process.

By contrast, the photograph is an image that is presented with little or no ostensible subjective bias other than light and shadow. It is an image of what the camera (and the photographer) captured and is open to interpretation by the viewer. Different viewers may choose to interpret the image differently, but the source they view is held in common. With a drawn plan, the image is simplified and the interpretation already made for the viewer. Photographs, of course, are normally oblique rather than orthographic and therefore contain

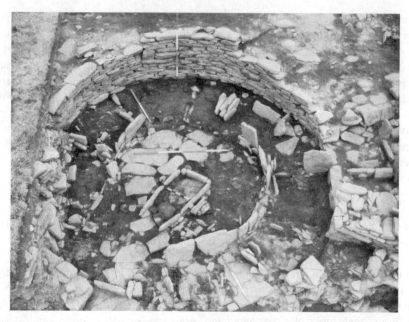

Figure 6.19   A photograph of the same archaeological features shown in Figure 6.17 during excavation.

distortion; they also lack the resolution of a small-scale drawing. However, they maintain a wider field of vision and offer a greater perception of context and depth than any plan. Photographs can be argued to be a 'real' representation of the site as opposed to a planned interpretation of the site. In many respects the two are complementary: the photograph presents an image of the site as seen visually in three dimensions and from different angles, and the drawn plan selects important aspects from the site and presents them in a stylised way for ease of representation and understanding. Figure 6.19 provides a photographic image that can be compared to the plan off the same site seen in Figure 6.17.

Standard scene of crime photography is geared to take both general views and details of features, exhibits and objects as directed. Plans, by contrast, tend to be specific to the grave or to the immediate grave environment and at a single scale. The photographic record needs to be comprehensive because, like archaeological excavation, crime scenes are systematically deconstructed by the very process of investigation. Scene of crime photographers are expert in taking photographs of high quality; they are not experts in pathology, blood spatter, archaeology, or anything else (although they tend to have a wide experience of which types of evidence require photographing, and how), and they are amenable to advice as to which specific images to take, the level of detail needed and the most rewarding angle. As in conventional archaeology, these images need to provide a sequential illustration of the archaeologist's 'story': each change of layer; the grave outline; the record of spit-by-spit removal; the exposure of the body; the empty grave and so forth. These are not random images: each captures events and sequences that the archaeologist believes to be significant and that allow the entire digging of the grave, burial and concealment to be reconstructed through a photographic record (Case Study 6.10). Sometimes, according to circumstance, it

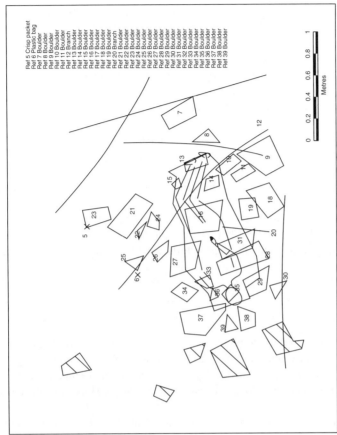

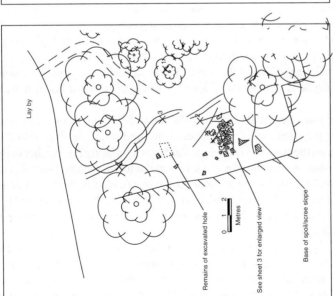

Figure 6.20 Recording of a crime scene using a total station instrument. The detailed plan on the right is incorporated into the wider plan on the left, which ties it into fixed points on the landscape. On the plan on the right, the body is visible under the numbered stones, and the curved lines represent breaks in slope.

may be beneficial to take a number of images from the same location and height throughout the excavation process, for example from one end of the grave. This allows the whole excavation process to be recorded from one place and allows sequences of events to be evidenced more clearly, especially to a jury.

Photographs taken of sections through a grave will be informative, but not as informative as a planned section of the same feature. The photograph will not show the same level of detail as the plan, or the boundaries between layers, but the two will be complementary and the photograph will provide some form of check on the accuracy of the drawn plan. Most scene of crime photographers use scales only for detail or for objects – these scales are normally at a macro-level (centimetres/inches); for wider images, scales are not normally used at all. This runs *contra* to standard archaeological convention that ideally requires photographic scales specifically aligned in order to demonstrate the general size of the site: a vertical marker to indicate depth, and two additional markers located at right-angles to indicate horizontal dimensions. This is equally important in relation to graves: relative measurement is self-evident on plans, but photographs require visual indicators of scale in order to minimise misinterpretation through distortion, and in order to be able to understand relative distance better.

Case Study 6.10

A dog walker had reported to the police what he thought was a lower leg of a buried body on a steep embankment, discovered by his dog. A forensic archaeologist was requested to assist at the scene, which lay on a steep wooded embankment with a pathway adjacent to top of the slope. Access to the bottom of slope was prevented by a high metal wired fence.

It was obvious that human remains were buried at the scene and the dog had discovered an exposed left lower leg, indicating that the body lay with the head towards the top of embankment and feet towards the bottom. The exposure of the leg allowed easy access for insects and required the services of an entomologist in order to assist in the PMI calculation. The burial was in a patch of flowering bluebells, which helpfully indicated the position of the burial. There was evidence of recently uprooted foxgloves and bluebells around the sides as a result of which a botanist was also called in.

The burial site had a large and obviously old tree branch lying along its left together with a large sawn log. There was no tree directly over the burial site and a visual search identified a mark on the embankment where this branch formerly lay. Further in respect of the sawn log, there was a pile of similar logs at the top of embankment. There was no natural physical explanation to account for the positioning of the two large pieces of wood; these were recorded as potential markers to enable the perpetrator(s) to walk along the pathway at the top embankment and to check on the security of the burial without approaching it.

The burial was half-sectioned commencing at the foot end, along with the taking of soil samples, with a static camera taking photographs of the stages of the excavation. The half section revealed a shallow burial of a fully clothed lower body, except that there were no shoes and the legs were bound together. Great care was taken not to

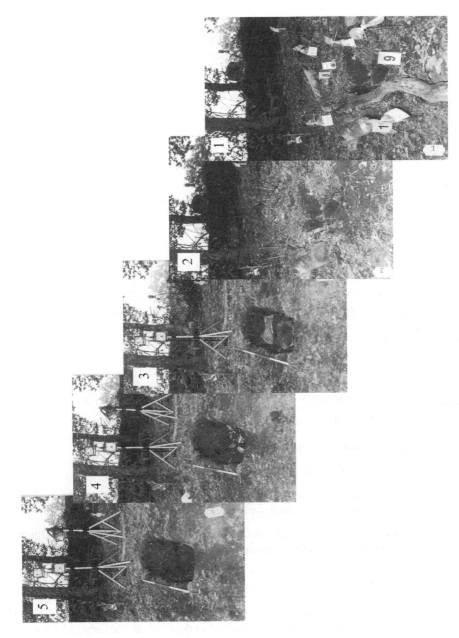

Figure 6.21 Stages of an excavation from a fixed camera position.

disturbed the binding and the knot as potential sources of trace evidence. The upper part of the grave was then excavated; this revealed that the upper body was covered in plastic sheeting and bound around the neck. The pathologist attended the scene to view the remains *in situ* and to advise on and supervise the removal of the body, underneath which the archaeologist recovered the missing shoes.

The steep slope appeared to have affected the digging of the grave causing the head end (higher up slope) to be deeper than the foot end (lower down the slope). This allowed easy access for scavengers to find and expose the burial. The crime assessment was able to provide a supported opinion as to the sequence of events of the burial: the grave was dug, and judging by the shallowness at the foot end and the bent up legs, probably not in advance; the shoes were placed in the grave followed by the already bound body; the grave was backfilled, and the branch and log markers were subsequently placed in position (Figure 6.21).

This case illustrates how a multidisciplined and sequenced approach to a clandestine grave can provide forensic opportunities to gain extra evidence. The static camera provided a photographic sequence of the excavation to assist in explaining to the Court the process of the excavation. The incident also utilised the services of a police vehicle collision examiner to plan the scene.

Appendix: The forensic archaeologist's report (taken from Section 7 of the Standards and Guidance for Forensic Archaeologists)

The forensic archaeologist must:

(a) Produce a formal report to record:

   (i) the information provided to them with regards to the history of the case

  (ii) that data justifying actions and decisions taken at the scene have been retained

 (iii) the excavation strategy and methods utilised and/or considered

 (iv) the results of the excavation

  (v) the justification for preferring one explanation over others, where findings may lead to more than one explanation

 (vi) conclusions and explanations for those conclusions, with reference to current and pertinent literature when appropriate

 (vii) the quantification of all records and samples kept by the forensic archaeologist, referring to police exhibit numbers where allocated

(viii) any additional information required, with reference to the Crown Prosecution Service guidance on expert witnesses' obligations on disclosure (Annex K of *The Disclosure Manual*, 2005).

(b) Ensure that the requirements outlined in the Criminal Procedure Rules (2010), Part 33 are met.

(c) Have in place a critical conclusions check.

(d) Produce the report as quickly as is practical within the specific circumstances of the case and within an agreed timescale.

(e) Be prepared to consider new information and produce supplementary reports as appropriate.

(f) Ensure that the report contains sufficient detail to comply with current and relevant guidance.

(g) Write the report in a fair and unbiased manner, taking into account all relevant issues.

7 Recovery, sampling and dating

7.1 Sieving

Retention of soils is a pre-requisite for subsequent sieving (screening) off-site and offers much potential depending upon the questions being asked by the investigation. The soils may also be required for defence examination. The sieving of soils is standard practice on archaeological sites, usually coarser sieving (5–10 mm) for recovering small items that may have been missed during excavation, and finer sieves (<1 mm) for recovering macro-remains (animal bones, insects and botanical evidence) in order to reconstruct a past environment. The various methodologies are well documented in most archaeological texts (e.g. Greene 2002; Grant *et al.* 2008; English Heritage 2002). In most cases, especially in environmental work, layers will be sampled for sieving, and much work has been undertaken on evaluating representation and bias according to sample volume and mesh size (e.g. Payne 1975) resulting in published recommendations for gaining the most effective and accurate results (English Heritage 2002, 21, table 3). 'Screening' tends to be undertaken in a more wholesale way in North America, where the evolution of archaeological techniques and the nature of the soils have combined to make it a standard on-site procedure on most excavations. The types of forensic material that can be recovered through visual sieving that may have been missed during excavation include small durable objects such as buttons, items of jewellery, glass fragments, projectiles, small elements of human remains (e.g. tarsals, phalanges, neonatal bones, nails, etc.), or less durable items such as paper, wrappers or cigarette ends. Survival of the latter items will be more heavily dependent on the soil environment, the time since burial and the level of human decay within the grave.

Only recently, however, has consideration been given to the value of sieving in a forensic archaeological context, not simply for the recovery of small bones that may have been overlooked during excavation (e.g. Cox and Bell 1999), but more specifically for trace evidence that may have been transferred from an offender, typically human hair, fibres and elements of clothing. There is now a relatively small literature available that considers sieving methodology *per se*, rather than seeing it as something incidental to scene recovery (e.g. Bunch 2010; Bailey 1990). The whole subject of forensic sieving has since been evaluated by Ross (2010) who has examined the methods available (wet sieving, dry sieving, flotation, etc.) in relation to the type of forensic evidence likely to be encountered and the potential for recovering it. To a large extent the methods of sieving employed depend

Forensic Approaches to Buried Remains, First Edition. John Hunter, Barrie Simpson and Caroline Sturdy Colls.
© 2013 John Wiley & Sons, Ltd. Published 2013 by John Wiley & Sons, Ltd.

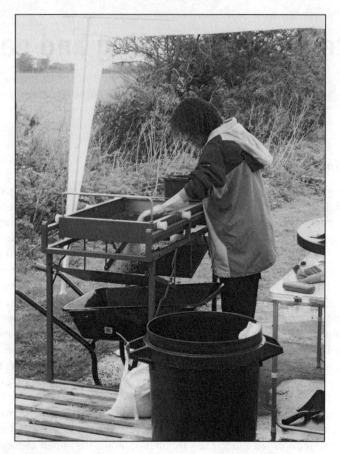

Figure 7.1 Wet sieving being undertaken using a hose pipe to break down heavy soils in looking for neonatal remains.

on two important factors: the nature of the soil in the grave and the type of material or objects being looked for. Dry sieving involves the mechanical agitation of the soil through an appropriately sized mesh and works effectively for lighter, dry soils, which are friable and easily broken down. Wet sieving, on the other hand, is the only option for heavier or wet soils where the soil mass needs to be disaggregated in water, usually through a jet over the sieve (Figure 7.1). Soils tend to be heavy in many parts of the UK and, on the basis of climate, wet sieving is often the only option. In archaeology a column of different sized sieves of decreasing mesh size is sometimes used, for example from 5 mm down to 300 microns to capture a range of evidential types as the soils are 'washed' down the column (Kenward *et al.* 1980). Flotation is another option: this requires the soil to be broken down in water, either by manual agitation or through moving water. Lighter bodies rise to the surface where they can be floated off, and the heavier bodies stay contained within the residue. Both can be sorted under a microscope. The collection can sometimes be aided by the addition of a little paraffin; this sits across the surface and allows the floating material to gather and be skimmed off more easily. All these methods are time consuming and require the soils to be processed a little at a time, which is one reason why sampling strategies are so important. However, in dealing with the fill of a clandestine grave, sampling is not normally an option. Unlike conventional archaeological capture, it requires 100% processing rather than strategic sampling in order to entertain any hope of a comprehensive recovery. Moreover, additional time is required in cleaning the equipment between the processing of each layer to avoid contamination, and in maintaining rigorous control of the numbering system for the various residues, slurries and exhibits, and a record of the processes, mesh sizes and sample volumes used. Ross has designed a pro forma that tabulates casework data for ease of record and synthesis (Ross 2010, 29–30; Figure 7.2 and Figure 7.3). A coarse estimation suggests that the fill of a typical grave would take approximately one working week to process.

Another question relates to the types of trace evidence that might survive forensically within a buried environment. Human hair, for example, which is shed daily as a natural course of events (Gaudette 2000, 1032) and more profusely during exercise, for example when digging a grave, has been shown to be a relatively good survivor in certain environments (e.g. Rowe 1997, 340, table 1) with a high potential for DNA extraction (Melton et al. 2005). Experiments by Gray (2006) have been successful in recovering hair from simulated burial sites and different buried conditions using wet sieving down to 0.5 mm mesh sizes. The presence and survival of fibres depends on the ease of transfer and the nature of the fibre itself, whether natural (e.g. cotton or wool, which are short survivors) or most synthetics (e.g. nylon or polyester, which are longer survivors, but see Rowe 1997, 345, table 2). Bulk fibres in the form of clothing are likely to have a greater degree of preservation than single fibres; both, however, may be vulnerable to body decay products (Rodriguez and Bass 1985). Experiments in non-buried environments have shown that during normal wear some 90% of transferred fibres are lost after sixteen hours, and that increased activity leads to a further increase in losses (Akulova et al. 2002). Activity involved in digging a grave will presumably generate a relatively significant loss, depending on fabric, and present the potential for at least some of those fibres to become trapped and sealed within the grave fill itself. The survival of fibres of different types under buried conditions has been discussed at length elsewhere (e.g. Janaway 2002; Rowe 1997) and need not be pursued further here.

One of the main drawbacks in the recovery of trace evidence is that of contamination, both at the crime scene and during any sieving recovery process. This can be minimized at the scene itself by adherence to standard scene protocols, typically: limited personnel access; wearing of 'whites', gloves and face masks; sealing of material immediately on recovery; and using clean equipment (see also Baldwin and May 2000). There is also the important issue regarding contamination of one layer to another during the excavation itself (Section 6.1): if this occurs within the sealed context of the grave it lessens the value of that evidence (the evidence is still retained in the sealed deposit of the grave but it relates to the total event of infilling as opposed to a specific part of it), but if the contamination occurs from outwith the grave (for example from uncleaned external surfaces that present the potential for local surface remains to enter the grave) then the problem is more fundamental (see Section 6.2; Steyn et al. 2000, 237).

Contamination is harder to avoid in the subsequent processing. Being a 'dirty' process, sieving usually takes place outdoors where, even with the best prophylactic care, airborne hair, fibres and insects can contaminate the material being processed. This can be partly prevented by sensible precautions – the use of tenting, or ensuring that the operation is

Job No:	
Customer:	
Date:	

MANLOVE
F O R E N S I C S
Sieving Report

Context No.:		Sample No:	
Soil Type:		Sample Size:	
Soil Condition:		Storage Method:	

Sample Collection Method			
Trowel	Spade	Machine	Other

Sieving Method		
Dry (Laboratory / Outdoors)	Wet (Laboratory / Outdoors)	Flot (Laboratory / Outdoors)

		Finds/Qty.	Finds/Qty.	Finds/Qty.	Finds/Qty.	Finds/Qty.
Size	Dry					
10mm						
5mm						
2mm						
1mm						
Size	Wet					
10mm						
5mm						
2mm						
1mm						
Flot Medium						

Processor:		Signature:	
Witnessed:		Signature:	

Page No.:

Figure 7.2 An example of a sieving record sheet for the recovery of forensic remains (after Ross 2010).

Job No:	
Customer:	
Date:	

MANLOVE
F O R E N S I C S

Summary of Finds

Sieving Method		
Dry (Laboratory / Outdoors)	Wet (Laboratory / Outdoors)	Flot (Laboratory / Outdoors)

Context	Finds/Qty.	Finds/Qty.	Finds/Qty.	Finds/Qty.	Finds/Qty.
Total					

Processor:		Signature:	
Witnessed:		Signature:	

Figure 7.3 An example of a summary finds (exhibits) record sheet for the recovery of forensic remains (after Ross 2010).

carried out upwind of potential contaminants – but it is still open to criticism in Court for the field recovery of anything other than small, solid objects such as bone fragments that are unlikely to have been airborne.

In an ideal world, sieving or the processing of soils for trace evidence requires controlled laboratory conditions, but even here there are difficulties. Wet sieving is not conducive to a clean laboratory environment – the options being either to spread out the material on a shallow tray to dry before it can be broken down or alternatively to freeze dry it, which allows it to be broken up easily into friable elements on defrosting. Given the quantity of soil likely to be investigated (typically around 0.75 cubic metres for an 'average' grave of proportions $1.8 \times 0.6 \times 0.7$ m) this can be a lengthy and painstaking operation. But it will allow the soil to be micro-sieved more easily, or small ferrous objects to be attracted using a magnet, and it may be the only that very small items are recovered. As far as recovering trace evidence is concerned, studies carried out to investigate the transfer of fibres in a clean room used for clothing examination found that airborne movement was such that it became necessary to monitor the background in order to create a standard against which recovered items could be measured (Roux *et al.* 2001). This would entail the use of adhesive tapes judiciously positioned within the room to measure any background contamination. Once this is achieved, however, the soils can be spread manually and sieved according to the evidence type looked for. It may also be possible, if the soils are spread out sufficiently thinly, to use a static wand manoeuvered systematically across the dried material to attract any fibres or hairs. It is as well to remember that recent graves dug out in lumps will also be returned as infill in much the same state. Fibres, hairs or other trace material will not lie *within* the lumps but will be caught between them. In other words breaking down the lumps will be an unnecessary exercise, but this only applies if the grave is recent and factors of water penetration, climate or consolidation have not occurred significantly. An experienced archaeologist should be in a position to advise on this.

7.2 Sampling and forensic ecology

Examination for trace evidence requires the full bulk investigation of the grave fill, but there are some sources of evidence that can be derived from strategic sampling. Whilst not directly archaeological *per se* these evidence sources reflect the contextual elements of a crime scene and event sequencing with which archaeology is strictly concerned and closely associated, hence the relevance here.

In conventional archaeology the importance of the living world is well known as a source of evidence types. These include insect remains, snails, pollen grains and soil micromorphs; study of these allows the archaeologist to recreate past environments (e.g. Evans and O'Connor 2000). The same evidence types can also be relevant in crime scenes irrespective of the interval defined by the word 'past', although the paradigm shift from conventional archaeology into forensics is far from straightforward (see Wiltshire 2006a). Contact with the environment is unavoidable, and some aspect of the physical world we inhabit (notably its fauna, flora and geology), whether macroscopic or microscopic, always surrounds human activity. It is these natural and unsolicited contacts with the environment that present the potential to supply forensic evidence.

The living world produces micro-ecofacts such as insects, pollen grains, diatoms, phytoliths, and soil micromorphs – all these present forensic opportunities. The chronology of insect life cycles, for example, is predictable and can be used to calculate at least part of the post-mortem interval (PMI) of recent victims; distributed pollen can reflect the flora of particular places or habitats, and soil types and their inclusions can be geologically specific. Their various morphologies allow identification into defined taxa which can be related to specific ecological or geological locations and can be of immense forensic value.

Moreover, trace evidence from both pollen and soils can easily transfer to persons or objects, as well as being highly resistant to mechanical and chemical destruction. Perhaps more importantly, because the evidence is sometimes microscopic, offenders are essentially unaware of the trace evidence present on clothing or footwear (Mildenhall *et al.* 2006; Walsh and Horrocks 2008; Wiltshire 2010). The generic term for the study of these evidence types. 'forensic ecology', might be defined as the interdisciplinary study involving the abundance and distribution of organisms and their interactions with their environment. The subject is variously described as being an under-utilised forensic resource (Bock and Norris 1997; Walsh and Horrocks 2008) and as being in its infancy (Wiltshire 2010).

Some aspects of forensic ecology have particular relevance here in that that they may need to be integrated into the excavation strategy of a clandestine grave, in particular the study of insects (entomology), pollen (palynology) and soils (pedology). On occasions, a suitably cross-trained archaeologist, while not a specialist in any of these fields, should, given specific and documented training, be sufficiently aware of the evidential theory and potential to be able to sample and record effectively in a manner that allows other scientific specialists to process, analyse and interpret these samples with confidence. In an ideal situation these other experts would be at the scene themselves, but this is not always possible in a forensic world constrained by logistics and imposed police spending restraints. The process separates scene from laboratory work but is acceptable providing the scene recording and sampling is of appropriate integrity; it can periodically place a new and significant onus on the archaeologist. It has to be stated that a caveat may be introduced from specialist scientists that they will only be able to interpret exhibits and data that is presented to them holistically in the same way as if they had attended the scene themselves.

7.2.1 Entomology

Forensic entomology is the use and interpretation of insect activity as evidence to assist the Court (Catts and Haskell 1999; Erzinçlioglu 2000; Byrd and Castner 2001; Gennard 2007). It requires a knowledge of insect species, species and their behaviour, inter- and intra-specific interactions and, where relevant, patterns of insect succession in relation to decomposing remains and insect life cycles. When taken together with scene environmental factors (e.g. temperature) this may allow an estimate of the post-mortem interval (PMI) to be made or provide intelligence that the body has been moved from one insect habitat to another (i.e. from an open to a closed environment, or *vice versa*). This is far from being a simple equation as the activity of insects is also affected by geographical location, seasonal variations, humidity, light and shade and availability of, and competition for, a food supply. It is to be noted that here PMI is in fact a misnomer and it is the age of the insects that is being calculated; the time the insects took to lay their eggs (pre-ovipositional period or POP) is unknown and may vary extensively in relation to a number of variables.

Establishing the PMI is the most frequent application of entomology. The species mostly likely to be encountered at the scene of a deposition site are those known to feed on

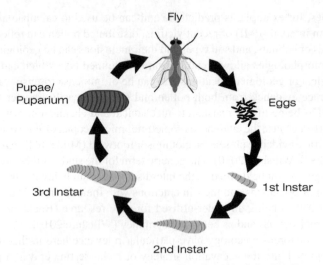

Figure 7.4 Outline life cycle stages (instar) of the blowfly.

dead bodies (necrophagus). Amongst the foremost of these are the blowflies, for example, the genera *Calliphora* (blue-bottles) and *Lucilia* (green-bottles) and their eggs, larvae and puparia. The general theory is well known: these flies are usually the first insects to deposit their eggs (oviposit) on an exposed body after death and, importantly for forensic purposes, the blowfly larvae grow at a rate that is roughly proportionate to the ambient temperature. Therefore, the age of these insects can allow an estimate to be calculated as to when a body was first exposed to insect activity, and thereby a minimum interval since death (PMI). The process of sampling of insects has some archaeological implications and merits outlining here.

Using the blowflies as a working example, the life cycle consists of a number of stages; eggs are laid, then hatch into first instar (stage) larvae. These then pass through two further stages into larger, third instar feeding larvae before, in most cases, leaving their food source as so-called post-feeding larvae. They then enter a resting phase as puparia and metamorphosise into the adult fly (Figure 7.4). The eggs of blowflies resemble miniature grains of rice, and these species will lay their eggs (oviposit) initially in the natural body orifices and the eyes, as well as on any wounds that have been created in a body. They can also occur at the interface of the body with the substrate, and under the body, and on any wrappings around the body itself. On hatching the larvae enter the first life stage (or first instar) and begin feeding. As they develop, they will form feeding masses and be able to consume, as a mass, large volumes of feeding material. Early stage larvae are not always apparent and may be feeding within folds of skin, eyes, the nasal cavity or other concealed areas; as such an apparent absence should not be taken as absolute and a more thorough search be undertaken. In the later stages of their development the larva may move to other parts of the body, perhaps still hidden from view within the body orifices, wounds or folds in the skin. The larvae develop through a second instar, and then into their final third instar, still feeding, so that the larvae are much larger and can be easier to find. It is during the second and third stages that these larvae, often but not always feeding at a concentrated area on a body, can form 'maggot masses' with implications for temperature measurements (below).

Once the feeding stage is complete, most species will leave their food source (usually the decomposing body, but bear in mind that it may be fluids that have seeped from the body) and migrate to find a place in which to pupate. They may pupate adjacent to the food source or travel several metres from the body to find a place hidden from view for this purpose. Recent research suggests that the depth within soils that the larvae might burrow to pupate is dependent on the compaction of the soil: in heavily compacted soils this can be as little as 0.5 cm; in uncompacted soils over 4 cm (Cammack *et al.* 2010). In indoor scenes the third instar larvae may often have to travel much further to find a place to pupate compared to an outside deposition scene (Anderson 2011). As far as graves are concerned, the maggots *may* have migrated before excavation commences and have penetrated through the grave walls at a deeper level from the surface than would otherwise be expected. Sampling needs to take this into account accordingly and on a systematic basis. This can best be achieved by using the scaled plan of the grave site (see Section 6.2) and marking out a small number of tangential transects for sampling at intervals of (say) 0.1 m, 0.5 m, 1.0 m and 2.0 m from the grave edge, where sample points can be excavated by an entomologist using a small hand trowel to a depth of around 0.25 m in order to identify and capture any migrants. Great care needs to be employed when taking these samples to avoid damaging these larvae. Depicting this data on the archaeological plan has the advantage of being able to present a coordinated and integrated log of events that can be returned to and interrogated later if required.

Blowflies themselves are unlikely to be able to access buried remains, and the presence of eggs or larvae on a buried victim is almost certainly the result of ovipositioning before the burial itself. However, there are insects that are capable of burrowing down to buried remains to lay their eggs, especially in loosely compacted soils, for example those from the fly family *Phoridae* ('scuttle flies') (Gun and Bird 2010); there may also be certain species of beetle (Coleoptera) associated with buried human remains, particularly in the later stages of decomposition (Kulshrestha and Satpathy 2001). There are also certain types of mite that are now beginning to play a more significant forensic role (Perotti *et al.* 2009).

Sampling, killing and preservation procedures are well documented elsewhere, notably by the European Association of Forensic Entomologists (EAFE; see Amendt *et al.* 2007), but some key elements are worth emphasising here in view of the differences inherent in buried as opposed to surface remains which constitutes the majority of the entomological literature. The main issue relates to temperature, given that the speed of the life cycle of an insect is temperature-dependent and therefore requires knowledge of the temperature at the scene. This is not only a matter of recording the ambient and ground surface temperatures, but also the soil temperature corresponding to the body's depth in the grave, as well as the temperature of the body itself. On exposure to oxygen and increased air temperature the decay process of the body will accelerate (according to state) and the environment will be more conducive to insect development. This means that temperature readings will need to be taken of the soil and the victim *during* excavation as soon as the body becomes exposed. Similarly, if maggot masses are discovered (maggot masses tend to have a higher temperature due to the activity within the maggot mass) they will also need to be measured on immediate exposure. Failure to recognise the effects of exposure during excavation can have a significant effect on the calculation of the PMI (Charabidze *et al.* 2011; Amendt *et al.*

2007). It makes good sense for the necessary entomological sampling to be integrated into the archaeological process; moreover, all measurement points taken within the grave can be denoted on the archaeological context sheets or plans and tied in with other data to provide a consistent and cross-referenced record. To obtain the most accurate PMI, minimum and maximum daily temperatures are needed for the period the body has been *in situ*. This is normally calculated by obtaining temperatures provided by the nearest meteorological station for about two weeks after recovery and comparing them to scene temperatures over the same two weeks taken from a judiciously place data logger, which can also be located on the archaeological plan. This can be reburied and recovered at a later date to allow any temperature differential between meteorological station and scene temperatures gathered over those two weeks to be extrapolated back from the time of recovery to give a more accurate scene temperature on which to base life cycle calculations.

7.2.2 Palynology

Palynology is concerned with the study of microscopic entities (palynomorphs) that have been scattered or moved from their natural source; in a forensic context this is mainly concerned with pollen grains and plant spores. There is an established taxonomy (the theory of final classification and systematics) that is fundamental for the identification of various plants, trees, mosses, ferns and fungi. In other words, each plant or tree species produces its own idiosyncratic pollen grains, although these are sometimes only identifiable to *genus* or family; these can become distributed by self-pollination, wind distribution, by water, or by insect or animal activities. In addition, the distances each type of pollen, spore or other ecofact would be expected to travel naturally are largely predictable.

In a forensic setting, one of palynology's key roles has been to corroborate or contradict testimony as to the presence of a person or an object at a crime scene on the basis of similarity or dissimilarity of comparative pollen profiles (Mildenhall *et al.* 2006). It allows, for example, the pollen profile from a specific assemblage of plants found at a crime scene to be compared to pollen grains found on a suspect's clothing. The more unusual the profile, or the rarer an individual species represented, the greater the likelihood of the suspect having visited that place. Hence, pollen from exotic flora in a municipal park presents strong evidence that the suspect was in that particular location, whereas more common pollen grains, for example from grasses, would be less specific. Pollen evidence is not in any way conclusive, but it provides strong evidence with which to confront a suspect, and can aid in creating a larger picture of events (see Case Study 7.1). It can even be specific to a season of the year as a result of dispersal (Szibor *et al.* 1998).

Research has also demonstrated the degree to which pollen in soil samples from the same localised areas, even with similar vegetation, can present significantly different assemblages (Horrocks *et al.* 1998a, 1998b). This had practical application in a rape case where the fine resolution of pollen patterns for two scenes only a few metres apart showed two distinctive vegetations. It was therefore possible to compare the pollen assemblages on both the claimant's and suspect's clothing to each other, and to the crime scene where the victim had been. It provided strong circumstantial evidence to support the fact that the suspect had been in the same spot as the victim and not just a few metres away as he had claimed (Walsh and Horrocks 2008). Pollen assemblages have also been used successfully in searching for missing victims, for example using pollen from a vehicle that had been used to transport a victim in order to locate a specific deposition site (Brown *et al.* 2002).

In many respects it makes sense to conduct pollen sampling as part of the archaeological strategy because, like the entomological sampling, it enables the sample mapping to be integrated with the archaeology (focused on the grave) as part of a composite planning exercise.

Within the grave itself the disturbed fill will contain an equally disturbed set of pollen profiles. The pollen species present are likely to be consistent per sample, but differ in proportion according to homogeneity of fill. A small soil sample provides an adequate indication of species present and can be taken on a spit-by-spit basis. However, once the excavation has been completed, the remains recovered and the archaeological examination and recording of the grave has been completed, there is some benefit in taking a complete vertical profile through the layers of the cleaned grave wall using a stainless steel monolith. This sample effectively provides a standard for the 'historic' environment of the grave itself to which the bulk sample of the fill may need to be compared. Pollen in the buried layers around the grave site may be distinctive, or different, from those on the current ground surface; their appearance on a suspect's clothes or shoes may indicate contact with buried deposits and provide a strong forensic argument. Neither the bulk sample nor the vertical profile may ever be used, but the effort expended in their collection is minimal in relation to problems encountered later when the evidence may suddenly be thought to be important and when the opportunity has been lost. Sampling during the excavation ensures proper forensic integrity and evidential continuity.

Sampling points in the vicinity of the deposition site also need to be considered, or those from any other location the suspect may have visited. Sampling around the deposition site itself *after* the excavation is effectively pointless as, by the end of the recovery exercise, the area around the grave will be heavily trampled. It makes sense to conduct it beforehand but practicalities, logistics and the focusing of others tend to inhibit this. Other sample locations might include the route (or likely route) taken by the suspect. This will often be obvious although sometimes, depending on the time lapse between the commission of the crime and the discovery of the crime scene, it will be overgrown. The 'common approach path' defined by the police is the defined route *least* likely to have been taken. Sampling along the suspected route to and from the scene can offer much potential and, as the pollens will be confined to surface material, there is no requirement to involve the lower levels when taking samples (for sampling collection methods see Wiltshire 2010, 76–77). The sampling process is a spatial one and lends itself to incorporation on a single site plan.

There is much advantage in recording the wider environment of the deposition site even if it seems pointless at the time. This can be carried out photographically in a 360° panorama (Mildenhall *et al.* 2006; Wiltshire 2010) with more detailed photographs of trees, shrubs, herbaceous plants and any unusual species. This is not a vegetation survey as such, nor is it a substitute for having a botanist on site, but it provides a starting point if a botanist is introduced later, or if botanical material is recovered subsequently from the grave fill. It keeps the investigative options open and provides 'comparator samples' for future reference (Wiltshire 2010, 76). Working at a forensic scene always involves 'standing around' time that can usefully be spent creating this type of general environmental record. It does no harm, and the information can be easily, if coarsely, integrated into a composite plan by simple measurement or, more rapidly, by using a total station system. The extent of the area covered will depend on the surroundings, but a circle of radius 20 m centred on the deposition would provide a useful preparatory record. The scale will need to be appropriate if the plan is to include this and other sampling strategies as well as the grave itself. This is why time spent thinking out exactly what may need to be planned and recorded is a good investment before any excavation commences.

One final area of sampling, and one to which the archaeologist is unaccustomed, is the pollen source lying within the hair and within the upper nasal cavities of the victim (Wiltshire 2006b; Wiltshire and Black 2006). Collection of both requires close cooperation with the pathologist. Pollen in the hair may be washed off and collected in the mortuary, although its collection may be at odds with other evidential sources (e.g. gunshot residue), but pollen in the nasal cavities can be collected from the body by the palynologist on site using a small nasal brush to collect the grains and preserve them in an airtight container. This pollen, and the profile it reflects, represents the last breaths of the victim and therefore of the immediate death environment. It can be of supreme importance to an investigation.

Case Study 7.1

In 1984, a 9-year old boy went missing while babysitting for his sister. Two days later his body was found by a dog walker in a local stream. The body was in a plastic carpet underlay bag weighted down by a brick. He had suffered head injuries and his clothing had been disturbed, suggesting he had been sexually assaulted. Despite an intensive investigation no one was charged with this murder. However, the police never close an unsolved murder and the case remained open and subject to regular reviews of the evidence. Some 18 years later an uncle of the boy became a suspect when allegations of child abuse, all occurring after the murder, relating to four different boys were levelled against him. The uncle was convicted in 2003 of a total of nine counts of sex offences involving children and jailed for seven-and-a-half years.

A further police review of the unsolved murder showed a strong circumstantial case against the uncle. He lived locally, he owned a car that fitted the description of a vehicle seen near the victim's house on the night, he did not have an alibi, he had previous knowledge of the stream where the body was dumped, he was shown to have lied to police about key issues in the case, he had a history of paedophilia, and an important piece of evidence was a bite mark on the deceased's buttocks that was consistent with the uncle's *modus operandi* in the other cases of child abuse. He was subsequently arrested in May 2006 in connection with his nephew's death but detectives were unable to gather conclusive evidence to charge him with the murder. Although he had the 'means and motive' the case against him lacked the final piece of the jigsaw – there was no scientific evidence against him.

However, the case still remained open and further review was undertaken to see if there was any scientific evidence available using the advances in forensic science. DNA could not assist but the police now turned to palynology to see if any pollen or spores on any of the exhibits would help. It transpired that there was enough pollen and other plant associated evidence on the boy's clothing, specific to the uncle's garden, to provide a scientific link between victim and suspect's garden. Further the brick that had been used to weight the body down in the stream was also scientifically linked to a water feature in the uncle's garden.

All hope of a confession ended when the uncle died in 2008, three weeks before he was due to be released from prison and arrested for this crime, and no charge was ever brought against him. However, in 2012 the police submitted the evidence they now had to the leading Counsel for an opinion. This opinion supported a view that, had the uncle been alive, there was sufficient evidence to charge him with a realistic chance of conviction. The police did not have the advantages of DNA and palynology in the original investigation. However, the case highlights two important points: the recovery of trace materials and its secure storage for future availability and review, and the longevity/survivability of microscopic pollen evidence.

7.3 Essential taphonomics

Whether or not a deposition has occurred recently or falls into the category of a 'cold case', the dynamic nature of the burial environment needs to be considered. Due to the very nature of buried or concealed depositions in an outdoor setting, there will be a series of interactions: there is a dynamic between the disturbance caused by digging a grave and the landscape into which it is dug; there is also a dynamic between the remains and their surrounding landscape, whether those remains are buried or not (Efremov 1940). These are both two-way processes. Such changes, known as taphonomic modifications, have to be considered during search, recovery and post-excavation analysis. Additionally, being aware of the potential for such modifications to occur is particularly important in instances where the time since deposition is unknown, as remains may have an 'older' or more 'recent' appearance in certain conditions (Section 7.5).

The presence, and in particular the decay, of human remains, means that a number of changes are likely to occur within the environment in which they are situated. These have been described in detail by Hochrein (2002) and Hunter and Cox (2005), and so need only be summarised here. The release of body fluids will fundamentally alter the chemistry of the surrounding soil, acting as a catalyst for changes in vegetation growth, making it more abundant or inhibiting growth, and modifying the species present. Depressions and/or compressions in the form of visible modifications in the topography above a grave as a result of the settling of the grave fill and the collapse of the rib cage during decomposition (Hochrein 2002) will be influenced by the speed and extent to which the body decomposes, and the size of the individual. These depressions may be detected through systematic ground searches, aerial imagery or using more recently developed technologies, such as digital kinematic GPS systems, capable of detecting sub-centimetre microtopographic change (Section 2.3). Additionally, given the changes to the properties in the soil, it is possible, aside from visual identification, to detect taphonomic change using an array of geophysical techniques (Nobes 2000; Buck 2003; Fenning and Donnelly 2004; Watters and Hunter 2004; Schultz 2012a). The moisture content of the top and sub-soil will also influence the extent to which sedimentation, that is the cracking of the grave edges, will occur. This effect may be seasonal and so the ability to detect this indicator will be largely dependent upon the time of year that the search takes place, or the weather conditions. Generally speaking, however, unlike the modifications that occur to the body itself (below), the modifications caused in the environment as a result of the deposition more often act as indicators; thus they assist in search, rather than hindering it (for vegetation change see also Section 2.3).

With regard to the body itself, the environment will interact with the body and the body with the environment, and this can result in changes in the appearance of both (Wilson *et al.* 2007). Such modifications can be seen to fall into three categories: those that are natural; those that are anthropogenic (including those that are incited by the perpetrator), and those that relate to animal activity. The first two are detailed here; animal activity is discussed in the following section (Section 7.4).

7.3.1   *Natural modifications*

In relation to human remains, the burial environment will impact on the speed and nature of decomposition, and on the post-mortem modification of the remains. This may be in the form of bone and/or soft tissue modification due to weathering, plant root activity or soil acidity/alkalinity. These factors have been succinctly summarised by Haglund and Sorg (2002a, 4). The climatic conditions during the period of deposition can also have serious implications in terms of the taphonomic modification of remains, particularly where they are partially or entirely exposed. Cases where bodies have effectively become mummified (Case Study 7.2), frozen or where bone weathering has taken place are well attested. Where the body has become preserved as a result of the environmental conditions, this may actually assist in analysis of trauma and identification, but degradation of the bone is likely to hinder its ability to be characterised and cause difficulty and confusion throughout search, recovery and post-recovery analysis.

With regards to burials, the moisture content of the soil at the deposition site needs to be assessed. As well as impacting on the recovery strategy (Case Study 6.4), the presence of high water content will influence the preservation of the remains, but not necessarily in a predictable manner. In some cases, waterlogging will result in better preservation of the corpse (Case Study 6.9) but in others, bone may erode more rapidly due to the presence of organic acids, micro-organisms or ions in ground or rain water (Mays 1998, 20–21). For deeper burials, the impact of contact with the water table also needs to be considered (Schultz 2012b, 72). As a secondary effect of high moisture content, plant roots are more likely to become established, causing damage to skeletal elements (Roderiguez 1997). Similarly, it has been noted that 'plant roots grow towards a decaying corpse, seeking rich organic nutrients produced by decomposition' (ibid, 460). Extreme temperature and moisture changes can in some cases lead to diagenesis and some instances have been recorded where remains have decomposed to the extent that only the grave itself is recognisable, due to total destruction of bone (Hunter *et al.* 1996; Clark *et al.* 1997; Mays 1998).

Remains deposited on the surface or partially concealed may *become* buried as a result of taphonomic processes whereby sedimentation occurs and the remains become sealed by soil or sand deposits. This may be as a result of rainfall, wind activity or other forms of ground movement as result of climatic conditions. Equally, bodies may become exposed as a result of the same processes, thus in turn increasing the likelihood of other taphonomic modification such as animal scavenging (see Section 7.4). As discussed above, determining (and defending) an interpretation as to whether remains have become buried or were deliberately buried can represent one of the main roles of a forensic archaeologist. It may have significant implications in terms of the findings at a Coroner's Inquest, in pursuance of a homicide investigation and in any subsequent sentencing of a suspect. An experienced archaeologist should be able to recognise the difference between sedimentation and deliberate burial.

There have also been instances where decomposition and taphonomic modification have varied on the same body. These have resulted from factors such as alterations in the temperature and moisture of the soil, the differential exposure of different parts of the body, the compaction of the strata and the depth of burial (Wilson *et al.* 2007, 9; see Case Study 7.2). Through experiments with porcine samples, Cunningham *et al.* (2011) have demonstrated that the extent of cortical flaking and the exposure of trabecular bone can also vary between skeletal elements; thus, estimates of the time since deposition may vary depending upon which bones are present at a scene.

Differential preservation and weathering in a variety of soil types has been well documented. As an example, Cardoso *et al.* (2011, 2) describe a case where it was unclear whether the bone destruction and discolouration was as a result of 'a very long post-depositional period or the result of the harsh burial conditions', owing to the highly acidic nature of the soil. Discolouration of bone may also be caused by the nature of the sub-soil in which it is buried. Moreover, the colour and consistency of surrounding geological deposits can alter the colour and friability of bone, as can the presence of specific chemical elements such as manganese or iron (Butler 2012). The likely cause of discolouration and friability may be evident when geological records are consulted (Section 2.2) but in some instances further laboratory testing may be required.

Some modification indicators will be more easily observed than others, for example, the presence of plant roots or soil composition; this may prompt the involvement of further experts such as botanists, geologists or chemists. Other indicators, such as those caused by climatic variation in humidity and temperature or by precipitation and snow fall, may be more difficult to quantify. But in all cases where bone modification is known to have occurred or is suspected to have occurred, it is prudent to consult local weather reports for the estimated period of deposition (this may already be in train if entomological data is being collected, see Section 7.2), as well as drawing on local hydrological and geological sources.

The collection of day-to-day climatic data, including that from the Meterological Office, often forms part of the routine police search log, but covers the period of search only, not the likely time of deposition, nor the interval since deposition. To this end some research may be necessary into the predicted extent and nature of vegetation cover at the time and season of disposal, or the occurrence of extreme weather conditions since disposal resulting in, for example, drought or flooding. Any extreme environmental conditions can impact not only on the offender's ability to dispose of the body in the first place, but also on the appearance of the deposition site over time and the nature and rate of decomposition and modification.

Case Study 7.2

A search of an area of farm land was instigated after new information was provided by a convicted perpetrator in relation to the location of a body. The post-burial interval exceeded four years and it was therefore deemed probable that the remains would be in an advanced state of decomposition, most likely skeletalised. The search area in question was characterised by a heavily compacted sand subsoil which overlaid natural compacted fragmented bedrock. The area was systematically stripped using a mechanical excavator under archaeological supervision and the grave was then excavated by hand once its location was determined. The grave construction reflected the difficulties faced by the perpetrator when he had attempted to dig into the heavily compacted ground surface; it was shallow at one end, where the compacted bedrock had been encountered closer to the surface, and almost one metre deep at the other, given the sloping topography of the site. The deposition of the body in this L-shaped grave, coupled with the hydrology of the area, meant that the body was saponified in the torso and head regions, located at the deeper end of the grave, whilst the legs and feet located at the shallower end were mummified. The position of the body and these varied states of decomposition made recovery extremely difficult and it was undertaken using the platform method (see Section 6.1 and Case Study 4.9) to allow the body to be removed intact. The spoil in and around the grave was also sieved to ensure any small bones, particularly those of the feet, were recovered. The recovery process took in excess of three hours. This case demonstrates the complexities caused by differential decomposition and highlights the need for pragmatism during the recovery process.

As an additional note, the area of interest was also searched systematically using ground penetrating radar (GPR). Although tree roots were detected, the grave was not identified. This might be explained by the fact that the process of mummification and saponification had provided the body with a density very similar to the local bedrock background. The grave itself, cut into sand and backfilled with sand, would also have been difficult to locate. The case also highlights how decompositional phenomena might impact on the effectiveness of search assets.

7.3.2 Anthropogenic modification

Anthropogenic modification of soft tissue and bone may be as a result of disinterment of the remains, as a result of, for example, ploughing, excavation works or, in some cases, the actions of the perpetrator. It is not uncommon for ploughing activity to lead to the serendipitous discovery of remains, thus giving forensic archaeologists a starting point to begin search. In such cases, and in other instances where bodies are recovered from a rural site, the potential for damage to have been caused by ploughing activity may need to be assessed. A much needed study by Haglund et al. (2002) identified how primary and secondary tillage, cultivators and fertiliser applicators can all impact on the location of buried remains in a variety of different ways, thus requiring forensic archaeologists to have at least some knowledge of farming methodology and machinery. Bone may be crushed and its level of exposure to fertilisers and chemical change increased (Ubelaker 1997). Also, remains may be moved from their original position by machinery, exposed and subsequently scavenged by animals, thus dispersing and removing evidence from, and connected to, the deposition site. Continuous ploughing over only a short period of time will also disguise the depression left by a grave and other taphonomic indicators that may be associated with the burial (see above).

Excavation works as a result of service installation or maintanance, building works or landscaping can also result in modification (also Section 5.2) by virtue of dispersal, crushing, fragmentation and re-deposition of remains (Case Study 7.3). Associated evidence needs to be considered, and search perimeters (re)defined accordingly, particularly with regard to redeposition at greater depth. As a result resource requirements, the priorities of the investigation, and health and safety factors may need review. Modifications may also result from actions of the perpetrator, and there are countless examples where perpetrators have attempted to hide their crimes. Notable cases cited here include the use of acid (Case Study 7.4), a domestic mincer (Case Study 5.12), burning and shredding (Case Study 6.7) and the feeding of the body or body parts to animals (*The Guardian* 2006).

However, despite television crime dramas and popularised representations of body disposals, the general public (including actual or would-be perpetrators) continue to be ill-informed concerning the ability to successful destroy a body, in its entirety and without trace (Case Study 7.4). Research in forensic and archaeological cremation studies has provided published examples demonstrating that even extremely high temperatures over a prolonged period of time can still result in small fragments of bone being recoverable and identifiable by suitably trained anthropologists (Brickley and McKinley 2004; Thompson 2004; Fairgreave 2008; see also Chapter 6.1.2 and Case Study 6.7). That said, the exposure of a body to fire will hinder recovery; sieving methods are likely to be employed, whilst trauma identification will be made more difficult or even impossible, depending upon the extent of the damage.

Recent research by Schotsmans *et al.* (2012) has dispelled the widely-held belief that lime destroys corpses and has demonstrated the opposite to be true: it actually delays decomposition. Consequently, as part of some attempt at taphonomic modification, perpetrators may unwittingly find themselves preserving the evidence of their crimes. Similarly, whilst other actions such as the freezing of a body may make estimating the post-mortem interval more difficult on recovery, such forms of taphonomic modification also preserve signs of trauma, trace evidence and indicators that can be used in the identification of the deceased (Micozzi 1997).

Case Study 7.3

Archaeologists were called to a scene where machine clearance work was taking place on an industrial site measuring approximately 75×75 m. The land in question was wasteland; three sides were open, but one edge was bounded by a line of scrub bushes and undergrowth against the wall of an industrial building. The development work was concerned with removing the upper consolidated surface of the site by machine and pushing the waste into mounds for disposal elsewhere before providing a new consolidated hard core surface for construction. The work was all but completed when, in removing the scrub bushes, the machine operator noticed the skull and upper skeleton of an individual leaning against the building (Figure 7.5).

The identity of the individual was relatively quickly ascertained (a pace-maker with an identifying code was recovered *in situ* from the body) but, despite careful excavation, no skeletal elements could be found below those of the lower vertebrae. Investigation showed that these had almost certainly been removed by machine action,

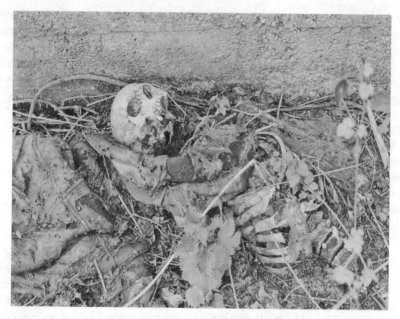

Figure 7.5 The exposure of the upper part of a human skeleton during building operations.

partially spread around the site as a result and then moved into the spoil heaps. Some may already have been disposed of. Initial examination of the immediate vicinity yielded one or two further bones, but the SIO was of the opinion that resources spent on significant further investigation of the site and the spoil would not be justified. The case illustrates the extent to which inadvertent anthropogenic activity can result in both the destruction and widespread distribution of remains.

Case Study 7.4

In 1949, John George Haigh was arrested for the suspected murder of nine people whose bodies had not been found, including an elderly widow who had gone missing from a hotel in London. Upon his arrest, Haigh announced 'Mrs Durand Deacon no longer exists. She has disappeared completely and no trace can ever be found of her again . . . How can you prove murder if there is no body?' (Radin 2008, 136). Haigh had dissolved the bodies of his victims in sulphuric acid and scattered the remnants in his garden. Whilst this appeared to be the 'perfect crime', when the soil in the garden was excavated by the lead pathologist on the case, 28 lbs (*c*. 13 kg) of human fat, along with a pair dentures and three gallstones were recovered. The identification of the dentures by a dentist as belonging to Mrs Durand Deacon resulted in Haigh being hung for his crimes (Paine 2012). This case demonstrates how, even in instances where the soft and hard tissue of a body is seemingly 'destroyed', in some instances traces can still be detected when innovative or thorough search methods are employed.

7.4 Physical anthropology, recovery and surface scatters

Some broad introduction to the role of anthropology was made in Section 1.3 together with comments on definition and its relationship with archaeology. There was also recognition of the overlap between the two disciplines. Many police forces not only continue to confuse the two, but are also unfamiliar with how they can be integrated within the same enquiry. There are a plethora of texts on anthropology, a discipline often prefixed by the word 'physical' (the preferred term here) or 'biological'. Key works include those by Krogman and Iscan (1986), Byers (2011) and Dirkmaat 2012. A further useful text by White and Folkens (2005) demonstrates the significant overlap with the field skills of the archaeologist in a North American context. In a UK forensic environment, physical anthropology is essentially concerned with the study of the human skeleton (hard tissue) in terms of identification (age, stature, sex and possibly race) and with trauma. Trauma can be both identification-related and cause/manner of death-related and is the subject of more specialist literature (e.g. Galloway 1999; Kimmerle and Baraybar 2008). Operationally, physical anthropologists can support an investigation in a variety of ways: by distinguishing between disarticulated animal and human bone typically encountered during surface searches or from construction work or gardening; by working at a scene in the recovery of human remains; by being integrated at the post-mortem stage, and by more specialised areas of knowledge such as bio-mechanics, the study of juveniles (Scheuer and Black 2000) or facial reconstruction (Wilkinson 2004). They have a particular role to play in the excavation of mass graves (Section 8.1). Moreover, in the same way that archaeologists are becoming accepted at the crime scene, physical anthropologists are being more routinely adopted by forensic pathologists both at the scene and also at the post-mortem stage. The two disciplines have developed simultaneously and have become mutually supportive.

The buried skeletal, or partly skeletonised, remains of victims are rarely found in anatomical order as a result of pressure of soil and post-depositional perturbation; they need to be recorded, recovered (seized) and logged on removal. Unlike the recovery of human remains in conventional archaeology, where the majority of individuals are in recognised burial positions (e.g. supine or crouched), the deposition character of murder victims is more random. It is rarely possible to uncover all the remains *in situ* before lifting. Some elements may need to be removed first in order to access those buried below, a problem often exacerbated by differential preservation and the survival, or partial survival, of clothing and wrapping. This poses a particular problem in mass graves where skeletal elements of individuals have become commingled during the decomposition process and compressed due to the weight of soil or mechanical excavator movement. Even in individual graves, the full configuration of the victim is often unclear when the first elements are uncovered: the body could be twisted, doubled up, spread out, bent or even dismembered, and the grave may have irregular sides or be deeper at one end than the other. In other words, the positioning of the various anatomical elements is not always predictable.

Configuration of the victim is important as it may have a bearing not only on the cause/manner of death, but also on the method of disposal. Sometimes the positioning of the remains can only be understood by excavating selectively, and by feeling around the body as it becomes exposed. Here, the physical anthropologist's knowledge of skeletal anatomy is fundamental, particularly in the recognition of smaller bones, notably those of the hands and feet, and those of children and neonates, and in supporting their lifting by advising on their character and weakness of fracture points. Essential too is an understanding of anatomical order, for example in the arrangement of the vertebrae or ribs, which may have become detached and spread as the body decomposes and collapses. Some bones in particular, notably the hyoid which can provide evidence for strangulation, not only need to be located in relation to the body's configuration, but also recovered without creating post-depositional damage. Similar issues apply with other evidential types, for example with the identification of projectiles in relation to the body.

There is a strong teamwork element here between archaeologist, anthropologist and pathologist, as each has their own evidential requirements and each will need to be aware of the requirements of others. Method and process will be by agreement, and by frequent review. In conventional archaeology, excavating human remains is a painstaking and slow exercise; in a forensic setting the process is even slower as a result of the robustness of the exhibit recording system (coordinated by an Exhibits Officer who becomes a further key member of the team), as well as by the need to recover trace evidence, record, bag and seal the excavated soils. These various elements of record all require cross-referencing.

The importance of recovering all the components of the skeleton is sometimes under-stated. If an individual is buried (i.e. sealed) in a grave, then all the body components are part of that sealed unit and are bounded and defined by the grave edges. Absence of even a small part of any human material within this might be explained on the basis of animal scavenging (which should be obvious archaeologically), but otherwise might have significant implications. For example, absence of the bones from a particular finger might have implications for identity, trophyism or torture. Or it might simply be the result of inadequate excavation. Equally, a process of diagenesis might have caused bone loss on the basis of extreme soil characteristics or burial environment; this is unlikely in most UK contexts (Cox and Bell 1999), but is more feasible with the buried remains of children and neonates where the bones are smaller and not fully calcified. Oddly, Courts never seem to ask about the totality of recovery, or even query it. Perhaps they should? Sieving (Section 7.1) is often an essential follow-up to excavation: it provides a second opportunity to recover material not visible during excavation, and is a further area where anthropological expertise is beneficial. Moreover, it further lessens the likelihood of even small elements being found in years to come and new enquiries having to be implemented.

There are also occasions when stray human bone is recovered scattered on the surface and where the likelihood of a full skeletal recovery is minimal. Apart from problems of recovery there are also issues of identification, and of dating the time of surface deposition (see Section 7.5 below). Many of these instances may be innocent (hypothermia victims, lost hill walkers, etc.) but they still require full investigation and maximum recovery. Some work has been undertaken in the United States regarding the spatial extent of scatter in relation to the passage of time (Morse et al. 1983; Haglund et al. 1989; Haglund 1997). The data suggests a direct relationship between length of exposure and the distance that the dislocated parts travelled from the initial point of deposition, but the case studies can only indicate general trends. It is a matter of common-sense to suppose that the greater the passage of time, the wider the extent of scatter as a result of scavenging. There is a corollary too which might indicate from the same data the degree of scatter that might be expected from a person who went missing X months or Y years earlier. But neither trend fully takes into account differences in climate, localised environment, level of concealment, the scavenging species present, nor the extent to which the body was deposited in a confined space. Turton's study into the habitats of typical UK scavengers (carnivores, rodents and avians) identified the areas of greatest scavenging potential to be gardens, parks, cemeteries, overgrown buildings and rubbish tips. Least likely places were considered to be moorland, sea cliffs and rock landscapes; embankments, cuttings, woodland and fields lay somewhere in between (Turton 2003, 161, table 4).

The size and strength of scavenger is also significant. Carson *et al.* noted that a bear could drag a carcass at least 25 m whereas a coyote could barely move a similar carcass until it had become disarticulated (2000, 525). Records taken over a seven-year period relating to the disarticulation pattern of a juvenile cow which fell off a cliff and landed in area of restricted access makes the point well (Andrews 1995): material was gradually moved from the deposition site only by those scavengers that could gain access and were strong enough to move individual elements, even after skeletonisation. In another instance, the main skeletal elements of the small boy described in Case Study 1.1 were substantially complete after 26 years despite being deposited on the ground surface during winter. In that case, however, he was wrapped and partly concealed under a layer of stones. By contrast, the body of a young girl who had been missing for six weeks, also in winter, had been heavily scavenged with most of the lower body reduced to a skeletal state (Case Study 7.5). Moreover, the species of scavenger differ in various parts of the world; the experimental work cited in most literature was undertaken in North America (e.g. Haglund *et al.* 1989; France *et al.* 1992, 1997), but with some exceptions, for example in Australia (Powell 2010). Different models are likely to apply in the UK where, instead of bears, coyotes, dingos and vultures, the main scavengers tend to be foxes (*vulpes vulpes*), badgers (*meles meles*) and rats (*rattus rattus*). They each have their characteristic mode of sourcing, addressing and consuming food both for individual survival and for feeding their young (Turton 2003).

All this has implications, partly for affecting the degree of scatter that might be anticipated, partly for recovery management purposes, and partly because the physical anthropologist may need to be able to distinguish hard tissue modification caused by animal teeth from ante-mortem trauma. In some instances these modifications may even mask or mirror bone trauma, and to this end certain idiosyncratic damage marks caused by gnawing and chewing have been defined in some detail (see Haglund *et al.* 1988, 986). In addition, there are an abundance of published case studies that highlight the propensity for animal scavenging to have a similar appearance to various types of trauma or pathologies, whilst actual insults on the bone may be obscured by the damage caused by gnawing, digestion or piercing of bone by animals (Haglund 1992; Berryman 2002; Byers 2003, 359–63; Steadman and Worne 2007; Moraitis and Spiliopoulou 2010). It should not be assumed that scavenging will always begin immediately after, or even close to, the time of death and disposal. An important study by Rothschild and Schneider (1997) has discussed the motivation of animals feeding on human remains and serves as a useful guide in terms of the factors that should be considered when attempting to determine the extent of scavenging in relation to the time since deposition. At the micro-level, insects, molluscs and marine creatures may also be responsible for bone modification, with the particular species responsible being dictated by location, climate and the proximity of the body to their habitat (Anderson 2010; Ubelaker and Scammal 1992). Bone modification can also be created by natural phenomena, through weathering, ice formation and thawing, exfoliation of surfaces and by root action (e.g. Marshall 1989, 20; see also Section 7.3); experienced physical anthropologists will be conversant with these phenomena.

Some mention needs to be made of the feeding habits of UK scavengers as this impacts on the character of bone dispersal, the expectancy of recovery, and on the likelihood of bone modification. Foxes (*vulpes vulpes*) live and scavenge in both urban and rural environments. Those in urban habitats survive substantially on discarded food and domestic rubbish and are thus less affected by winter than their rural cousins whose main food source of small animals becomes diminished in the colder weather. Consequently, there is a greater chance that a body disposed of in winter will be more quickly scavenged in the countryside than elsewhere. Foxes tend not to feed in groups, unless the food source (e.g. the human body) is large enough. They tend to eat at the place of kill or discovery, unless feeding a gestating vixen or cubs, in which case food will be taken back to the den. The breeding season for foxes is typically from late December to February, gestation is around two months, and cubs become self-sufficient for food by five months of age. This means that during the period between approximately January to June the likelihood of skeletal elements being moved away from the focal source is greater than during the rest of the year, especially in rural areas. The size of the elements being removed will be dictated by the strength of the animal and the state of decay of the individual. To some extent this might be counteracted by the victim wearing thicker winter clothes, or the lower temperature slowing down the rate of decomposition. Scavenging is optimised when the victim is at the end of the autolysis stage of decay; but this is probably at its most extensive at the putrefaction stage when some elements become more easily transportable by smaller animals.

In the UK the largest carnivores are badgers (*meles meles*) (Clark 1988). They could be argued to be gatherers, whereas foxes are hunters. Having stronger jaws than foxes they can transport larger elements of a human body, or even whole carcasses of animals (see Case Study 7.5; Neal 1986), but they tend to be much more restricted to woodland and arable areas than to urban environments. Badger teeth are stronger and more damaging than those of foxes; their cubs, like fox cubs, belong to a breeding season in the early part of the calendar year but, unlike fox cubs, are less dependent on their parents for food, their diet being more usually concerned with worms, grubs and beetles once they are weaned. Breeding is not, therefore, necessarily associated with the increased potential for the transportation of body elements back to the sett as it is with foxes. Moreover, there is a tendency for badgers to be semi-dormant during the colder months before the cubs are born and therefore the emphasis of foraging at that time is reduced.

Rats (*rattus rattus*) appear to be less contained in either feeding or breeding. They have no specific breeding time during the year, they can reproduce from eleven weeks of age, the gestation period is around four weeks, and young rats leave the nest to fend for themselves after only three weeks from birth. In scavenging, rats appear to prefer soft tissue (Case Study 7.6), the organs in particular, especially if there is ante-mortem trauma allowing them easier access; they are only capable of moving small body components, notably from the areas of the hands and feet. They will not travel anything like the distances travelled by foxes and badgers, and there appears to be little in the way of seasonal variation in their feeding habits.

Overall, surface scatters can require a number of factors to be brought into consideration: the nature of habitat of deposition; the season of deposition; the date of deposition; the scavenging species in the locality, and recognition of bone modification. There are then attendant problems of logistics for the Senior Investigating Officer (SIO) or Crime Scene Manager (CSM) in trying to determine how large an area to search and using which assets.

Realistically, the greater the spread of material on discovery, the lower the potential for finding anything approaching a complete set of remains. But there will be some pointers: different types of bone modification may lead to a determination of scavenging species and hence to more directed searching; any defined search area may then need to take into account fox dens and badger setts in order to plot likely transport routes. A defined search area can range from a few square metres to a few hundred square metres according to landscape and the nature of initial discovery. Some of the larger bones may be recovered by a close contact line search, but this will also serve to trample in smaller, unseen material. A primary systematic search using free roam dogs is probably optimum, thereafter it becomes the decision of the SIO as to how best to continue and at which point to stop. S/he needs to be able to demonstrate that all reasonable steps had been taken, including the deployment of a physical anthropologist, to provide a strategy designed to ensure the fullest possible recovery.

Case Study 7.5

A young girl had been reported missing during the winter and her body was eventually found less than half a mile from her house on a steep slope among brambles and scrub. Despite the proximity to the place of last sighting and the almost total absence of leaf or tree cover, the body was not located for almost six weeks when it was found in a relatively open part of the scrub. This was despite a number of searches throughout the eventual area of discovery by police search teams, the military, helicopters, dogs and members of the public. The assumption was that the child's body must have been moved by predators, in this case badgers. This was reflected in the almost complete stripping of soft tissue from the lower limbs, the abdomen and parts of the arms, teeth marks on the bone and the presence of badger hair caught on an adjacent wire fence. It is unlikely that foxes would have been sufficiently strong to move the body. On this occasion the police saw fit to bring an expert on badgers into the enquiry. The case demonstrates the importance of taking animal activity into account in the search for small children deposited on the ground surface.

Case Study 7.6

In one instance where a victim had been buried hurriedly his left elbow had been left partly exposed above the ground. When he was excavated some two weeks later, the three protruding bones of the arm were almost completely devoid of soft tissue while the rest of the body was intact. The exposed bones exhibited gnawing marks associated with rats. There was no evidence for either foxes or badgers, although the environment was amenable to both. It would seem that the remains were insufficiently decayed for their immediate attentions. Nor had any attempts been made by either species to unearth or scavenge the buried remains.

This particular case was interesting for a number of other reasons. The earth was thick and could only be moved in clods for which a garden fork had been used, the impression of the implement's tines being clearly visible in the sides of the grave.

Additionally, the grave was located in a copse dominated by a rare species of tree, the pollen of which was easily detectable on both the ground and the footwell of the vehicle used to dispose of the body. Whilst not conclusive evidence in its own right, it provided the police with important avenues of enquiry.

7.5 Dating

There are two key questions which have to be asked by police when human remains, usually skeletal, are unearthed during building operations or gardening, or when encountered on the surface by dog walkers or ramblers. One is 'How old are these remains?' and the other is 'What is the identity of the individual?' The first of these is the subject of this section; it also generates a string of ancillary questions thus:

- Are the remains disarticulated, or do they belong to a definable burial?

- In either case, do they have an identifiable context in the ground (i.e. associated layers or features) (see also Case Study 7.7)?

- Do any of the associated layers or features have fixed dates (e.g. are they associated with foundations of structures or do they lie under floors or patios where the date of building is known)?

- If so, can the remains be allocated a *terminus ante quem* or a *terminus post quem* (see also Section 5.7)?

- If the remains do not belong to a definable burial, or have an identifiable context, how can their presence be explained, however broadly, in that particular place?

Knowing the date of original deposition (as opposed to the age of the individual at death) is necessary to determine whether or not remains are of forensic significance. In the UK this is taken to mean that an individual needs to have died within approximately the last 70 years (i.e. living memory) (Scheuer and Black 2006, 200). In other countries this time period may differ considerably; in Portugal, for example, after only 15 years a crime will no longer be deemed important from an investigative perspective (Cardoso *et al.* 2011, 1). In the UK human remains that can be demonstrated as being deposited more than 70 years ago are not seen to justify an enquiry on the basis that appropriate evidence for a conviction is unlikely to be forthcoming. Moreover, the age of criminal responsibility in the UK is 10 years, meaning that a potential offender would be over 80 years of age. There is a grey area here, given that it is virtually impossible to date human remains or a buried context in which they were discovered to the accuracy of one year over that timescale. Seventy years is normally seen as a guide rather than a strict rule, and the distinction between remains of 'forensic interest' and those that are earlier is usually relatively clear cut. The problems arise when a greater degree of dating precision is required, for example in instances where the digging of the grave needs to be tied in with the movements of a suspect or with the last sightings of a missing person, or when a human femur is found in a ditch. In most respects problems of dating graves are easier than dating non-buried or surface remains.

As far as burials are concerned, in the field there are a number of pointers that might be used as indicators for burials lying within a forensic timeframe. These indicators tend to result from the interaction between the burial and its environment, but are mostly arbitrary and based on personal experience and opinion. Without solid evidence they are unlikely to stand up in Court, but they can have the effect of providing an investigation with additional information. Pointers might include the presence of surface spoil, depressions, vegetation change (inhibited or increased growth), the extent of interface or merging between the grave fill and the grave walls, or even the extent to which the sides of a grave have slumped inwards (see Case Study 6.2). Others may carry more scientific weight, such as the extent or density of vegetation succession, or the renewed growth of roots cut during the original digging of the grave (Dupras *et al.* 2008, 72; Forbes 2008, 207). If remains are found scattered on the surface there can be some deduced correlation between spatial extent of scatter and elapsed time since deposition (Haglund *et al.* 1989; Haglund 1997) but this can depend on season, climate, geographical location and species of scavenger (see also Turton 2003; also Section 7.4). In most of these instances this kind of 'dating' can be expressed in a broad sense only and not in the more precise way that an investigation wants, or that a Court normally requires.

Levels of decomposition are sometimes alluded to as indicators of the post-mortem and post-burial interval. Decomposition of a cadaver occurs when a number of intrinsic processes occur: the depletion of oxygen in tissue; the destruction of cells; the production of organic acids and gases, autolysis, putrefaction and decay (Forbes 2008, 204; Dix 2000). However, particularly with regard to buried remains, decomposition is far from the 'sequential and somewhat predictable process' that has been suggested in the past (Nafte 2000, 39). The presence of soft tissue, for example, is not necessarily indicative of a recent deposition. Countless archaeological examples can be cited where soft issue or saponified material was still present after a considerable elapsed time (for an overview of the discovery of bog bodies dating to the Iron Age and Middle Ages, see Peska *et al.* 2010; for soft tissue preservation in crypts, see Cox 2001b; for the preservation of organs in an archaeological context, see O'Connor *et al.* 2011). The factors that can complicate interpretation of the interval between death/deposition and discovery can be seen to fall into two categories: those that are intrinsic (i.e. relating to the body itself and the circumstances of burial), and those that are extrinsic (i.e. relating to the environment in which the body is deposited) (also Section 7.3). The former includes, for example, the body mass and health of the individual and any injuries sustained. The latter includes plant and animal activity, the composition, acidity/alkalinity of the soil, hydrology, depth and weather conditions to name but a few, as well as any wrapping or clothing (Wilson *et al.* 2007; Tibbett and Carter 2008; see Section 7.3).

Assessment of the speed of degradation of associated grave materials presents the same subjective problems as that of the human body. Some research has been carried out which indicates that, under certain circumstances, it may be possible to establish the post-burial interval of other types of buried remains. These include hair and textiles (Janaway 2002 and 2008, and Wilson 2008), but again the variables of the buried environment also apply.

Many human remains are discovered in a skeletal state, both buried and on the surface. Here, similar judgement calls apply to the visual dating of human bone on the basis of its 'old' appearance. In general, human bone loses its greasiness and dries out over time becoming brittle. This can be a useful guide to date, but no more than that and the difficulties in interpreting the weathering of bone have been well emphasised (Lyman and Fox 1997). When bone dries it loses its vitality and also its ability to support organic growth, thus any remains bearing moss or fungi are more likely to be recent (L. Hackman pers. comm.). Conversely, excessive wear on teeth is likely to be indicative of an individual from further back in antiquity (see also Case Study 7.7) on the basis that ancient teeth wear patterns tend not to correspond to contemporary wear patterns as a result of modern diet.

7.5.1 Relative dating

Remains discovered from a buried environment often have the potential to be dated on a relative basis, that is in relation to other layers or features lying in the ground. Any archaeological site (including a grave) can be determined as a stratigraphic sequence in which the process of layer superimposition presents a relative chronology, i.e. one layer occurs before another, or after another, and so on. But this chronology floats in time. It has no fixed points unless specific layers in that sequence can be identified with defined chronological events or, alternatively, unless objects recorded from layers in the sequence can be given known dates. In more conventional archaeology, relative dating has been the basis of understanding pottery seriations, typologies and general artefact development through time. For example, certain types of artefact tend to occur stratigraphically before other types or forms of artefact, which in turn may be associated with particular types of structure or different types of object. This allows the archaeologist to build up a picture of how the material past changed through time. Little by little this picture becomes more detailed as more stratified evidence comes to light. Objects can be cross-referenced from one site to another, occasionally firmed up by the discovery of coins or similar objects of known specific date. Coins do not date layers, but they can help create *termini* for the layers above and below. The more datable material there is in adjacent layers, the more precisely the date of deposition of each layer can be established. This is well illustrated by Philip Rahtz in his excavations at the Anglo-Saxon Royal Palace at Cheddar, Somerset (Rahtz 1979) (Figure 7.6). His excavations of the surrounding ditch, which had silted and been re-cut, found a number of coins stratified in the silting and re-cutting deposits. These allowed a fairly tight chronology of the activities to be determined, and hence facilitated dating of the palace itself to which the ditch and its later re-cutting was directly associated.

Clandestine graves are usually less interesting stratigraphically, but the same principles apply. Coins are rarely discovered, but the presence of man-made fabrics or other modern materials seized from stratigraphically significant positions can serve to eliminate archaeological timescales and point to potential forensic relevance. A good example was where building works uncovered skeletal human remains during re-development of an urban centre. The remains were kept *in situ* and archaeological examination demonstrated that they related to a grave which had been cut into the fill of a pipe trench carrying sewage. The top of the grave had then been overlain by hardcore for the foundations of a municipal swimming pool. Reference to the local planning applications showed that the sewage pipe was inserted in 1958 and that the swimming pool had been constructed in 1962, thus giving a date of between 1958 and 1962 for the digging of the grave, a date within forensic timescales. Sometimes further honing is required, for example by the presence of wrappers, packaging or containers which often have 'sell by' or 'best by' dates (see Case Study 1.2), or even graphic designs which can, by research, be attributed to known manufacturing production

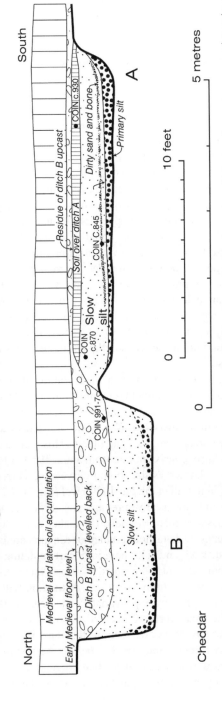

Figure 7.6 Simplified section through a ditch and ditch re-cutting at Cheddar, Somerset showing value of the *terminus ante quem* and *terminus post quem* based on coin evidence (after Rahtz 1979, 84).

spans. Depending on stratified context these may demonstrate that a grave was dug *before* or was dug *after* a certain date, but not *at* a specific point in time.

7.5.2 Absolute dating

Relative dating is not applicable, however, in instances where there is no direct stratigraphic association, for example: remains discovered on the ground surface, remains in suitcases in ditches, or skeletons of neonates in attics. These require some form of *absolute* dating in order to ascertain their relative antiquity; this is another matter entirely.

A small number of dating methods exist but by far the most commonly applied is that of radiocarbon dating. This can provide a date range in years based on the depletion of the ^{14}C isotope following the death of an organism, in this case the living body. The isotopic decay rate is known and is predictable, and the values can be converted into calendar years (Libby 1952). In theory this can be applied to all organic matter including wood and plants as well as bone. Unfortunately, the concept is not quite that simple. Libby's discovery assumed that the amount of radiocarbon in the atmosphere was consistent throughout time and that its absorption by living matter was therefore equally consistent. This proved not to be the case and derived dates had to be corrected by radiocarbon dating of the individual annual rings of ancient trees (dendrochronology) in order to produce corrected values, producing what became known as a 'calibration curve'. It works well in archaeological timescales: 'raw' radiocarbon dates are calculated in years 'bp' (bp = before present, 'present' being 1950); calibrated (i.e. corrected) values are calculated in years 'BP'. The concept is based on the half-life decay of the ^{14}C isotope (5730 +/− 40 years) which means that, because of statistical issues in counting this decay rate, the dating becomes less accurate the closer it comes towards the present.

However, in recent years there has been a proliferation of research into the uses of artificial radiocarbon data for dating human remains (Ubelaker 2001; Ubelaker *et al.* 2006; Lynnerup *et al.* 2010). The increased amount of ^{14}C released into the atmosphere as a result of nuclear testing during the Cold War (1950–63) led to a subsequent increased uptake of this element by humans, animals and plants. This increase in radioactivity in the atmosphere occurred at a fairly consistent rate from about 1950 to 1963 and then fell away, but less steeply, in what is known as the 'bomb curve'; the current level at the time of writing (2012) still being higher than the pre-1950 level (Figure 7.7). In general terms this means that the remains of individuals alive pre- and post-1950 can be readily distinguished from each other on the basis of this difference (Ubelaker *et al.* 2006). This has become a coarse, but effective means of determining whether remains are of forensic significance or not (see also Case Studies 5.7 and 7.7 where radiocarbon dating was used to determine whether buried human bones, which presented no observable relative dating, required further investigation). However, as time passes this distinction will become progressively less meaningful in forensic terms: by approximately the year 2020 (70 years after 1950) it will cease to possess the clear 'forensic interest' factor that it currently holds. Equally, there is a grey area in that any death occurring in the years immediately preceding 1950 (i.e. within the period of 'forensic interest' but *before* the bomb curve) will be largely indistinguishable statistically from earlier dates that are not of forensic interest. However, if a sample contains the higher measurement of radiocarbon that would place it within the

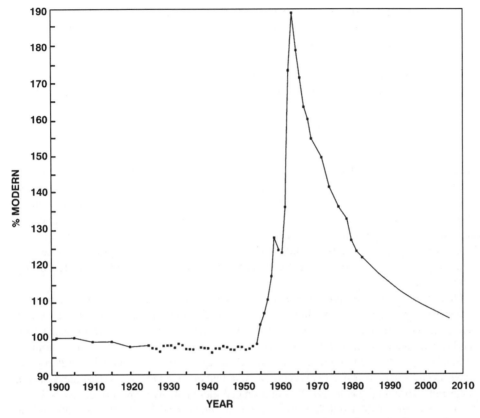

Figure 7.7 Diagram illustrating the 'bomb curve' and its value in identifying whether remains are of forensic interest or not (after Arner *et al.* 2011).

last 70 years, there are further problems in trying to position it within that 70-year period. This is because the amount of ^{14}C can sit on either side of the slope of the curve (pre-1963 or post-1963). To some extent this ambiguity has meant that it has yet to become the *de facto* dating method used in forensic scenarios, other than for ascertaining general forensic relevance (Ubelaker *et al.* 2006, 484).

However, different parts of the body are known to remodel at different stages in the life course: some tissue ceases to absorb radiocarbon at an early stage in life, while other tissue continues to absorb it through until death. In terms of establishing the date of an early stage in life, dental enamel has been considered one of the most useful parts of the body, given the fact that it does not remodel following the final formation of enamel (roughly at the age of 12) and ceases to absorb radiocarbon at that point; it is also highly durable under buried conditions (Ubelaker *et al.* 2006, 485). Spalding *et al.* (2005, 333) have argued that analysis of ^{14}C in tooth enamel offers the possibility of accurately determining an individual's year of birth within 1.6 years, compared to 5–10 years for traditional anthropological methods. Conversely, soft tissue, including hair and nails (if they survive), undergoes faster turnover and is favourable for age at death estimations (Lynnerup *et al.* 2010). Most useful here in view of its greater survival potential is bone, particularly trabecular bone, such as that found at the end of long bones. In view of its porosity, trabecular bone absorbs radiocarbon right up until the day of death (Ubelaker *et al.* 2006). Hence, by dating those body parts for which absorption ceases at an early age and at death (typically teeth and trebecular bone respectively), it increases the chances of identifying on which side of the curve, and where on the curve, the span of dates is likely to sit.

Bones or material selected for radiocarbon dating need to be bagged and secured as soon as possible after recovery and maintained in an environment that is unlikely to support bacterial or fungal growth. Sampling from the bone will be carried out under laboratory conditions to prepare it for pre-treatment processes. Analytical techniques have developed over recent years and most commercial dating laboratories use mass spectrometry systems, which not only provide a more convenient and cost-effective means of analysing samples (Spalding *et al.* 2005), but also utilise much smaller sample sizes. Advertised sample sizes are typically 2–10 g for bone or a single tooth, although smaller samples may be feasible. Turn around time is normally around three weeks, and this may cause problems if security of a site is to be maintained throughout this period. Some companies offer a faster service, but at a cost.

Of course not all cases present the desirable teeth and long bones, usually as a result of scavenging or dismemberment. In those cases a single date can only demonstrate forensic relevance (or not) and other methods of dating refinement are needed. Here recent work has begun to demonstrate the value of other ingested man-made isotopes, notably strontium (^{90}Sr), lead (^{210}Pb) and Polonium (^{210}Po) which have extremely short half-lives (29.5 years, 22 years and 138 days respectively) compared to that of ^{14}C (5730 years) (Froidevaux *et al.* 2006 and 2010; Schrag *et al.* 2012). Additionally, these half-lives are further reduced since the nuclear tests of the Cold War, for example in the case of ^{90}Sr to 10–13 years (Schrag *et al.* 2012). This means that the statistical counting error involved with ^{14}C in determining modern dates is massively reduced, and that a much higher degree of accuracy can be achieved (Swift *et al.* 2001). Similarly, the extraction of these isotopes from a variety of skeletal elements, including vertebrae, teeth and long bones, has been successful. A new method proposed by Schrag *et al.* (2012), tested on vertebrae of individuals who died in Switzerland between 1960–2001 and in Italy in 1990, appears to overcome the issues with contamination of skeletal elements during diagenesis that have been noted in previous studies (Price *et al.* 1992; Budd *et al.* 2000; Zapata *et al.* 2006) and suggests that the combined analysis of ^{210}Po and ^{90}Sr more accurately defines the PMI.

A number of other dating methods are now being researched and are beginning to appear in the literature, but all can still be seen to be in the early stages of development and have not yet been deemed reliable enough for practical forensic application. Examples include: the examination of what has become known as a Cadaveric Decomposition Island (CDI) (Forbes 2008), the use of various blood detection methods to discriminate between archaeological and recent bone (Ramsthaler *et al.* 2011), RNA analysis (van Doorm *et al.* 2011) and the measurement of the Crystallinity Index of bone (Thompson *et al.* 2011, 168). These are mentioned here in terms of their potential rather than their current application. Radiocarbon dating, despite its limitations, continues to be the main well-proven technique.

Case Study 7.7

During the construction of an area of new housing in the south Midlands the mechanical excavator that was being used to strip topsoil disturbed a number of bones. These lay

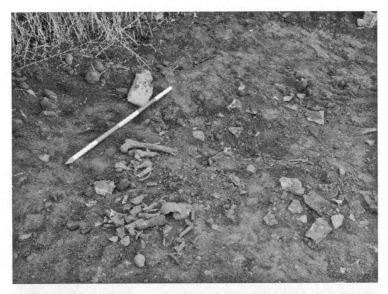

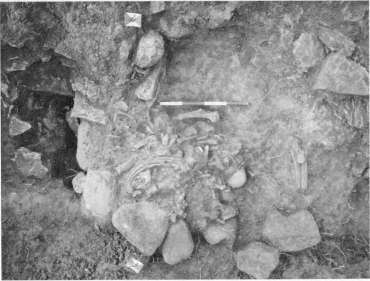

Figure 7.8 Top, human remains unearthed by a mechanical excavator during building operations. Bottom, archaeological investigation of their context together with an anthropological assessment pointed to a date well before forensic timescales. Image by courtesy of Albion Archaeology (project funded by Taylor Wimpey + Bucks CC).

just below the topsoil, at a depth of no more than 30 cm below the present ground surface at the edge of a field. Work ceased and the police were called, the bones photographed with an appropriate scale, emailed to anthropologists in Dundee, and established as being human. Police then called in archaeologists to undertake a detailed excavation. On arrival the archaeologists found that the disturbed bones had been collected by building workers and piled up adjacent to a disturbance in the ground (Figure 7.8). The disturbed area in question measured little more than 2 × 2 m and also contained a number of slab-like stones which had been dislocated by the digger.

The initial process of excavation involved the collection of further bones and fragments and the on-site sieving of loose soil removed from around the disturbance. During this process more bone material was recovered and it soon became clear that a number of individuals, and of different ages, were represented. After cleaning, it was also clear that a substantial number of other bones were present, and that they were not in anatomical order. In an attempt to clarify this rather unusual situation a trial section was cut across the disturbance. This showed that the slab-like stones appeared to have been part of a long, narrow structure some 0.4 m wide and of unknown length. The slabs had been used to provide upright sides to the 'grave' which had been capped by further slabs.

At this point the investigation took pause to review the position and asked for the local authority archaeologist to attend and give opinion on the nature of archaeological monuments in the area. Further human material, including jaw bones containing teeth, was photographed and sent to Dundee for further comment. The Dundee anthropologists reaffirmed the likely antiquity of the bones on the basis of their dryness and brittleness, supported by substantial wear evident on the teeth. The local authority archaeologist was familiar with similar 'cist' constructed burials in the vicinity dated to the Romano-British period, although not one with this level of commingling. The overall weight of opinion from all concerned was that the remains were of archaeological as opposed to of forensic interest. Relative dating was not possible as there were no related layers or features. Radiocarbon dating on a sample of the bones demonstrated that the assemblage belonged to the mid-fourth millennium BC.

8 The investigation of multiple burials

8.1 Diversity and challenges

Forensic archaeologists and anthropologists are now regularly engaged in the investigation of mass burials, and this chapter reviews some of the issues involved. Most commonly, these mass burials result from the relatively recent disposal of victims of genocide, usually during a period of conflict, the disappearance of whom has been undertaken covertly to prevent discovery. Only in recent years have the developments in this field been reported in the literature, but there is now a plethora of texts that consider the essential mechanics employed in these scenarios (e.g. Haglund 2002; Schmitt 2002; Skinner and Sterenberg 2005; Tuller and Djuric 2006; Cox *et al.* 2007); these reflect the growing specialism of mass grave investigation and the diverse environments in which archaeologists can find themselves. Additionally, the recognition of the humanitarian, as well as judicial, rationale for the recovery of human remains as result of homicide, genocide and war crimes has led to an emergence of literature dealing with ethical and sociological implications (Blau 2009; Sterenberg 2009; Steele 2008). This burgeoning momentum has also impacted on the practical developments of search and recovery methodologies: investigations in the Balkans, for example, have set a precedent for the use of non-invasive survey techniques to identify sites, and published literature is slowly beginning to address the contribution that such techniques can offer in socio-historical as well as forensic contexts (Saunders 2001; Gilchrist 2003; Juhl 2005; Sturdy Colls 2012a). There is a good argument to suggest that the relationship between growing intervention into contemporary genocide and the development of these practical methodologies is almost certainly symbiotic.

What actually constitutes a mass burial has been a pedantic point of discussion among some practitioners. Debate has tended to centre around the number of victims interred (Skinner 1987; UN 1991; Hunter and Simpson 2007), or on burial classification according to the nature of concealment or formation (Mant 1987). All scenarios are different and require different investigative responses; categorisation has the effect of over-simplifying more complex issues and often bears little relevance to the methodologies employed. Moreover, as in the recovery of all buried remains, the essential elements are the interrogation of evidence and the application of methods appropriate to answering the questions posed. Schmitt's view of a multiple burial being one which 'contains the remains of more than one victim who share some common trait connected with the cause and manner of death'

Forensic Approaches to Buried Remains, First Edition. John Hunter, Barrie Simpson and Caroline Sturdy Colls.
© 2013 John Wiley & Sons, Ltd. Published 2013 by John Wiley & Sons, Ltd.

(2002, 2) takes a more pragmatic approach. It recognises that, apart from individualisation, the key elements that require addressing in any mass burial are likely to be generic to the full complement of victims rather than individual to each. This applies irrespective of whether the burial results from genocide, battle or natural disaster, or indeed whether it occurred in the 21st century or the Middle Ages.

Conflict of any type provides the necessary cover for genocidal acts, motivated by race, religion, social class, politics, cultural affiliation or other personal attributes (Komar 2008) including, (usually) in more historical timescales, factors of gender, age and disability. It may be undertaken by a specific group, political party or nation; national governments may commit atrocities against their own people, or it may be perpetrated across several nations. Mass murder may also occur both during and outside of war time, against civilians, the military and, less commonly, as part of so-called 'neighbourhood genocide' (Zawodny 1962; Field 2007; Komar 2008). Disposals may be undertaken by the perpetrators or their associates, by those who would later become victims themselves or by the families of the deceased (IMTN 1947; Perera and Briggs 2008). Understanding the social context within which a mass burial might occur appears increasingly complex but is required homework for those involved: it underpins and configures the questions that need to be addressed in the investigation of the grave. Circumstances and considerations can vary, not least being the time elapsed between death, disposal, search and recovery (e.g. Paperno 2001 for Russia; Ballbé and Steadman 2008 for Spain).

Multiple burials involve a greater number of bodies and consequently a need for increased resources. In theory, the sheer magnitude of these depositions should make them easier to detect; even after lengthy periods of time this 'footprint' of activity is observable unless specific measures were taken at the time to disguise it (Komar and Buikstra (2008, 252). In one instance in the Balkans five small mass graves of various depths were deliberately buried under 25,000 tonnes of rubble spread across a large area in a manner that presented difficulties not only for detection, but also for recovery of the remains (Sterenberg pers. comm.). Equally, even large graves can be temporarily disguised, for example in fields that were subsequently put under crop (e.g. Wright 2005) or had been recently ploughed and where the vegetation effects may not have been immediately obvious.

Many of the relevant search methodologies have already been discussed in Chapters 2 and 3 with respect to individual (criminal) graves. For example, developments in Geographical Information Systems (GIS) offer opportunities for almost all types of spatial information about an investigation to be assimilated into a central resource for interrogation. However, the greater magnitude of mass graves presents additional impacts, for example in tapho-nomics where the six taphonomic indicators identified by Hochrein (2002) – stratification, tool marks, bioturbation, sedimentation, compression-depression and internal compaction – are all likely to be exacerbated, therefore potentially making graves easier to detect both from the ground and the air (Figure 8.1 and Figure 8.2).

There have also been significant developments in certain remote sensing technologies particularly well-suited to the identification of larger targets. Not least of these is the new generation of available satellite and shuttle imagery through space programmes such as IKONOS, SPOT and QUICKBIRD. These represent an important landmark in allowing landscape assessment in advance of ground operations: the images are up-to-date and are of sufficient pixel size and resolution to identify ground cover for designing search strategies and establishing priorities (USGS 2010; De Vos *et al.* 2008; Trier *et al.* 2009). Many mass graves are investigated by international organisations or governments supported by

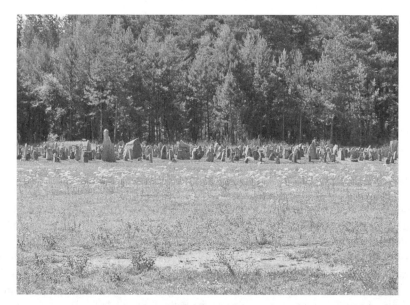

Figure 8.1   Vegetation change evidenced by tall weeds in the middle ground over a mass grave.

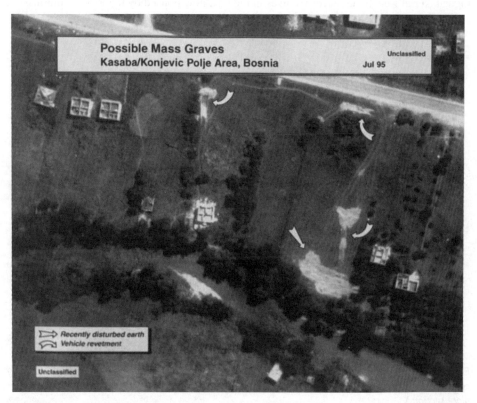

Figure 8.2   Aerial image showing ground scarring caused by a mass grave in Bosnia and Herzegovina. (PA 16578336 – Mark Lennihan/AP/Press Association Images.)

military hardware with access to state-of-the-art technology, including satellites. Military-grade imagery is well suited to targets the size of mass graves, notably the application of spectral analysis, a method long used by geologists to identify geological change through the use of colour bands (including IR and NIR) relating to different geological materials. This has been particularly beneficial in identifying gypsum, a mineral common in desert regions in Iraq, exposed in the large scale disturbance of the ground, including the construction of mass graves. Moreover, a large grave requires the removal of considerable quantities of earth; not only does this create a commensurate scale of scarring when the grave is infilled, it also creates a significant micro-floral impact where the spoil was stored temporarily, and compression where earth moving machinery consolidated the surrounding ground surface. These physical effects lend themselves well to interpretation from airborne LiDAR which has now been developed to overcome problems caused by obstructive vegetation, given the ability of the laser pulses emitted to propagate through trees and other obstacles (Jones *et al.* 2007; see also Section 2.3), and to subsequent digital terrain modelling (DTM). The latter also has the potential to analyse the geology, vegetation, distance from settlements and accessibility of a given area for the purposes of comparison with intelligence about the perpetrators and their victims (Figure 8.3). Moreover, in mass disaster environments, DTM has the potential for assessing the likely location of victims in relation to points of impact, e.g. the site of a plane crash, an explosion or the path of a tornado.

For socio-historic conflicts, the availability of historic imagery, such as the recently cata-logued Aerial Reconnaissance Archives in the UK, now housed by the Royal Commission

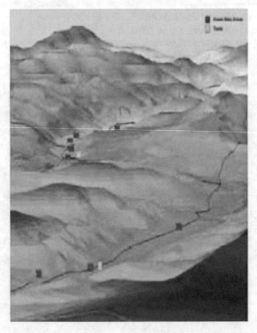

Figure 8.3 A digital terrain model (DTM) showing the location of mass graves in Bosnia. Image by courtesy of the International Commission on Missing Persons. (*For colour details please see colour plate section*.)

on Ancient and Historic Monuments of Scotland (RCAHMS) in Edinburgh (a collection formerly known as TARA, now NCAP – the National Collection of Aerial Photographs) or CORONA data can also aid analysis, subject to image quality. Comparisons between this and modern imagery can allow site histories to be generated and landscape change better understood. Unlike individual criminal graves, physical size is not the constraining factor; limitations are those of finance (some images are expensive), the availability of the equipment in certain areas and, perhaps most commonly, the quality and availability of mapping data for the country in question. The use of LiDAR suffers from similar constraints, not least being the logistics of completing flyovers in restricted airspace. These issues may go some way to explain why obvious methods of approach are seemingly under-deployed.

As noted in Section 3.1, geophysical survey methods have been significantly developed for use in forensic scenarios and their successful application has been demonstrated in both casework (Ruffell 2005; Nobes 2000) and research (Watters and Hunter 2004). However, it seems there has been little progress from Cheetham's observations (2005, 63) that GPR was the 'de-facto geophysical technique' in grave detection, despite studies demonstrating the potential of electrical imaging (ICMP 2007) and resistance survey (Watters and Hunter 2004). However, in mass burial scenarios, the use of any of the geophysical techniques available has not become widespread. In 2004, trials carried out by Scott and Hunter as to the suitability of resistance and electrical tomography methods to mass grave environments resulted in the production of advanced three-dimensional models of the site in advance of excavations (Figure 3.4). However, this study is unique and represents one of the few research projects conducted in such environments. The speed and additional pressures placed on practitioners involved in such cases, as well as the specialised nature of these methods (often unavailable at local level) probably represent some of the reasons that geophysical methods are not as widespread as might be expected. Further valuable lessons regarding this can also be drawn from archaeological examples, which have explored state-of-the-art three-dimensional presentations of geophysical data and the various means of assimilating them (Papadopoulos *et al.* 2006; Kvamme 2006). This includes data fusion, rarely used in the detection of mass graves, where geophysical images of the shallow sub-surface can be combined with high resolution aerial and satellite imagery. The innovation here is not in utilising these techniques individually, but in fusing the data spatially. This allows the growing science of GIS to be optimised: sites and buried features can be modelled in three dimensions, according to subtle contour and aspect, and virtual landscapes can be generated.

However, not all mass graves are intended to avoid detection. Some graves may have a more sinister purpose: making known the location of a mass grave through anecdotal means can act as a deterrent, preventing a community from returning to an area which has been 'cleansed'. Moreover, levels of intelligence about crimes are likely to vary on a case by case basis depending on a number of factors, such as the availability of witnesses, the cooperation of local investigators and the ability to detect other forensic evidence relating to the activities of perpetrators. The scale of the crimes and underlying threats of retaliation often discourage witnesses from coming forward. This provides the archaeologists with an unwelcome distraction in searching for graves, and one they can well do without – a dimension rarely discussed in literature but one, again, fundamental to their homework.

In addition, archaeologists, anthropologists, cadaver dog handlers, forensic scientists and search advisors are increasingly being consulted in mass disaster scenarios (Leclair *et al.* 2007; Rutty *et al.* 2007). Here, the victims have *become* buried, as opposed to being deliberately buried, as the result of 'open' events such as tsunamis, hurricanes, earthquakes and terrorist attacks, or of 'closed' events such as aircraft incidents (Interpol 2009). In the former, the numbers and identities of the victims tend to be unknown; in the latter there will be specific individuals to recover. Both present an undoubted role for physical anthropologists. Events over the last decade have done much to emphasise the contribution of anthropologists, particularly in establishing biological identity and in developing new skills. The archaeologists' contribution is slightly less pronounced but equally valid in the assessment of depositional sequences and in applying location methods. These are relatively new arenas for both disciplines; they present novel issues and potential problems in a challenging new range of circumstances.

8.2 Developments

The value of both archaeologists and anthropologists in the investigation of mass burials is now well recognised. This has been closely connected to the international response provided in places such as the western Balkans, Iraq, Rwanda and South America, and in the subsequent establishment of protocols and surge in publications (see below). The recognition of the need to investigate such occurrences accompanied by the development of entirely new subject areas (including forensic archaeology) in the last few decades, has significantly increased the evidential importance of excavating mass graves, as well as providing a source of employment for numerous specialists (Hunter and Cox 2005). One ancillary effect has been a somewhat predictable emergence of burgeoning numbers of 'forensic' degree programmes in Western universities; this reflects a more open coverage of events by the world media coinciding with a time of public enthusiasm for television crime fiction and forensic matters generally. However, it also has the advantage of illustrating the contribution that archaeologists and anthropologists can make to a society that has traditionally viewed them as being solely concerned with the distant past. For the first time they find their disciplines being acted out on a world stage, although as individuals they remain anonymous players. However, whilst their work within the context of mass graves is now mostly accepted as being necessary and commonplace, their position stems from a long and complex history of investigating war crimes that merits review here.

Since the time of German policies in World War II, which entailed the Holocaust killing of Jews and Gypsies on an industrial scale, the act of making people disappear has been used as a 'tool of war and repression' at state level (Juhl 2005, 3). Later, during the Nuremberg War Crimes Trials, the terms 'crimes against humanity' and 'genocide' became used to describe mass murder of this type. Much of the legislation governing the forensic investigation of these crimes was a direct result of the persecutions undertaken by Nazi Germany and stemmed from the establishment of the United Nations in 1945 and the acceptance of the Convention on the Prevention and Punishment of the Crime of Genocide (UN 1948; IMTN 1947). Although limited by the techniques available at that time, the searches aimed at locating victims of genocide represent the first international investigations with regards to mass burials; these searches also involved medico-legal professionals, in some cases initiating and developing many of the taphonomic and environmental processes central to modern forensics today (Zawodny 1962; Mant 1950, 1987; Auerbach 1979). Mant's work, for example, with the British War Commission, is significant not only because he was the first (and to this day one of the few) practitioners who attempted to identify victims from the Holocaust, but also because he offered new insights into the process of human decomposition at mass grave sites. He also emphasised the value of the pathologist as a witness of the Court, and the importance of victim identity (1950, 6); these were both novel at the time, but now fundamental to modern mass grave investigations.

The application of forensics and archaeology to human rights investigations occurs later, probably in South America in the 1980s following Argentina's re-transition into democracy (Juhl 2005, 24). There, the formation of the CONADEP Truth Commission (The National Commission on the Disappearance of Persons) marked a major landmark in cementing the role of the forensic archaeologist in mass grave investigations, although this was initially limited to exhumation as opposed to a full analysis of the grave contents (Doretti and Fondebrider 2001; CONADEP 1986). Developing technologies, together with increasing calls at international level for the conviction of the perpetrators of genocide, eventually led to the permanent creation of the International Criminal Tribunal for the Former Yugoslavia (ICTY) in 1993. Prior to this, various *ad hoc* courts had been established in the Former Yugoslavia, Rwanda, Sierre Leone, East-Timor, Cambodia and various other locations (Steele 2008). The same social momentum saw the creation of various forensic investigative units to locate mass grave sites in other parts of the world for the purpose of gathering evidence for both prosecution and humanitarian repatriation (Haglund 2002). These included both national organisations (the Argentine Forensic Anthropology Team (EAAF), the Guatemalan Team, the Peruvian Forensic Anthropology Team (EPAF) and the Independent Commission For The Location of Victims' Remains in Northern Ireland), and those providing an international response including the International Forensic Program (IFP) at Physicians for Human Rights (PHR), INFORCE, and the Centre for International Forensic Assistance (CIFA). In many cases these provided the platforms for experience and for the development of methodologies in what were essentially new disciplines.

A considerable number of investigations over the last decade have been undertaken under the auspice of the International Commission on Missing Persons (ICMP), which has shown a commitment to the identification of victims of genocide across the world and encouraged 'appropriate expressions of commemoration' to the 'missing' for humanitarian, as opposed to legal, purposes (ICMP 2008), although the two can often be closely linked. Established by US President Clinton at the G7 summit in Lyon (1996) the Commission has facilitated the largest identification programme in the world, based on the use of an innovative DNA database alongside traditional osteological assessments. The ICMP has devised a series of guidelines on the recovery of human remains based on its work in Bosnia (2008); as of September 2012 it had taken 89,068 samples from relatives of the missing and identified 16,289 individuals (ICMP 2012). Similar investigative units have also been established to assess South America, Rwanda and Iraq, where the need to locate the victims of war crimes has also been acknowledged (e.g. AFAT 2007; Hunter and Simpson 2007). Many of these organisations have also begun to provide both national and international responses in the aftermath of mass disasters.

However, many groups possess their own priorities and aspirations, and the absence of a set of universal guidelines to which practitioners might work has sometimes been a point of criticism (e.g. Cox *et al.* 2007, 17). Some general guidelines are available in the form of the *United Nations Manual on the Effective Prevention and Investigation of Extra-Legal, Arbitrary and Summary Executions* (1991) but no one text can ever hope to be generic either to mass graves in their many forms and political circumstances, or to the various scenarios of disaster recoveries, yet alone to both. To the contrary, there is a strong argument to maintain minimum standards across the board (which is another issue altogether), but not 'guidelines' which tend to assume a 'tick box' mentality and which may fail to take into account fundamental local differences of environment, practical methodologies and political circumstance on a case by case basis.

Archaeologists and anthropologists have tended to respond by complying with the respective guidelines in their own countries, for example the AAFS guidelines in Argentina, the codes devised by INFORCE or the former CRFP criteria in the UK, but many have noted that these are often inappropriate for mass grave scenarios and may be seen as flawed in Court (Steele 2008). Whilst in some countries practitioners may be forced to comply with a variety of local and national legislation, in others, such as Iraq and in some early investigations in Bosnia and Rwanda, a lack of procedures and facilities has meant that international intervention has been essential to facilitate and complete the work (Stover et al. 2003). Without this involvement it is doubtful whether either judicial or humanitarian ends would have been met; however, it is a thin wedge that separates international intervention from international interference. Surfacing quietly here, but rarely touched upon, is a certain arrogance that the values of Western governments, their legislations and social codes are the only ones that count.

A surge of papers between 2001 and 2007 began to address these issues, in particular the need for guidelines and Standard Operating Procedures (SOPs) (Skinner et al. 2003). Practitioners had also begun to debate the ethical and practical responsibilities of forensic archaeologists and anthropologists (Tuller and Duric 2006; Williams and Crews 2003; Skinner and Sterenberg 2005), whilst a few reflected on the extrinsic factors involved in operating within the difficult conditions of mass grave investigations and on the need for capacity building in order to obviate criticisms of colonialism (Hunter and Simpson 2007; Sterenberg 2009). This has occurred in Iraq, where local communities were encouraged to become involved in excavations where legal proceedings would not follow, and several individuals were sent to Bournemouth University for training (Steele 2008, 423). In Bosnia, unskilled workers were drafted in to assist with excavations, and training programmes were developed locally to facilitate studies in both archaeology and anthropology (ICMP 2007). To the archaeological purist this may seem to contravene the principles of competency, yet in those places deeply affected by conflict this programme not only represents an important resource, but also a significant reconciliatory and regeneration tool between local communities and investigators.

Only recently have practitioners begun to summarise the developments and case work over time (Anðelinoviæ et al. 2005; Juhl 2005), with the majority of papers focusing on individual case studies from Bosnia (Keough et al. 2000; Skinner et al. 2002), Iraq (Hunter and Simpson 2007) and Kosovo (Rainio et al. 2001). In the last few years, a handful of papers have begun to be published concerned with burials in mass disaster situations, for example the Asian Tsunami (Perera and Briggs 2008) and the World Trade Center (Leclair et al. 2007). This is a sensitive area and the investigation of such incidents at international level is still in relative infancy. In order to move the discipline forward, there is some need not only for more dissemination and comparison of techniques, but also for openness and honesty in admitting where mistakes may have been made. In the same way that the excavation of mass graves was forced to utilise and develop untried techniques and logistics 20 years earlier, so disaster recoveries may need a similar period of gestation inhibited perhaps by restrictions on information in situations involving terrorism. For example, experience of disasters in the UK has caused a new incident management structure since the *Marchioness* sinking in the Thames in 1989; now the disaster investigation itself is handled by a Senior Investigating Officer (SIO) with an equally ranked Senior Identification Manager (SIM) in overall charge of the victims. In some senses this epitomises the levels of change that have occurred. The investigation of mass graves and disasters is now multidisciplinary and not simply the concern of pathologists and police: experts from numerous fields are now regularly drawn in and coordinated – archaeologists, anthropologists, botanists, forensic scientists, entomologists, surveyors, chemists, biologists and legal experts, to name but a few. As with searches in domestic cases, their role is likely to differ in terms of scale and scope on a case by case basis, owing to the specific requirements of the lead investigators and the various logistical, judicial and humanitarian issues involved.

8.3 Interrogating the evidence

Some useful reasons for examining mass graves have been summarised by Haglund: to collect evidence to prosecute offenders; to identify victims; to 'create a document that should stand up to historical revisionists'; to prevent such crimes from happening again, and to provide 'basic dignity for the victims and for human life' (2002, 245). Few would disagree with this. However, the emphasis granted to each of these strands may vary depending on whether the focus of the exercise is more heavily weighted towards the prosecution of offenders, to the identification of victims, or to a balance of both. Moreover, given the multiplicity of organisations and agendas active in the field, archaeologists may find themselves faced with additional challenges according to the level of operational freedoms allowed to them. These 'freedoms' have been usefully summarised by Skinner and Sterenberg (2005) who outlined the various pressures and difficulties according to whether the archaeologist is able to have full control, work 'within the tapes', or merely fulfil the role of observer.

The legal rationale for the location and analysis of mass graves is significant owing to the evidential value of disposal sites for revealing information about the nature, scale and intent of killings. As with any forensic investigation, the scene provides the link between the victim(s) and the offender. This can be complex: in the Balkans many victims were executed, buried in primary graves, exhumed by the same perpetrators when the political heat became too great, and were subsequently buried in secondary graves in a different location. Some may even have been buried in tertiary graves. Archaeologists have been faced with the problem of correlating evidence that would link the various locations together, not only to demonstrate the nature and extent of the crime but also to identify the victims, some of whose body parts had been transported to different secondary graves (Figure 8.4). Archaeologists involved in this type of investigation may be called to testify as expert witnesses and may even be held accountable for the conduct of the excavations, including excavation records, even if they were operationally restricted (Wright *et al.* 2005, 139). Under these circumstances it would be easy to become duped into becoming 'unwitting apologists for criminals' (Vanezis 1999, 242).

Any emphasis on prosecuting perpetrators for large scale offences, such as 'crimes against humanity', also has the effect of relegating the personal tragedy of each individual

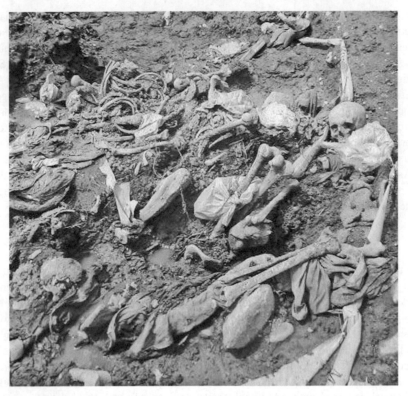

Figure 8.4   Part of a secondary mass grave containing commingled remains and personal belong-ings. Photo by courtesy of Cecily Cropper.

victim of the crime to a lower level of importance (Schmitt 2002). This is particularly true with regards to genocide where, given the sheer number of victims involved, the resources and attention paid to the investigation (for example) of a single murder victim in the UK is unlikely to be multiplied by the number of victims excavated from a mass grave. The simple existence of the mass grave itself may be enough to secure a conviction (Hunter and Simpson 2007, 271). In a case like this, archaeologists may be tasked (and pressured) only with the search for the grave, rather than its excavation. In a rather sanguine way, locating the grave may become more important than an analysis of its contents. In other instances, the removal of the bodies for reburial may be the priority. Such instances act as a timely reminder of the distinction between the 'excavation' and the 'exhumation' of victims, the former being conducted systematically, analytically and evidentially with the latter providing a less rigorous approach, sometimes using machinery, in order to recover bodies quickly (Sterenberg 2009).

In many instances the passage of time can preclude the need for judicial investiga-tion, or indeed there may be no legal mechanisms available for the prosecution of war crimes (Scheuer and Black 2006, 201). However, most investigations involving the exami-nation of mass graves are usually a direct response to specific allegations. For example, in 1990, graves in Serniki and Ustinovka in the Ukraine were the first, and to date the most comprehensively examined, mass graves of the Holocaust to be excavated by someone with archaeological experience (Dr Richard Wright). This was a direct result of the implementation of the War Crimes Amendment Bill (1998) in Australia, and specific allegations concerning a particular individual. Although the bodies of the victims at Serniki were not exhumed, the age, sex and cause of death were determined *in situ* (Dr Richard Wright pers. comm.). Another excavation carried out as a pragmatic response to an allegation, as opposed to forming part of a structured search programme, was that at Jedwabne in Poland. Poland's Institute of National Remembrance (IPN) carried out investigations of a mass grave in response to the publication of Gross' book *Neighbours* that controversially suggested that parts of the local community had assisted with the killings (Gross 2002; Polonsky and Michlic 2004). The investigation team focused on determining the number of victims but noted 'we did not conduct a full exhumation since we did not pull out the bones from the graves' (CNN 2001). Polonsky and Michlic have argued that the confusion regarding the number of victims at Jedwabne has actually been *caused* by this investigation given that 'what has been called an exhumation . . . lasted all of 5 days', and no prosecutions were made (Gross 2004, 359). In other cases relating to socio-historic events, such as the investigation of the Spanish Civil War victims, symbolic legal proceedings were mounted for the purpose of forcing the government to acknowledge the crimes (Ballbé and Steadman 2008), but the conviction of the perpetrators was not sought given that they were either deceased or of very advanced years.

In some cases, mass grave investigation for humanitarian purposes may represent the sole rationale. Here the pursuance of legal proceedings may be impossible given the time elapsed since the crimes were committed, or where the events in question represent natural disasters as opposed to criminal acts. With respect to relatively recent genocides, over the course of the last decade humanitarian responsibilities have become increasingly well recognised internationally (UN 1974). 'Genocide' as a term has achieved new heights of understanding and significance in moral vocabulary (Lang 1999, 15), and both media coverage of events and international pressure placed on governments to ensure appropriate investigation have generated a wider understanding of its implications. As a result, affording basic dignity to the victims through identification, and the provision of an appropriate burial, has been central to many investigations, as indeed has the recognition that 'the desire to know the fate of loved ones lost in armed conflicts is a basic human need which should be satisfied to the greatest extent possible' (Haglund 2002, 245). Notably, whilst the reasons for the individuals' deaths were most likely grounded in racial or religious intolerance, international protocols have generally endeavoured to ensure that no such prejudice exists within any subsequent investigations, spelled out clearly by the ICMP as the 'necessity of resolving the fate of missing persons without discrimination on the basis of ethnic affiliation, gender, race, language, religion, political or other beliefs, social origin, financial status, or their roles in armed conflicts or other hostilities, or the like' (2007, 6, 1).

Increased understanding of mass graves and their social implications also offers increased benefits to relatives of the victims, and even whole communities, in terms of the importance of the identification of victims. The difficulty of the grieving process, without a body to bury or confirmation of death, is increasingly being acknowledged: the women are 'not even widows, but widows waiting to happen' (Williams and Crews 2003, 252). Living relatives can be offered some element of closure when a mass grave is identified. Speaking before giving evidence in Court, Holocaust survivor Pepe Cohen felt that this was 'the day I bury my mother' (Bevan 1994, 107). Although the mass grave in which her mother's body was purported to have been buried was not fully excavated, nor her mother's specific remains identified, this survivor felt that the simple acknowledgement of this mass grave and the legal proceedings that followed its examination finally offered a sense of closure on events that had occurred 50 years earlier. It epitomises sentiments echoed in other accounts during which genocide has occurred. In other instances, the location of mass graves has been undertaken to provide the physical evidence to confirm witness testimonies, not in a legal sense but in order to provide verification for individuals and communities. One such instance was in Gnivan in the Ukraine where exhumation and reburial of the victims who were massacred in 1942 took place at the request of a local survivor of the incident; as stated by Dr Richard Wright (pers. comm.) 'that way, he [the survivor] said, his neighbours would now believe what he had told them over the decades' (Figure 8.5).

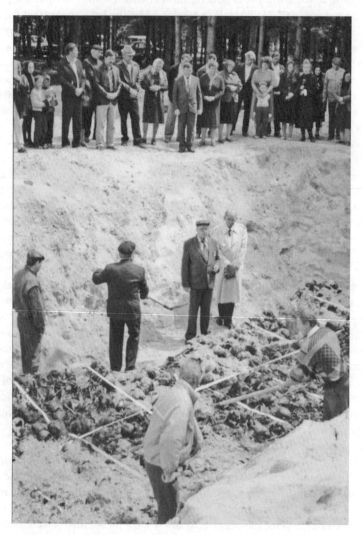

Figure 8.5 A memorial service at a mass grave in the Ukraine. Image by courtesy of Dr Richard Wright.

There will, of course, also be considerable variation in the extent of anthropological analysis of the individual, whatever the rationale for the search. Identification of each individual is the 'ethical, professional, and humanitarian ideal', although it depends on both necessary economic resources and ante-mortem data (Komar and Buikstra 2008, 245). The latter will be limited by a number of factors, such as the existence of medical records, the time since disposal and the traceability of relatives of the deceased. Stover *et al.* (2003) have noted the issues involved in obtaining DNA comparators when victims have been transported thousands of miles from their homes, the exact location of which is unclear. Other problems of identification arise when victims have been transported from primary to secondary deposition sites, not least being the separation of body parts of a single individual from a primary grave into different secondary graves. There are also situations where bodies have been exhumed by local communities and buried anonymously in cemeteries, as in Argentina (Egaña *et al.* 2008), and with many victims of the Holocaust. The condition of the remains will also be influential; scenarios involving commingled or burnt remains present a unique set of problems and may limit analysis to the designation of general biological identity, as opposed to assigning names to individuals, such as in El Mozote (El Salvador) and during investigations in Zimbabwe (Egaña *et al.* 2008).

8.4   The aftermath of conflict

Many investigations of mass burials will be undertaken in the immediate aftermath of conflict. In some communities the identification of gravesites and victims may be seen as an important part of the grieving and rebuilding process, but in others they may be seen as a hindrance to moving on and putting aside the past (Stover *et al.* 2003). Feelings may surface in the form of political tensions, impacting on the ability to undertake search and recovery, and resulting in confusion or disagreement between local, national and international authorities as to what should be done, when, and how. Those who shout loudest may end up with greatest influence, and there may be delicate balances between local concepts of justice and revenge (Steele 2008, 418). At such times the ill-considered imposition of Western values may be neither appropriate nor welcome. In all this the role of the archaeologist has to remain constant: objective, scientific and competent, albeit piggy-in-the-middle.

Archaeologists may find themselves working in a physically hostile environment, under tight security and with limited resources. This may be exacerbated in theatre: Hunter and Simpson (2007) have recounted the logistics involved of searching for mass graves in Iraq together with an outline of the personal danger involved, prohibitively high life insurance cover essential for those with families, and the potential for daily disruption or cancellation of operations on the basis of intelligence or perceived threats.

It is unlikely that access to the remains will occur immediately after cessation of hostilities, not least as a result of security issues caused by the ongoing nature of the conflict or instability in its wake. Other issues such as local politics, landscape change, availability of resources or the scale of the search and recovery operation may also have an impact not only on the time lapse between burial and recovery, but also on the commensurate state of decomposition of the remains. Moreover, the longer the elapsed time since burial, the greater the potential of post-burial disturbance such as looting or animal scavenging.

Changes of this nature are difficult to estimate, particularly in some earlier conflicts (e.g. World War I) where almost a century has passed since disposal.

Oddly, the lessons learnt and techniques developed in the course of modern war crime investigations have not always been adopted in the examination of graves from socio-historic conflicts, despite similarities between the issues involved in both. There is a strange dichotomy here that cannot simply be waved aside by the absence of any potential legal proceedings due to the interval of time concerned. Victims from earlier battle graves are archaeological and anonymous, those of modern genocide are contemporary and identifiable. Others sit somewhere in between, in some no-man's land of cultural memory, not quite history yet, but too far back in time to be remembered properly.

Examples are not uncommon, particularly among the large number of serendipitous discoveries of multiple burials made throughout Europe relating to the massacres of World War II. Many of these occurred as a result of natural or man-made landscape changes which tend to go hand in hand with large construction programmes. As such the fate of the disturbed burials lies in the hands of local communities and politicians, and among the interests of developers. There is no international body that takes responsibility for their investigation because the remains do not belong to a conflict that is contemporary. Nor is there any guarantee that appropriate archaeological or anthropological provision will be applied. Remains discovered in Poland at Gvozdavka-1 were 'immediately shovelled back into the ground', whilst at Malbork, also in Poland, skeletal elements were recovered using shovels and transported in wheelbarrows (BBC 2007). In Menden-Barge, Germany, remains were subject to DNA analysis and identification, whilst in Budapest, Hungary, although the remains were not recovered archaeologically during building work, an anthropological analysis was carried out nonetheless (Reuters 2006; Susa 2007). In none of these was more than forensic or humanitarian lip-service given to the victims, and it is difficult to understand why. Perhaps the remains were just too old? There are also those who would wish to forget the war, or who have no interest in, or affiliation to, the events and who resent the repeated references to crimes against humanity and view attempts to examine burial sites with contempt. For example, Paperno (2001, 107) cites the comments of Maryna Shleimovych, a local resident interviewed in the course of archaeological investigations into World War II Soviet atrocities:

> Here you are again with your graves! History has stuffed the whole earth with corpses! What do we have to do with this? Yes, I know that they shot people here once upon a time, but this was a long time ago, and I like strolling here.

This stands in sharp contrast to feelings in some other places, notably in the Ukraine where, in the course of a recent survey of mass grave sites it was observed that 'people talk as if these things happened yesterday, as if 60 years didn't exist' (Faith in Focus 2008, 1). In areas such as this where the desire to locate victims is most prominent, the means and resources to do so are unlikely to be available, as such it may fall to external organisations or individuals to carry out such investigations. Equally, the recent exhumations in Fromelles, of victims of World War I, gained a prolific reaction from members of the public, whilst relatives of those identified were able to gain answers to questions that had remained for the past 80 years (CWGC 2009).

Of course, for some it is often simply the case that 'the past is too near and too painful' (Polonsky and Michlic 2004, 43). They are unable, or not yet ready, to confront the events that occurred. In some instances the nature of the crimes committed has led to fear amongst witnesses with regards to identifying perpetrators, even though a considerable amount of time has elapsed (Bevan 1994). The locations of many mass graves may be known but not divulged; retaining their secrecy also serves to repress the memories that accompany them (Schmitt 2002, 2). Similarly, the lawyers involved in the Serniki case were attacked with acid, whilst the defendant was shot in the street, demonstrating the resonance that the Holocaust still has in modern society (Bevan 1994). It seems that the victims are still remembered, the survivors are still witnesses and the perpetrators are still feared. Conversely, when Ratko Mladic, known as the 'Butcher of Bosnia' and the army commander allegedly responsible for the murder of 7000 Bosnian males at Srebenica, was arrested in May 2011, he was given public demonstrations of support in Serbia. The war of the 1990s may have been long over but the ethnic differences still remained.

8.5 Politics and Religion

Where there has been state involvement in acts of genocide or human rights abuse, political pressure can often constrain the level of investigation or even prevent it altogether. In Zimbabwe, the current government has refused to acknowledge its involvement in atrocities and has prevented the implementation of thorough search strategies (Egaña *et al.* 2008). In Spain, criticism has been levied at the government for manipulating the results of a Civil War excavation for the purpose of proving that identification of victims was impossible. This has resulted in severe restrictions being placed on exhumations of other Civil War grave sites (Ballbé and Steadman 2008). Nor is there often a transparent process of responsibility: do the graves simply fall under the jurisdiction of a municipal planning authority, are they viewed as a legal evidential resource, or are they embraced as a new component of the cultural heritage landscape? Who presides and who decides?

As well as direct restrictions on the activities of field teams, the results of such investigations have also been used in political campaigns. For example, it has been argued that exhumations lend themselves to propaganda and, in the case of the former Yugoslavia, the memorial to Holocaust victims placed upon one mass grave led to the conflict in the 1990s (Skinner *et al.* 2002, 297). In the past, in Poland, any attempts to recover victims of the Holocaust who were not of a Catholic affiliation have been deemed 'anti-Polish' by the government (Polonsky and Michlic 2004, 9). These issues are clearly far beyond the control of archaeologists or anthropologists, but awareness of them is needed in order to be able to function effectively.

That said, political factors can also incite the search for mass graves. In Russia, the first systematic search to locate the victims of Stalin's purges using archaeological techniques was undertaken in the 1990s to mark the end of the old political regime. Paperno suggests that the end of the Communism allowed people to finally express sensitivities which may previously been suppressed – 'a deeply ingrained cultural tradition that associates the remains of the dead with a sense of collective identity, collective memory, and a promise of redemption' (2001, 90). A similar trend can be noted with reference to Holocaust mass graves in the Ukraine, where the end of Soviet domination led to an upsurge in interest in identifying graves before knowledge of their location passed from living memory (Faith in Focus 2008; Wright *et al.* 2005; see also Section 8.6 below). In many socio-historical cases, significant political controls such as these may go some way to explain the time lapse between disposals and exhumation. Even when political restrictions are lifted, a further delay still seems to occur before it is deemed acceptable to examine the physical evidence. Several organisations have recently been established in former eastern bloc countries to investigate the crimes against humanity that occurred during the 20th century, in particular during World War II. These include: the Commission of the Historians of Latvia; the Commission on Concealed Mass Graves in Slovenia; the Estonian International Commission for Investigation of Crimes against Humanity, and the Institute of National Remembrance in Poland. However, in some cases, for example in Latvia, it was not until 1998 that it was finally deemed suitable to conduct historical research into the occupation by the Soviets and the Nazis (Commission of the Historians of Latvia 2001). It is likely to be a long time before initiatives are taken to locate the mass graves relating to these events.

In other cases, issues such as the economic and social climate, as well as religious attitudes towards the dead, may influence field methodologies, not only in terms of the exhumation of victims but in terms of their reburial after the investigations have been completed (Sturdy 2008 and Sturdy Colls 2012b). For example, the examination of Holocaust Jewish burials has been limited owing to the restrictions on the disturbance of the dead set out in Halacha Law. The statutes of Hinduism in India with regards to burning the body immediately after death resulted, in some cases, in an inability of post-Tsunami investigators to provide formal identity of the victims according to international protocols (Perera and Briggs 2008; Pan American Health Organisation 2006). Additionally the involvement of local communities in burying victims from the Tsunami, in Sri Lanka and Thailand, in shallow mass burials close to settlements inhibited identification on the basis of public health concerns (Tsokos *et al.* 2006; Perera and Briggs 2008).

8.6 Archives for history

What is clear from the above is that the investigation of mass graves involves a complex of political, cultural and strategic issues; it is also clear that the longer the time interval between deposition and recovery, the harder it is to draw together the strands that place the event in a wider historical context. By contrast, the investigation of individual criminal graves is logistically more straightforward and unilaterally administered: in most UK police forces crime scene operations slide smoothly into place; facilities, equipment and specialists are organised, and well-rehearsed processes are followed. But within mass grave investigations there may be inherent problems through a combination of political tensions, bureaucracy, difficulties in communication and some lack of awareness. Unsurprisingly, therefore, some modern technical developments widely used in other relevant fields are likely to be under-utilised as a result of resourcing, or may not even be recognised as appropriate. The implications of this are considerable: not only does it incur delay, it can also limit the efficacy of the recovery programme and affect the accuracy of the historical record. During victim recovery the need to create archival records is hardly at the forefront of priorities, but it is the records that survive and that serve to underpin the history when all else is forgotten. There are clear lessons to be learnt from earlier crimes against humanity, even recent ones, where prosecutions are now unviable, investigations incomplete, witness accounts lost, and where events have slid out of memory.

The best example is undoubtedly the Holocaust. Millions of individuals from specific ethnic groups and other social minorities, as well as political prisoners, are known to have been systematically murdered across Europe around the time of World War II (Marrus 2000; Friedlander 1997). The debates are well embedded in the historical discourse of the period with a multitude of texts focusing on the nature of the 'Final Solution', Nazi political and social policy, and especially on assessing the scale of, and responsibility for, genocide (Goldhagen 1996). Discussion has also permeated a range of other disciplines, from psychology (Yehuda *et al.* 1997) and demography (Gilbert 2002) to heritage management (Young 1994; Beech 2000) and modern politics (Skinner *et al.* 2002), thus offering new insights into the crimes that took place.

Yet, the totality of different sites from this period has never been fully identified, mapped, recorded or examined; in fact they have never been integrated into the documented history of the 20th century. This physical evidence consists of hidden remains of concentration, labour and transit camps, ghettos and mass graves, totalling thousands. Despite the fact that a substantial number of Holocaust sites exist, only a handful of fieldwork investigations have ever been undertaken. At mass grave sites, many investigations have been incomplete, often utilising inappropriate techniques and seldom integrated with archaeologists.

Immediately after the Holocaust, a number of War Crimes Commissions were set up across Europe to investigate the extent and nature of the atrocities. These commissions were required to collect evidence for use at the International Military Tribunal at Nuremberg where the intention was the prosecution of offenders, regardless of their domicile (IMTN 1947). Such investigations were often carried out by local authorities or by a specially assembled group of medico-legal professionals but, given the scale of the atrocities, the purpose of these investigations was to compile a general report for each area about the likely scale of the killings and potential perpetrators (Arad *et al.* 1999). The majority of these investigations had a regional or even national remit but the reports were often based on a sample of smaller, localised areas. The work conducted was a response to immediate issues of generality for the purposes of conviction, not the detailed records of places and events that might serve to mould history. These investigations have undoubtedly contributed to the perception that this period has been 'dealt with' in terms of an examination of the physical evidence relating to it. This offers one explanation as to why relatively few examinations have been carried out since.

More recently, whilst an increased number of investigations by archaeologists have been carried out at Holocaust sites (Golden 2003; Gilead *et al.* 2009; Schute and Wijnen 2010; Theune 2010; Sturdy Colls 2012a), investigations of mass grave landscapes are few in number. The need to comply with Jewish Halacha Law, which discourages the disturbance of human remains (and thus the use of invasive methods), has seen only a handful of isolated grave sites across Europe being examined (Kola 2000; Bevan 1994; Gross 2004; Desbois 2008). The latter were most commonly in response to potential legal proceedings, hence why invasive work was permitted, although these activities have sometimes heightened hostility with the Jewish community. More commonly, mass graves have been excavated as a result of serendipitous discoveries due to man-made or natural landscape modification and, only occasionally, have archaeologists been contacted to excavate them (Susa 2007). Some studies of Holocaust sites have leapt straight from historical research to excavation;

few have utilised the range of available techniques now employed as standard practice in archaeological or forensic archaeological investigations (Hunter and Cox 2005, 28; Sturdy Colls 2012c; Sturdy Colls and Colls in press). The majority have one thing in common – they were reactive investigations, either to political events, land development, or legal pressure. Given the enormity of the genocide and suffering witnessed at these sites, it remains a salutary reflection of modern society that such little investigation has taken place.

On a different front, absence of any proper understanding of these sites, and lack of relevant scientifically derived data, has served to fuel the claims of Holocaust deniers who suggest that these events never happened. The sociological justification for application is well-founded: although Haglund's criteria for identifying mass grave sites from modern conflict look towards invasive action in the collection of evidence to prosecute offenders and identify victims, they also recognise the need to 'create a document that should stand up to historical revisionists' (2002, 245; also Section 8.3 above).

Finally, there is a further issue – the commemoration of the dead. There is considerable diversity in the way that Holocaust sites are commemorated (Sturdy 2012a). For example, whilst Auschwitz-Birkenau is well-maintained, managed as a tourist site hosting over one million visitors a year, and is designated a World Heritage site, the majority of other sites are poorly maintained, receive only a handful of visitors and have modest memorial plaques (Sweibocka 1995). In a significant number of cases sites are not marked at all, mass graves remain unlocated, and knowledge of these events slowly disappears from living memory (Figure 8.6). Whether or not this situation changes in the future remains to be seen and will likely be influenced by politics, economics and generational shifts in the

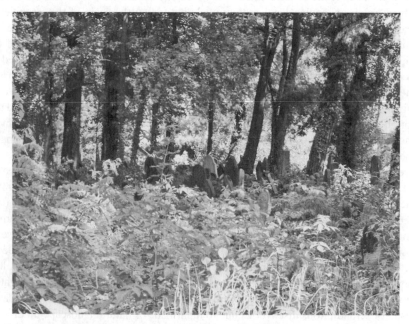

Figure 8.6 A dilapidated Jewish cemetery in Poland – one of thousands used as an execution site by the Nazis during the Holocaust.

perceived importance of sites. Non-invasive archaeological methods offer new possibilities for the location of sites in the future. However, if the number of investigations is to increase, methodologies must account for the complexities of the context in which they are being undertaken.

Elsewhere, the memorial at Srebrenica provides some reassurance that conflict and genocide can be recorded for posterity, in the same way that the American cemetery in Normandy or the Argentinean cemetery in the Falkland Islands focus on a collective event rather than the single elements of which they are composed. But it is, of course, the individual physical components – the graves, camps, execution sites and prisons – that provide the physical historical detail, and that is where the archaeological fieldwork, both non-invasive and invasive, has a key role to play in contributing to historical narratives and facilitating commemoration. When examining socio-historic events, archaeologists may no longer be forensic pioneers in a legal sense, but they have a responsibility to record such crimes and to create an archive for future generations.

Bibliography

ACPO (Association of Chief Police Officers). 2006. *Practice Advice on Search Management and Procedures*. Bramshill, Hook: NPIA (National Centre for Policing Excellence). Restricted.

ACPO (Association of Chief Police Officers). 2010. *Guidance on the Management, Recording and Investigation of Missing Persons*. Bramshill, Hook: NPIA (National Centre for Policing Excellence). Restricted.

ACPO (Association of Chief Police Officers). 2011a. *Police Search Management – Missing Persons*. Bramshill, Hook: NPIA (National Centre for Policing Excellence). Restricted.

ACPO (Association of Chief Police Officers). 2011b. *Police Dogs Manual of Guidance*. Powys: ACPO.

AFAT (Argentine Forensic Anthropology Team: Equipo Argentino de Anthropologia Forense). 2007. *Annual Report: Covering the Period January to December 2006*. Buenos Aires: EAAF.

Ainsworth, S. and Thomason, B. 2003. *Where on Earth are We?* Swindon: English Heritage.

Akulova, V., Vasiliauskiene, D. and Talaliene, D. 2002. 'Further insights into the persistence of transferred fibres on outdoor clothes', *Science & Justice* 42, 165–71.

Albicht, M. J. 2010. 'Using wartime aerial photographs to locate lost grave sites', in Cowley, D. C. *et al.* (eds.) 2010b, 263–65.

Amendt, J., Campobasso, C. P., Gaudry, E., *et al.* 2007. 'Best practice in forensic entomology - standards and guidelines', *International Journal of Legal Medicine* 121, 90–104.

ANBG (Association of Natural Burial Grounds). 2011. *Code of Conduct*. Winchester: The Natural Death Centre.

Anderson, G. S. 2010. 'Decomposition and invertebrate colonization of cadavers in coastal marine environments', in Amendt, J., *et al.* (eds.), *Current Concepts in Forensic Entomology*. Springer: Netherlands, 223–72.

Anderson, G. S. 2011. 'Comparison of decomposition rates and faunal colonisation of carrion in indoor and outdoor environments', *Journal of Forensic Sciences* 56:1, 136–42.

Andrews, P. 1995. 'Experiments in taphonomy', *Journal of Archaeological Science* 22:2, 147–53.

Arad, Y., Gutman, I. and Margaliot, A. (eds.). 1999. *Documents on the Holocaust: Selected sources on the destruction of the Jews of Germany, Austria, Poland, and the Soviet Union* (8th edition). London: University of Nebraska Press.

Arner, P., Bernard, S., Salehpour, M., *et al.* 2011. 'Dynamics of human adipose lipid turnover in health and metabolic disease', *Nature* 478, 110–13.

Anđelinoviæ, S., Sutloviæ, D., Ivkošiæ, I. E., *et al.* 2005. 'Twelve-year experience in identification of skeletal remains from mass graves', *Croatian Medical Journal* 46:4, 530–39.

Auerbach, R. 1979. 'In the fields of Treblinka' in Donat, A. (ed.), *The Death Camp Treblinka: A Documentary*, New York: Schocken Books, 19–73.

Bailey, J. W. 1990. 'The archaeological water separation machine in fire investigation', *Journal of Forensic Sciences* 35:1, 1201–06.

Baldwin, H. B. and May, C. P. 2000. 'Crime scene investigation and examination: Contamination', in Siegel, J. A., *et al.* (eds.), 412–16.

Ballbé, E. G. and Steadman, D. W. 2008. 'The political, social and scientific contexts of archaeological investigations of mass graves in Spain', in Starzmann, M. T., Pollock, S., and Bernbeck, R. (eds.), Imperial Inspections: Archaeology, War and Violence. *Archaeologies: Journal of the World Archaeological Congress* 4:3, 429–44.

BBC. 2007. British Broadcasting Corporation. 'Ukrainian mass Jewish grave found', [WWW] http://news. bbc.co.uk/1/hi/world/europe/6724481.stm (Accessed January 2008).

Beck, A. 2011. 'Archaeological applications of multi/hyper-spectral data – challenges and potential' in Cowley, D. C. (ed.) 2011b, 87–97.

Beder, J. 2002. 'Mourning the unfound: how can we help', *Families in Society: The Journal of Contemporary Human Services* 83:4, 400–3.

Beech, J. 2000. 'The enigma of holocaust sites as tourist attractions - the case of Buchenwald', *Managing Leisure* 5:1, 29–41.

Berryman, H. E. 2002. 'Disarticulation pattern and tooth mark artifacts associated with pig scavenging of human remains: a case study' in Haglund, W. D. and Sorg, M. H. (eds.) 2002a, 487–96.

Bevan, B. 1994. *A Case To Answer: The Story of Australia's First European War Crimes Prosecution.* Adelaide: Wakefield Press.

Bewley, R. H. 2006. 'Aerial survey for archaeology', in Hunter, J. R. and Ralston, I. B. M. (eds.), 276–91.

Bewley, R. H., Crutchley, S. P. and Shell, C. 2005. 'New light on ancient landscape: lidar survey in the Stonehenge World Heritage Site', *Antiquity* 79, 636–47.

Bianco, C. and Monckton, L. 2006. 'Ecclesiastical buildings in use' in Hunter, J. R. and Ralston, I. B. M. (eds.), 110–30.

Blackledge, R. D. (ed.). 2007. *Forensic Analysis on the Cutting Edge: New Methods or Trace Evidence Analysis.* New Jersey: Wiley.

Blau, S. 2009. 'More than just bare bones: Ethical considerations for forensic anthropologists' in Blau, S. and Ubelaker, D. (eds.), 457–67.

Blau, S. and Ubelaker, D. (eds.). 2009. *Handbook of Forensic Archaeology and Anthropology.* World Archaeological Congress Research Handbooks. Walnut Creek: Left Coast Press.

Bock, J. H. and Norris, D. O. 1997. 'Forensic botany: An under-utilised resource', *Journal of Forensic Sciences* 42:3, 364–67.

Bonnichsen, R. 1973. 'Millie's Camp: An experiment in archaeology', *World Archaeology* 4, 277–91.

Brickley, M. B. 2007. 'A case of disposal of a body through burning and recent advances in the study of burned human remains', in Brickley, M. and Ferlini, R. (eds.), 69–85.

Brickley, M. and Ferlini, R. (eds.). 2007. *Forensic Anthropology: Case Studies From Europe.* Springfield: Charles C. Thomas.

Brickley, M. and McKinley, J. I. (eds.) 2004. *Guidelines to the Standards for Recording Human Remains.* IfA Paper No. 7. Southampton: BABAO.

Brooks, S. and Brooks, R. H. 1997. 'The taphonomic effects of flood waters on bone' in Haglund, W. D. and Sorg, M. H. (eds.), 553–57.

Brothwell, D. and Gill-Robinson, H. 2002. 'Taphonomic and forensic aspects of bog bodies' in Haglund, W. and Sorg H. (eds.) 2002a, 119–32.

Brown, A. G., Smith, A. and Elmhirst, O. 2002. 'The combined use of pollen and soil analyses in a search and subsequent murder investigation', *Journal of Forensic Sciences* 47:3, 614–18.

Buck, S. C. 2003. 'Searching for graves using geophysical technology: Field tests with ground penetrating radar, magnetometry, and electrical resistivity', *Journal of Forensic Sciences* 48:1, 5–11.

Budd, P., Montgomery, J., Barreiro, B. and Thomas, R. G. 2000. 'Differential diagenesis of strontium in archaeological human dental tissues', *Applied Geochemistry* 15:5, 687–94.

Bunch, A. W. 2010. 'Indoor wet screening of exhumed skeletal remains: A suggested procedure for the preparation of fragile evidence for anthropological analysis', *Journal of Forensic Sciences* 55:4, 1102–4.

Burrough, P. and McDonnell, R. 1998. *Principles of Geographic Information Systems.* Oxford: Oxford University Press.

Butler, K. 2012. *Determining the Presence of Manganese in Discoloured Skeletal Remains from St James Church, Stoke on Trent, Using Scanning Electron Microscope Techniques.* Unpublished BA Thesis, Staffordshire University.

Byers, S. 2003. *Introduction to Forensic Anthropology.* London: Pearson.

Byers, S. N. 2011. *Introduction to Forensic Anthropology.* London: Pearson.

Byrd, J. H. and Castner, J. L. (eds.). 2001. *Entomological Evidence: The Utility of Arthropods in Legal Investigations.* Boca Raton: CRC Press.

Cabalk, M. E. and Sagebiel, J. C. 2011. 'Field capability of dogs to locate individual human teeth', *Journal of Forensic Sciences* 56:4, 1–7.

Caccianiga, M., Bottacin, S. and Cattaneo, C. 2012. 'Vegetation dynamics as a tool for detecting clandestine graves', *Journal of Forensic Sciences*. DOI: 10.1111/j.1556-4029.2012.02071.x.

Cammack, J. A., Adler, P. H., Tomberlin, J. K., *et al.* 2010. 'Influence of parasitism and soil compaction on pupation the green bottle fly, Lucilia sericata', *Entomologia Expermentalis et Applicata*. 136, 134–41.

Canter, D. 2000. 'Offender Profiling and Criminal Differentiation', *Legal and Criminal Psychology* 5, 23–46.

Canter, D. 2003. *Mapping Murder*. London: Virgin Books.

Canter, D. 2004. 'Geographical Profiling of Criminals', *Medico-Legal Journal* 72:2, 53–66.

Cardoso, H. V., Puentes, K., Monge Soares, A., *et al.* 2011. 'The value of radiocarbon analysis in determining the forensic interest of human skeletal remains found in unusual circumstances', *Journal of Forensic and Legal Medicine* 30, 1–4.

Carson, E. A., Stefan, V. H. and Powell, J. F. 2000. 'Skeletal manifestations of bear scavenging', *Journal of Forensic Sciences* 43:3, 515–26.

Carver, M. O. H. 2009. *Archaeological Investigation*. London: Routledge.

Catts Jr., E. P. and Haskell, N. H. (eds.). 1999. *Entomology & Death – A Procedural Guide*. Clemson, South Carolina: Joyce's Print Shop.

Chainey, S. and Ratcliffe, J. 2005. *GIS and Crime Mapping*. Chichester: Wiley.

Challis, K., Howard, A. J., Kincey, M. and Carey, C. 2008. *Analysis of the Effectiveness of Airborne Lidar Backscattered Laser Intensity for Predicting Organic Preservation Potential of Waterlogged Deposits*. ALSF Project 4782, Institute of Archaeology and Antiquity, University of Birmingham.

Ch'ng, E., Stone, R. J. and Arvanitis, T. N. 2005. 'A virtual reality archaeological framework for the investigation and interpretation of ancient landscapes', *European Internet and Multimedia Systems and Applications* 462, 144–46.

Chapman, H. 2006. *Landscape Archaeology and GIS*. Stroud: Tempus.

Charabidze, D., Bourel, B. and Gosset, D. 2011. 'Larval mass effect: characterisation of heat emission by necrophagus blowflies (Diptera: Calliphoridae) larval aggregates, *Forensic Science International* 211:1–3, 61–6.

Cheetham, P. 2005. 'Forensic geophysical survey', in Hunter, J. R. and Cox. M, 62–95.

Cheetham, P. and Hanson, I. 2009. 'Excavation and recovery in forensic archaeological investigations' in Blau, S. and Ubelaker, D. (eds.), 141–49.

Chudley, R. and Greeno, R. 2004. *Building Construction Handbook* (5th edition). Oxford: Elsevier Butterworth-Heinemann.

Chudley, R. and Greeno, R. 2005. *Construction Technology* (3rd edition). Harlow: Pearson Education.

Clark, A. J. 1996. *Seeing Beneath the Soil: Prospecting Methods in Archaeology* (2nd edition). London: Batsford.

Clark, M. A. 1988. *Meles meles*. London: Whittet Books.

Clark, M. A., Worrell, M. B, and Pless, J. E. 1997. 'Postmortem changes in soft tissues' in Haglund, W. and Sorg, H. (eds.), 151–64.

Clarke, M. D. 2011. 'Toolmark identification of a mattock to a clod of soil from a grave', *Journal of Forensic Sciences* 56:1, 241–43.

CNN. 2001 Cable News Network. 'Polish mass grave dig ends'. [WWW] http://edition.cnn.com/2001/WORLD/europe/06/04/poland.grave/index.html?_s=PM:WORLD (Accessed April 2013).

Commission of the Historians of Latvia. 2001. *The Progress Report of Latvia's History Commission: Crimes against Humanity Committed in the Territory of Latvia from 1940 to 1956 during the Occupations of the Soviet Union and National Socialist Germany*. Latvia: Wakefield Press.

CONADEP (Comisión Nacional sobre la Desaparición de Personas/The National Commission on the Disappearance of Persons). 1986. *Nuncas Más (Never Again): Report of Conadep (The National Commission on the Disappearance of Persons)*. London and New York: CONADEP.

Conyers, L. B. and Goodman, D. 1997. *Ground-Penetrating Radar: An Introduction for Archgaeologists*. Walnut Creek: Alta Mira Press.

Cook, T. and Tattersall, A. 2008. *Blackstone's Senior Investigating Officer's Handbook*. Oxford: Oxford University Press.

Cooke, R. A. and Ide, R. H. 1985. *Principles of Fire Investigation*. Leicester: Institution of Fire Engineers.

Corns, A., Fenwick, J. and Shaw, R. 2008. 'More than meets the eye', *Archaeology Ireland* 22: 3 (85), 34–8.

Cowley, D. C. 2011a. 'Remote sensing for archaeology and heritage management – site discovery, inter-pretation and registration' in Cowley, D. C. (ed.), 43–55.

Cowley, D. C. (ed.). 2011b. *Remote Sensing for Archaeological Heritage Management*. Occasional Publi-cation of the Aerial Archaeology Research Group No. 3. Brussels: Europae Archaeologiae Consilium.

Cowley, D. C., Standring, R. A. and Albicht, M. J. 2010a. 'Landscapes through the lens, an introduction', in Cowley, D. C. *et al.* (eds.), 1–6.

Cowley, D. C., Standring, R. A. and Albicht, M. J. (eds.). 2010b. *Landscapes through the Lens: Aerial Photography and Historic Environment*. Oxford: Oxbow.

Cox, M. 2001a. 'Forensic Archaeology in the UK: Questions of socio-intellectual context and socio-political responsibility' in Buchli, V. and Lucas, G. (eds.), *Archaeologies of the Contemporary Past*. London: Routledge, 145–57.

Cox, M. 2001b. *Crypt Archaeology: An Approach*, IFA Technical Paper No. 3. Reading: Institute of Field Archaeologists.

Cox, M. 2009. Forensic archaeology and anthropology: Past and Present – A United Kingdom perspective' in Blau, S. and Ubelaker, D. (eds.), 29–41.

Cox, M., and Bell, L. 1999. 'Recovery of human skeletal elements from a recent UK murder enquiry: Preservational signatures', *Journal of Forensic Sciences* 44:5, 945–50.

Cox, M., Flavel, A., Hanson, I., *et al.* (eds.). 2007. *The Scientific Investigation of Mass Graves: Towards Protocols and Standard Operating Procedures*. Cambridge: Cambridge University Press.

Coyle, H. M. 2004. *Forensic Botany: Principles and Applications to Criminal Casework*. Boca Raton: CRC Press.

Coyle, T. 2010. 'Trace and contact evidence', in White, P. (ed.), 106–26.

Crow, P., Benham, S., Devereux, B. J. and Amable, G. S. 2007. 'Woodland vegetation and its implications for archaeological survey using LIDaR', *Forestry* 80, 241–52.

Crutchley, S. and Crow, P. 2009. *The Light Fantastic: Using Airborne Laser Scanning in Archaeological Survey*. Swindon: English Heritage.

Cullingworth, B. and Nadin, V. (eds.). 2002. *Town and Country Planning in the UK* (13th edition). London: Routledge.

Cunningham, S. L., Kirkland, S. A. and Ross, A. H. 2011. 'Bone Weathering of Juvenile-Sized Remains in the North Carolina Piedmont' in Ross, A. H. and Abel, S. M. (eds.), *The Juvenile Skeleton in Forensic Abuse Investigations*. New York: Humana Press, 179–96.

CWGC. 2009. Commonwealth War Graves Commission. [WWW] http://www.cwgc.org (Accessed April 2013).

Davenport, G. C. 2001. 'Remote sensing applications in forensic investigations', *Journal of Historical Archaeology* 35:1, 87–100.

Davis, J., Heginbottom, J., Annan, A., *et al.* 2000. 'GPR surveys to locate 1918 Spanish flu victims in permafrost', *Journal of Forensic Sciences* 45:1, 68–76.

DCLG (Department for Communities and Local Government). 2004. Planning Policy Statement 23: Plan-ning and Pollution Control (PPS 23). London: HMSO.

DCLG (Department for Communities and Local Government). 2007. The Validation of Planning Applica-tions: Guidance for local planning authorities. London: HMSO.

DCLG (Department for Communities and Local Government). 2008. Planning Policy Statement 12: Local Spatial Planning (PPS 12). London: HMSO.

DCLG (Department for Communities and Local Government). 2010. Planning Policy Statement 5: Planning for the Historic Environment (PPS 5). London: HMSO.

DCLG (Department for Communities and Local Government). 2011a. Planning Policy Guidance (PPG) and Planning Policy Statements (PPS). London: HMSO.

DCLG (Department for Communities and Local Government). 2011b. Planning Policy Statement 3: Hous-ing (PPS 3). London: HMSO.

DCLG (Department for Communities and Local Government). 2011c. [WWW] DCLG corporate site homepage. http://www.communities.gov.uk/corporate/ (Accessed August 2011).

DCLG (Department for Communities and Local Government). 2012. National Planning Policy Frame-work. Available online: [WWW] http://www.communities.gov.uk/planningandbuilding/planningsystem/planningpolicy/planningpolicyframework (Accessed April 2013).

De Vos, H., Jongerden, J. and Van Etten, J. 2008. 'Images of war: Using satellite images for human rights monitoring in Turkish Kurdistan', *Disasters* 32:3, 449–66.

DEFRA (Department for Environment, Food and Rural Affairs). 1996. *Waste Management - The Duty of Care - A Code of Practice*. London: HMSO.

DEFRA (Department for Environment, Food and Rural Affairs). 2008. UK Data required by EU Waste Statistics Regulation (EC 2150/2002) for 2006 compiled by DEFRA on behalf of the United Kingdom; sent to Eurostat in June 2008. [WWW] Available online: http://archive.defra.gov.uk/evidence/statistics/environment/waste/wreuwastestats.htm (Accessed April 2013).

DEFRA (Department for Environment, Food and Rural Affairs). 2010. *The Environmental Permitting (England and Wales) Regulations*. London: DEFRA.

Dehaan, J. D. and D. J. Icove. 2012. *Kirk's Fire Investigation* (7th edition). New Jersey: Pearson.

Desbois, P. 2008. *The Holocaust by Bullets: A Priest's Journey to Uncover the Truth behind the Murder of 1.5 Million Jews*. Basingstoke: Palgrave Macmillan.

Devereux, B. J., Amable, G. S., Crow, P. and Cliff, A. D. 2005. 'The potential of airborne LIDaR for the detection of archaeological features under woodland canopies', *Antiquity* 78, 648–60.

Dickson, G. C., Poulter, R. T. M., Maas, E. W., *et al.* 2011. 'Marine bacterial succession as a potential indicator of post-mortem submersion interval', *Forensic Science International* 209:1–3, 1–10.

Dilley, R. 2005. 'Legal Matters' in Hunter, J. R. and Cox. M., 177–203.

Dirkmaat, D.C. (ed.) 2012. *A Companion to Forensic Anthropology*. Chichester: Wiley-Blackwell.

Dix, J. 2000. *Time of Death, Decomposition and Identification: An Atlas*. Boca Raton: CRC Press.

DOE and DNH (Department of the Environment and Department of National Heritage). 1994. Planning Policy Guidance Note 15: Planning and the Historic Environment. London: DoE and DHN.

Doneus, M. and Briese, C. 2011. 'Airborne laser scanning in forested areas – potential and limitations of an archaeological prospection technique' in Cowley, D.C. (ed.) 2011b, 59–76.

Donnelly, L. J. and Harrison, M. 2010. *Geomorphological and Geoforensic Interpretation of Maps, Aerial Imagery, Conditions of Diggability and the Colour Coded RAG Prioritisation System in Searches for Criminal Burials*. 3rd International Workshop on Criminal & Environmental Soil Forensics, 2-4 November 2010, Long Beach, California.

Doretti, M. and Fondebrider, L. 2001. 'Science and human rights: Truth, justice, reparation and reconciliation, a long way in Third World Countries' in Buchli, V. and Lucas, G. (eds.), *Archaeologies of the Contemporary Past*. London: Routledge, 138–44.

Dupras, T. L., Schwartz, J. J., Wheeler, S. M. and Williams, L. J. 2008. *Forensic Recovery of Human Remains: Archaeological Approaches*. Boca Raton: CRC Press.

Efremov, I. 1940. 'Taphonomy: New branch of paleontology', *Pan American Geologist* 74, 81–93.

Egaña, S., Turner, S., Doretti, M., *et al.* 2008. *Commingled Human Remains and Human Rights Investigations*. Totowa: Humana Press, 57–80.

English Heritage. 2002. *Environmental Archaeology: A guide to the theory and practice of methods, from sampling and recovery to post-excavation*. Swindon: English Heritage.

English Heritage. 2011. *Paradise Preserved: Registered cemeteries in date order with notes on principal reasons for designation and designers and architects*. Available online: http//:www.english-heritage.org.uk/professional/advice/advice-by-topic/parks-and-gardens. (Accessed April 2013).

English, J. and Card, R. 1999. *Butterworth's Police Law* (6th edition). London: Butterworths.

Erzinçlioglu, Y. Z. 2000. *Maggots, Murder and Men: Memories and Reflections of a Forensic Entomologist*. Colchester: Harley Books.

EU (European Union). 2002. *Official Journal of the European Communities L332/1 – Regulation (EC) No. 2150/2002 of the European Parliament and of Council (of 25 November, 2002) on Waste Statistics*. Brussels: European Parliament.

Evans, J. and O'Connor, T. 2000. *Environmental Archaeology: Principles and Methods*. Stroud: Sutton Publishing.

Faith in Focus. 2008. [WWW] http://faithinfocus.wordpress.com/2008/02/22/french-priesthelps-find-800-mass-graves-from-holocaust-in-ukraine/ (Accessed 23rd June 2008).

Fairgreave, S. I. 2008. *Forensic Cremation: Recovery and Analysis*. Boca Raton: CRC Press.

Farren, T. M. 2004. *A Study into how Behavioural Science might focus the Search for Human Remains*. Unpublished MPhil thesis, University of Birmingham, UK.

Fenning, P. J. and Donnelly, L. J. 2004. 'Geophysical techniques for forensic investigation', in Pye, K. and Croft, D. J. (eds.), 11–20.

Ferguson, L. 2011. 'Aerial archives for archaeological heritage management: The aerial reconnaissance archive – a shared European resource', in Cowley, D. C. (eds.) 2011b, 205–12.

Fiedler, S., Illich, B., Berger, J. and Graw, M. 2009. 'The effectiveness of ground-penetrating radar surveys in the location of unmarked burial sites in modern cemeteries' *Journal of Applied Geophysics* 68, 38–385.

Field. S. 2007. '"No-one has allowed me to cry": Trauma, memorialisation and children in post-genocide Rwanda', in Purbrick, L. Aulich, J. and Dawson, G. (eds.), *Contested Spaces: Sites, Representations and Histories of Conflict*. Basingstoke: Palgrave Macmillan, 211–32.

Forbes, S. L. 2008. 'Decomposition chemistry in a burial environment', in Tibbett, M. and Carter, D. O. (eds.), 203–46.

France, D. L., Griffin, T. J., Swanburg, J. G., *et al.* 1992. 'A multidisciplinary approach to the detection of clandestine graves', *Journal of Forensic Science* 37:6, 1445–58.

France, D. L., Griffin, T. J., Swanburg, J. G., *et al.* 1997. 'Necrosearch revisited: Further multidisciplinary approaches to the detection of clandestine graves' in Haglund, W. and Sorg, H. (eds.), 497–509.

Francis, B., Barry, J., Bowater, R., *et al.* 2004. *Using Homicide Data to Assist Murder Investigations*. London: HMSO.

Fraser, D. 1978. *The Evolution of the British Welfare State*. London: MacMillan.

Friedlander, S. 1997. *The Years of Persecution, 1933–1939*. London: Harper Collins.

Froidevaux, P., Geering, J. J. and Valley, J. F. 2006. 'Sr-90 in deciduous teeth from 1950 to 2002: The Swiss experience', *Science of the Total Environment* 367, 596–605.

Froidevaux, P., Bochud, F. and Haldimann, M. 2010. 'Retention half times in the skeleton of plutonium and Sr-90 from above-ground nuclear tests: A retrospective study of the Swiss population', *Chemosphere* 80, 519–24.

FSS (Forensic Science Service). 2006a. 'Operation Advance – A joint initiative with the Home Office Police Standards Unit (PSU)' [WWW] www.forensic.gov.uk (Accessed 14 July 2006).

FSS (Forensic Science Service). 2006b, [WWW] www.forensic.gov.uk/forensic_t/inside/news/list_press_release.php?case+35&y (Accessed 12 August 2006).

Gaffney, C. and Gater, J. 2003. *Revealing the Buried Past: Geophysics for Archaeologists*. Stroud: Tempus.

Gaffney, C. and Gaffney, V. 2011. 'Through an imperfect filter: Geophysical techniques and the management of archaeological heritage' in Cowley, D.C. (ed.) 2011b, 117–27.

Galloway, A (ed.). 1999. *Broken Bones: The Anthropological Analysis of Blunt Force Trauma*. Springfield: Charles C. Thomas.

Galloway, A., Birkby, W. H., Jones, A. M., *et al.* 1989. 'Decay rates of human remains in an arid environment', *Journal of Forensic Sciences* 34:3, 607–16.

Gaudette, B. D. 2000. 'Hair: Hair transfer, persistence and recovery' in Siegel, J.A., *et al.* (eds.), 1032–34.

Gennard, D. E. 2007. *Forensic Entomology: An Introduction*. Chichester: Wiley.

Gibb, G. J. and Woolnough, P. 2007. *Missing Persons*. Grampian Police.

Gilbert, M. 2002. *The Routledge Atlas of the Holocaust* (3rd edition). London: Routledge.

Gilchrist, R. 2003. 'Introduction: Towards a social archaeology of warfare', *World Archaeology* 35:1, 1–6.

Gilead, I., Hamai, Y. and Mazurek, W. 2009. 'Excavating Nazi Extermination Centres', *Present Pasts* 1, 10–39.

Golden, J. 2003. 'Remembering Chelmno:Heart-wrenching finds from a Nazi death camp' *Archaeology* 56:1, 50–54.

Goldhagen, D. 1996. *Hitler's Willing Executioners: Ordinary Germans and the Holocaust*. London: Little, Brown & Company.

Grant, J., Gorin, S. and Fleming, N. 2008. *The Archaeology Coursebook: An Introduction to Themes, Sites, Methods and Skills* (3rd edition). London: Routledge.

Gray, V. 2006. *The Recovery of Hairs From a Grave Fill*. Unpublished MSc dissertation, University of Bournemouth.

Greene, K. 2002. *Archaeology: an Introduction* (4th edition). London: Routledge.

Greig, C. 2006. *Cold Cases: Criminals Finally Brought To Justice*. London: Capella.

Gross, J. 2002. *Neighbours: The Destruction of the Jewish Community in Jedwabne, Poland*. London: Arrow.

Gross, J. 2004. 'Critical remarks indeed' in Polonsky, A. and Michlic, J. B. (eds.), *The Neighbours Respond: The Controversy Over The Jedwabne Massacre In Poland*. Princeton: Princeton University Press, 344–70.

Gruber, S. and Myers, P. 1995. *Survey of Historic Jewish Monuments in Poland: A Report to the United States Commission for the Protection of America's Heritage Abroad* (2nd edition). United States: World Monuments Fund.

Gun, A. and Bird, J. 2010. The ability of blowflies Calliphora vomitoria (Linnaeus), Calliphora vicina (Rob-Desvoidy) and Lucilia sericata (Meigan) (Diptera: Calliphoridae) and the muscid flies Muscina stabulans (Fallén) and Muscina prolapse (Harris) (Diptera: Muscidae) to colonise buried remains, *Forensic Science International*, 207:1–3, 198–204.

Haglund, W. D. 1992. 'Contribution of rodents to postmortem artifacts of bone and soft tissue', *Journal of Forensic Sciences* 37:6, 1459–65.

Haglund, W. D. 1997. 'Dogs and coyotes: Postmortem involvement with human remains', in Haglund, W. D. and Sorg, M. H. (eds.), 367–81.

Haglund, W. D. 2002. 'Recent mass graves: An introduction' in Haglund, W. and Sorg, M. H. (eds.) 243–62.

Haglund, W. D. and Sorg, M. H. (eds.). 1997. *Forensic Taphonomy: The Postmortem Fate of Human Remains*. Boca Raton: CRC Press.

Haglund, W. D. and Sorg, M. H. (eds). 2002a. *Advances in Forensic Taphonomy: Method, Theory and Archaeological Perspectives*. Boca Raton: CRC Press.

Haglund, W. D. and Sorg, M. H. 2002b. 'Human remains in water environments' in Haglund, W. D. and Sorg, M. H. (eds.), 201–18.

Haglund, W. D., Connor, M. and Scott, D. D. 2001. 'The archaeology of contemporary mass graves', *Historical Archaeology* 35, 57–69.

Haglund, W. D., Connor, M. and Scott, D. D. 2002. 'The effect of cultivation on buried human remains' in Haglund, W. and Sorg, M. H. (eds.) 2002a, 133–50.

Haglund, W. D., Reay, T. and Swindler, D. R. 1988. 'Toothmark artifacts and survival of bones in animal scavenged human skeletons', *Journal of Forensic Sciences* 33:4, 985–95.

Haglund, W. D., Reay, D. T. and Swindler, D. R. 1989. 'Canid scavenging/disarticulation sequence of human remains in the Pacific Northwest', *Journal of Forensic Sciences* 34:3, 587–606.

Hanson, I. D. 2004. 'The importance of stratigraphy in forensic investigation', in Pye, K. and Croft, D. J. (eds.), 39–47.

Harris, E. 1979. *Principles of Archaeological Stratigraphy*. London: Academic Press.

Harrison, K. 2008. *An Investigation into the Relationships between the Archaeology of Burnt Structures and Fire Science as Employed in a Forensic Context*. Unpublished PhD thesis, University of Reading.

Haskell, N. H., McShaffrey, D. G., Hawley, D. A., *et al.* 1989. 'Use of aquatic insects in determining submersion interval', *Journal of Forensic Sciences* 34:3, 622–32.

Hinkes, M. 2006. 'Forensic anthropology in cold cases' in Walton, R. H. (ed.) *Cold Case Homicides: Practical Investigation Techniques*. Boca Raton: CRC Press.

Hirschfield, A. and Bowers, K. 2001. *Mapping and Analysing Crime Data: Lessons from Research and Practice*. New York: Taylor and Francis.

HMSO (Her Majesty's Stationery Office). 1861. Offences Against the Person Act. [WWW] http://www.legislation.gov.uk/ukpga/Vict/24-25/100/contents (Accessed April 2013). London: HMSO.

HMSO (Her Majesty's Stationery Office). 1864. Registration of Burials Act 1864. [WWW] www.legislation.gov.uk. London: HMSO.

HMSO (Her Majesty's Stationery Office). 1926. Births and Deaths Registration Act. London: HMSO.

HMSO (Her Majesty's Stationery Office). 1929. Infant Life (Preservation) Act. London: HMSO.

HMSO (Her Majesty's Stationery Office). 1938. Infanticide Act. London: HMSO.

HMSO (Her Majesty's Stationery Office). 1947a. Town and Country Planning Act. London: HMSO.

HMSO (Her Majesty's Stationery Office). 1947b. Town and Country Planning (Scotland) Act. London: HMSO.

HMSO (Her Majesty's Stationery Office). 1972. The Local Government Act (as amended). London: HMSO.

HMSO (Her Majesty Stationery Office). 1977. Local Authorities' Cemeteries Order Statutory Instrument No. 204 – Burial England and Wales (as amended). London: HMSO.

HMSO (Her Majesty's Stationery Office). 1984a Police and Criminal Evidence Act 1984. London: HMSO.

HMSO (Her Majesty's Stationery Office). 1984b. The Building Act, 1984. London: HMSO.

HMSO (Her Majesty's Stationery Office). 1985. Prosecution of Offences Act 1985. London: HMSO.

HMSO (Her Majesty's Stationery Office). 1988. The Town and Country Planning (Applications) Regulations, 1988. London: HMSO.

HMSO (Her Majesty's Stationery Office). 1989. The Control of Pollution (Amendment) Act, 1989. London: HMSO.

HMSO (Her Majesty's Stationery Office). 1990a. Town and Country Planning Act 1990. London: HMSO.

HMSO (Her Majesty's Stationery Office). 1990b. Planning Policy Guidance 16: Archaeology and planning. London, HMSO.

HMSO (Her Majesty's Stationery Office). 1991. The Controlled Waste (Registration of Carriers and Seizure of Vehicles) Regulations, 1991 (as amended). London: HMSO.

HMSO (Her Majesty's Stationery Office). 1996a. Criminal Procedure and Investigations Act 1996. London: HMSO.

HMSO (Her Majesty's Stationery Office). 1996b. Treasure Act 1996. London: HMSO.

HMSO (Her Majesty's Stationery Office). 1998. Human Rights Act. London: HMSO.

HMSO (Her Majesty's Stationery Office). 1999. The Pollution Prevention and Control Act 1999. London: HMSO.

HMSO (Her Majesty's Stationery Office). 2000a. The Building (Approved Inspectors etc.) Regulations, 2000 (S.I. 2000/2532) (as amended – 2001). London: HMSO.

HMSO (Her Majesty's Stationery Office). 2000b. The Pollution Prevention Control (England and Wales) Regulations, 2000 (as amended). London: HMSO.

HMSO (Her Majesty's Stationery Office). 2003. Sexual Offences Act. London: HMSO.

HMSO (Her Majesty's Stationery Office). 2004a. Human Tissue Act. London: HMSO.

HMSO (Her Majesty's Stationery Office). 2004b. Domestic Violence, Crime and Victims Act. London: HMSO.

HMSO (Her Majesty's Stationery Office). 2004c. Planning and Compulsory Purchase Act, 2004. London: HMSO.

HMSO (Her Majesty's Stationery Office). 2004d. The Town and Country Planning (General Development Procedure) (Amendment) (England) Order, 2004. London: HMSO.

HMSO (Her Majesty's Stationery Office). 2006. Human Tissue (Scotland) Act. London: HMSO.

HMSO (Her Majesty's Stationery Office). 2010a. The Building Regulations (as amended). London: HMSO.

HMSO (Her Majesty's Stationery Office). 2010b. The Building (Approved Inspectors etc.) Regulations. London: HMSO.

HMSO (Her Majesty's Stationery Office). 2012. Domestic Violence, Crime and Victims (Amendment) Act. London: HMSO.

Hobischak, N. R. and Anderson, G. S. 2002. 'Time of submergence using aquatic invertebrate succession and decompositional changes', *Journal of Forensic Sciences* 47:1, 142–51.

Hochrein, M. J. 1997. 'The dirty dozen: The recognition and collection of toolmarks in the forensic geotaphonomic record', *Journal of Forensic Identification* 47:2, 171–98.

Hochrein, M. J. 2002. 'An autopsy of the grave: Recognising, collecting and preserving forensic geotaphonomic evidence', in Haglung, W. D. and Sorg, M. H. (eds.), 45–70.

Home Office. 2005, [WWW] http://police.homeoffice.gov.uk/operational-policing/technology-equipment/forensic-science.html (Accessed 14 July 2006).

Honig, J. W. and Both, N. 1996. *Srebrenica: Record of a War Crime*. Harmondsworth: Penguin Books.

Horrocks, M., Coulson, S. A. and Walsh, K. A. J. 1998a. 'Forensic palynology: variation in the pollen content of soil surface samples', *Journal of Forensic Sciences* 43, 320–23.

Horrocks, M., Coulson, S. A. and Walsh, K. A. J. 1998b. 'Forensic palynology: Variation in the pollen content of soil on shoes in shoeprints in soil', *Journal of Forensic Sciences* 44:1, 119–22.

Houck, M. M. (ed). 2001. *Mute Witnesses: Trace Evidence Analysis*. London: Academic Press.

Houck, M. M. (ed). 2003. *Trace Evidence Analysis: More cases in mute witnesses*. London: Elsevier, Academic Press.

HTA (Human Tissue Authority). 2009. *Codes of Practice*. [WWW] www.hta.gov.uk/legislationpolicies andcodesofpractice/codesofpractice.cfm (Accessed April 2013).

Hunter, J. R. 1994. 'Forensic Archaeology in Britain', *Antiquity* 68, 758–69.

Hunter, J. R, 1999. 'Research for the detection of clandestine graves using controlled animal burials' *Proceedings of the International Association of Forensic Sciences 15th Triennial Meeting, Los Angeles 1999*, 45.

Hunter, J. 2009. 'Domestic Homicide Investigations in the United Kingdom' in Blau, S. and Ubelaker, D. (eds.), 363–73.

Hunter, J. and Cox, M. 2005. *Forensic Archaeology: Advances in Theory and Practice*. London: Routledge.

Hunter, J.R. and Ralston, I.B.M. (eds.). 2006. *Archaeological Resource Management in the UK*. Stroud: Sutton Publishing.

Hunter, J. and Simpson, B. 2007. 'Preparing the ground: archaeology in a war zone' in Ferlini, R. (ed.), *Forensic Archaeology and Human Rights Violations*. Springfield: Charles C Thomas, 266–92.

Hunter, J. R., Karaska, J. B. T., Scott, E. A., *et al*. 2005. *The Identification of Mass Graves in Former Yugoslavia Using Geophysics and Remote Sensing*. Sarajevo: International Commission on Missing persons.

Hunter, J., Roberts, C. and Martin, A. 1996. *Studies in Crime: An Introduction to Forensic Archaeology*. London: Batsford.

ICCM (Institute of Cemetery and Crematorium Management). 2004. *Policy Relating to Shallow Depth Graves*. London: ICCM National Office, City of London Cemetery.

ICMP (International Commisssion on Missing Persons). 2007. *3rd Meeting of the Steering Committee on Forensic Science Programs*. Sarajevo: ICMP.

ICMP (International Commisssion on Missing Persons). 2008. 'Mandate', [WWW] www.ic-mp.org/mandate (Accessed 29 July 2011).

IMTN (International Military Tribunal at Nuremberg). 1947 *Trial of the Major War Criminals before the International Military Tribunal Nuremberg 14 November 1945 – 1 October 1946. Nuremberg*, [WWW] http://www.loc.gov/rr/frd/Military_Law/NT_major-war-criminals.html (Accessed April 2013).

Interpol. 2009. *Disaster Victim Identification Guide*. Lyon: Interpol.

Isser, N. K. and Schwartz, L. L. 2001. 'Neonaticide: An appropriate application for therapeutic jurisprudence'. *Behavioral Sciences and the Law* 19, 703–18.

Jackson, M. 2002. *Infanticide: Historical Perspectives on Child Murder and Concealment, 1550-2000*. Guildford: Ashgate.

Janaway, R. C. 1996. 'The decay of buried human remains and their associated materials' in Hunter, J. *et al.*, 58–85.

Janaway, R. C. 2002. 'Degradation of clothing and other dress materials associated with buried bodies of archaeological and forensic interest' in Haglund, W.D. and Sorg, M. H. (eds.) 2002a, 379–402.

Janaway, R. C. 2008. 'The decomposition of materials associated with buried cadavers' in Tibbett, M. and Carter, D. O. (eds.), 153–202.

Jones, A. F., Brewer, P. A., Johnstone, E., and Macklin, M. G. 2007. 'High-resolution interpretative geomorphological mapping of river valley environments using airborne LIDaR data', *Earth Surface Processes and Landforms* 32, 1574–92.

Jones, D. M. (ed.). 2011. *3D Laser Scanning for Heritage*. (2nd edition). Swindon: English Heritage.

Juhl, K. 2005. 'The contribution by (forensic) archaeologists to Human Rights investigations of mass graves', *Arkeologisk museum i Stavanger* 5, 1–67.

Kahana, T., Almog, J., Levy, J., Shmeltzer, E., Spier, Y. and Hiss, J. 1999. 'Marine taphonomy: adipocere formation in a series of bodies recovered from a single shipwreck', *Journal of Forensic Sciences* 44:5, 897–901.

Kalacska, M., Bell, L. S., Sanchez-Azofeifa, G. A. and Caelli, T. 2009. 'The application of remote sensing for detecting mass graves: An experimental case study from Costa Rica', *Journal of Forensic Science* 54:1, 159–66.

Kenward, H. K., Hall, A. R. and Jones, A. K. 1980. 'A tested set of techniques for the extraction of plant and animal macrofossils from waterlogged archaeological deposits', *Science and Archaeology* 22, 3–15.

Keough, M. E. Kahn, S. and Andreievic, A. 2000. 'Disclosing the truth: informed participation in the antemortem database project for survivors of Srebrenica', *Health and Human Rights* 68:5, 68–87.

Kerr, B. 2008. 'Windsor Castle: Destruction and salvage' in Rakoczy, L. (ed.), *The Archaeology of Destruction*. Cambridge: Cambridge Scholars Publishing. 152–75.

Killam, E. W. 2004. *The Detection of Human Remains* (2nd edition). Springfield: Charles C. Thomas.

Kimmerle, E. H. and Baraybar, J. P. 2008. *Skeletal Trauma: Identification of Injuries Resulting from Human Rights Abuse and Armed Conflict*. Boca Raton: CRC Press.

Kola, A. 2000. *Bełżec: The Nazi Camp for Jews in the Light of Archaeological Sources, Excavations 1997-1999*. Warsaw and Washington: The Council for the Protection of Memory of Combat and Martyrdom.

Komar, D. 1999. 'The use of cadaver dogs in locating scattered, scavenged human remains: Preliminary field test results', *Journal of Forensic Sciences* 44:2, 405–08.

Komar, D. 2008. 'Variables influencing victim selection in genocide', *Journal of Forensic Sciences* 53:1, 172–77.

Komar, D. A. and Buikstra, J. E. 2008. *Forensic Anthropology: Contemporary Theory and Practice*. Oxford: Oxford University Press.

Krebs, C. J. 1999. *Ecological Methodology* (2nd edition). California: Benjamin Cummings.

Krogman, W. M. and Iscan, M. Y. 1986. *The Human Skeleton in Forensic Medicine* (2nd edition). Springfield: Charles C. Thomas.

Kulshrestha. P. and Satpathy, D. K. 2001. 'The use of beetles in forensic entomology', *Forensic Science International* 120:1–2, 15–17.

Kvamme, K. 2006. 'Integrating multidimensional geophysical data', *Archaeological Prospection* 13:2, 91–102.

Lane, B. and Gregg, W. 1995. *Encyclopaedia of Serial Killers*. New York: Headline Publishing.

Lang, B. 1999. *Between History and Memory: The Future of the Holocaust*. Ithaca: Cornell University Press.

Lasseter, A. E., Jacobi, K. P., Farley, R. and Hensel, L. 2003. 'Cadaver dog and handler team capabilities in the recovery of buried human remains in the southeastern United States', *Journal of Forensic Sciences* 48:3, 617–21.

Laukkanen, M-S., Pekka, J. and Patrick-Sandnabba, K. 2008. 'Predicting offender home location in urban burglary series', *Forensic Science International* 174:2–3, 224–35.

Leclair, B., Shaler, R., Carmody, G., *et al.* 2007. 'Bioinformatics and human identification in mass fatality incidents: The World Trade Center disaster', *Journal of Forensic Sciences* 52:4, 806–19.

Lewis, M. E. 2007. *The Bioarchaeology of Children*. Cambridge: Cambridge University Press.

Libby, W. 1952. *Radiocarbon Dating*. Chicago: Chicago University Press.

Listi, G. A., Manhein, M. H. and Leitner, M. 2007. 'Use of the global positioning system in the field recovery of scattered human remains', *Journal of Forensic Sciences*, 52:1, 11–15.

Lit, L. and Crawford, C.A. 2006. 'Effects of training paradigms on search dog performance', *Applied Animal Behaviour Science* 98, 277–92.

Locard, E. 1920. *L'Enquete Criminelle et les Methodes Scientifiques*. Paris: Flammarion.

Lorenzo, N., Wan, T., Harper, R. J., *et al.* 2003. 'Laboratory and field experiments used to identify *Canis lupus* var. *familiaris* active odor signature chemicals from drugs, explosives, and humans', *Analytical and Bioanalytical Chemistry* 346:8, 1212–24.

Lyman, R. L. and Fox, G. L. 1997. 'A critical evaluation of bone weathering as an indication of bone assemblage formation', in Haglund, W. D. and Sorg, M. H. (eds.), 223–47.

Lynam, J. T. 1978. *Techniques of geophysical prospection as applied to near surface structure determination*. Unpublished PhD thesis, University of Bradford, UK.

Lynnerup, N., Kjeldsen, H., Zweihoff, R., *et al.* 2010. 'Ascertaining year of birth/age at death in forensic cases: A review of conventional methods allowing for absolute chronology', *Forensic Science International* 20, 74–78.

Mant, A. K. 1950. *A Study of Exhumation Data*. London: Unpublished MD thesis, London University.

Mant, A. K., 1987. 'Knowledge Acquired from Post-War Exhumations' in Boddington, A. Garland, N. A. and Janaway, R. C. (eds.), *Death, Decay and Reconstruction*. Manchester: Manchester University Press, 65–78.

Marshall, L. G. 1989. 'Bone Modification - "The Laws of Burial"' in Bonnischen, R. and Sorg, M. H. (eds.), *Bone Modification*. Orono: Thompson-Shore Inc, 7–24.

Marquez-Grant, N., Litherland, S. and Roberts, J. 2012. 'European perspectives and the role of the forensic archaeologist' in Dirkmaat, D. C. (ed.), *A Companion to Forensic Anthropology*. Chichester: Wiley-Blackwell, 598–625.

Marrus, M. R. 2000. *The Holocaust in History*. London: Penguin.

Mays, S. 1998. *The Archaeology of Human Bones*. London: Routledge.

Mays, S. 2000. 'The archaeology and history of infanticide, and its occurrence in earlier British populations', in Derevenski, J. (ed.), *Children and Material Culture*. London: Psychology Press, 180–99.

McGann, N. 2002. 'Still waiting to bury my child', [WWW] http://news.bbc.co.uk/1/hi/england/ 2499991.stm (Accessed 19 August 2006).

McKinley, J. 2000. 'The analysis of cremated bone', in Cox, M. and Mays, S. (eds.), *Archaeological and Forensic Science*. Greenwich Medical Media: London, 403–21.

Melton, T., Dimick, G., Higgins, B., *et al.* 2005. 'Forensic mitochondrial DNA analysis of 691 casework hairs', *Journal of Forensic Sciences*, 50:1, 1–8.

Metropolitan Police. 2006, [WWW] http://met.police.uk/scd/units/homicide_support.htm (Accessed 12 August 2006).

Micozzi, M. S. 1997. 'Frozen Environments and Soft Tissue Preservation' Haglund, W. and Sorg, H. (eds.), 171–80.

Mildenhall, D. C., Wiltshire, P. E. J. and Bryant, V. M. 2006. 'Forensic palynology: Why do it and how it works', *Forensic Science International* 163:3, 163–72.

Millar, M. L., Freeland, R. S. and Koppenjan, S. K. 2002. 'Searching for concealed human remains using GPR imaging of decomposition', *Ninth International Conference on Ground- penetrating Radar*, *Proceedings of SPIE*, 4758, 539–44.

MOJ (Ministry of Justice). 2007. *Burial Law and Policy in the 21st Century - The Way Forward*. London: Coroners Unit Ministry of Justice.

MOJ (Ministry of Justice). 2009. *Natural Burial Grounds - Guidance for Operators*. London: Ministry of Justice, Coroners and Burials Division.

MoLAS (Museum of London Archaeology Service), 1994. *Archaeological Site Manual* (3rd edition). London: Museum of London.

Moraitis, K. and Spiliopoulou, C. 2010. 'Forensic implications of carnivore scavenging on human remains recovered from outdoor locations in Greece', *Journal of Forensic and Legal Medicine* 17:6, 298–303.

Morse, D., Duncan, J. and Stoutamire, J. 1983. *Handbook of Forensic Archaeology and Anthropology*. Tallahassee: Rose Printing.

Nafte, M. 2000. *Flesh and Bone: An Introduction to Forensic Anthropology*. North Carolina: Carolina Academic Press.

Nawrocki, S. P., Pless, J. E., Hawley, D. A. and Wagner, S. A. 1997. 'Fluvial transport of human crania' in Haglund, W. D. and Sorg, M. H. (eds.), 529–52.

Neal, E. 1986. *The Natural History of Meles Meles*. London: Croom Helm.

Newiss, G. 2005. 'A study of the characteristics of outstanding missing persons: Implications for the development of a police risk assessment', *Policing and Society* 15:2, 212–25.

Newiss, G. 2006. 'Understanding the risk of going missing: Eliminating the risk of fatal outcomes in cancelled cases', *Policing* 29:2, 246–60.

Nichol, C., Innes, M., Gee, D. and Feist, A. 2004. *Reviewing Murder Investigations: An Analysis of Progress Reviews from Six Police Forces*. London: Home Office.

Nobes, D. C. 2000. 'The Search for "Yvonne": a case example of the delineation of a grave using near-surface geophysical methods', *Journal of Forensic Sciences* 45:3, 715–21.

Notter, S. J. and Stuart, B. H. 2012. 'The effect of body coverings on the formation of adipocere in an aqueous environment', *Journal of Forensic Sciences* 57:1, 120–25.

Novo, A., Lorenzo, H., Rial, I. F. and Solla, M. 2011. '3-D GPR in forensics: Finding a clandestine grave in a mountain environment', *Forensic Science International* 204:1–3, 134–38.

Noy, E. A. 1998. *Public Health Acts and Building Regulations in the Nineteenth Century*. London: New Millennium.

O'Connor, S., Ali, E., Al-Sabah, S., *et al.* 2011. 'Exceptional preservation of a prehistoric human brain from Heslington, Yorkshire, UK', *Journal of Archaeological Science* 38:7, 1641–54.

Oesterhelweg, L., Kröber, S., Rottmann, K., *et al.* 2008. 'Cadaver dogs - A study on detection of contaminated carpet squares', *Forensic Science International* 174, 35–39.

Orengo, H. A. 2008. 'Detection of body dump sites and clandestine burials: A GIS-based landscape approach', in Clark, J. T. and Hagemeister, M. (eds.), *Digital Discovery, Exploring New Frontiers in Human Heritage*. Computer Applications and Quantitative Methods in Archaeology. Proceedings of the 34th Conference, Fargo, United States, April 2006, 185–90. Budapest: Archaeolingua.

Ozin, P., Norton, H. and Spivev, P. 2010. *PACE: A Practical Guide to the Police and Criminal Evidence Act 1984*. Oxford: Oxford University Press.

Paine, D. 2012. *John Haigh: The Acid Bath Murderer*. [WWW] www.tba.org/journal/john-haigh-the-acid-bath-murderer. (Accessed April 2013).

Palmer, R. 2011. 'Knowledge-based aerial image interpretation' in Cowley, D. C. (ed.) 2011b, 283–91.

Pan American Health Organization. 2006, World Health Organization, International Federation of Red Cross and Red Crescent Societies, International Committee of the Red Cross. *Management of Dead Bodies After Disasters: A Field Manual for First Responders*, [WWW] http://www.ifrc.org/docs/idrl/I967EN.pdf (Accessed April 2013).

Papadopoulos, N. G., Tsourlos, P., Tsokas, G. N. and Sarris, A. 2006. 'Two- dimensional and three-dimensional resistivity imaging in archaeological site investigation', *Archaeological Prospection* 13, 161–81.

Paperno, I. 2001. 'Exhuming the bodies of Soviet terror', *Representations* 45, 89–118.

Parker, R., Ruffell., A., Hughes, D. and Pringle, J. 2010. 'Geophysics and the search for freshwater bodies: A review', *Science and Justice* 50:3, 141–49.

Payne, S. 1975. 'Partial recovery and sample bias' in Clason, A. T. (ed.), *Archaeozoological Studies*. Oxford: North-Holland, 7–17.

Perera, C. and Briggs, C. 2008. 'Guidelines for the effective conduct of mass burials following mass disasters: post-Asian Tsunami disaster experience in retrospect', *Forensic Science, Medicine and Pathology* 4, 1–8.

Perotti, M. A., Goff, L. M., Baker, A. S., *et al*. 2009. 'Forensic acarology: An introduction, *Experimental and Applied Acarology* 49:1–2, 3–13.

Polonsky, A. and Michlic, J. B. 2004. *The Neighbours Respond: The Controversy Over The Jedwabne Massacre In Poland*. Princeton: Princeton University Press.

Powell, K. 2010. *Grave Concerns: Locating and Unearthing Human Bodies*. Bowen Hills: Australian Academic Press.

PPG 16. 1990. *Planning Policy Guidance Note 16: Archaeology and Planning*. Department of the Environment. London: HMSO.

PPS 5. 2010. *Planning Policy Statement 5: Planning for the Historic Environment*. Department of the Environment. London: HMSO.

Prangnell, J. and McGowan, G. 2009. 'Soil temperature calculation for burial site analysis', *Forensic Science International* 191: 1–3, 104–09.

Preuss, J., Strehler, M., Dressler, J., *et al*. 2006. 'Dumping after homicide using setting in concrete and/or sealing with bricks – six case reports', *Forensic Science International* 159, 56–60.

Price, T. D., Blitz, J., Burton, J. and Ezzo, J. A. 1992. 'Diagenesis in prehistoric bone: problems and solutions', *Journal of Archaeological Science* 19:5, 513–29.

Pringle, J. K. and Jervis, J. R. 2010. 'Electrical resistivity survey to search for a recent clandestine burial of a homicide victim, UK', *Forensic Science International* 202, 1–3, e1–e7.

Pringle, J. K., Jervis, J. R., Hansen, J. D., *et al*. 2011. 'Geophysical monitoring of simulated clandestine graves using electrical and Ground Penetrating Radar methods: 0-3 years after burial'. Extended abstract for a presentation at the 16th European Meeting of Environmental & Engineering Geophysics of the Near Surface Geoscience Division of the EAGE, Leicester, 12th-14th September, 2011.

Pringle, J. K., Ruffell, A., Jervis, J. R., *et al*. 2012. 'The use of geoscience methods for terrestrial forensic searches', *Earth-Science Reviews* 114, 108–23.

Pye, K. and Croft, D. J. (eds.). 2004. *Forensic Geoscience: Principles, Techniques and Applications*. Geological Society Publication 232. London: Geological Society.

Radin, E. D. 2008. *The Deadly Reasons*. Rockville: Wildside Press LLC.

Rahtz, P. 1979. *The Saxon and Medieval Palaces at Cheddar. Excavations 1960-62*. British Archaeological Reports, British Series 65. Oxford: BAR.

Rainio, J., Hedman, M., Karkola, K., *et al*. 2001. 'Forensic osteological investigations in Kosovo', *Forensic Science International* 121, 166–73.

Ramsthaler, F., Ebach, S. C., Birngruber, C. G. and Verhoff, M. A. 2011. 'Postmortem interval of skeletal remains through the detection of intraosseol hemin traces. A comparison of UV-fluorescence, luminol, Hexagon-OBTI®, and Combur® tests', *Forensic Science International* 209, 59–63.

Rebmann, A. Undated. 'Cadaver Dogs: A Search Tool for Locating Human Remains', [WWW] www.barksar.org/Cadaver_Dogs_A_Search_Tool_for_Locating_Human_Remains.pdf (Accessed 18 November 2010).

Rebmann, A., David, E. and Sorg, M. H., 2000. *Cadaver Dog Handbook*. Florida: CRC Press.

Reddick, A. J. 2005. *The Use of Spatial Techniques in the Location and Excavation of Contemporary Mass Graves*. Unpublished MPhil thesis, University of Birmingham, UK.

Reuters 2006. 'Germany uncovers Nazi-era mass grave' [WWW] http://www.msnbc.msn.com/id/15147988/ns/world_news-europe/t/germany-uncovers-nazi-era-mass-grave/ (Accessed 21 October 2007).

Reynolds, J. M. 2011. *An Introduction to Applied and Environmental Geophysics*. (2nd edition). Chichester: Wiley.

Reynolds, P. J. 1989. 'Sherd movement in the ploughzone', *British Archaeology* 6, 24–27.

Reynolds, P. J. and Schadla-Hall, R. T. 1980. 'Measurements of plough damage and the effect of ploughing on archaeological material', *Directorate of Ancient Monuments and Historic Buildings, Occasional Papers 3*, 114–19.

Rezos, M. M., Schultz, J. J., Murdock, R. A. and Smith, S. A. 2010. 'Controlled research utilizing a basic all-metal detector in the search for buried firearms and miscellaneous weapons', *Forensic Science International*, 195, 121–27.

Rodriguez, W. C. and Bass, W. M. 1985. 'Decomposition of buried bodies and methods that may aid in their location', *Journal of Forensic Sciences* 30:3, 836–52.

Rooney, N. J., Bradshaw, J. W. S. and Almey, H. 2004. 'Attributes of specialist search dogs -a questionnaire survey of UK dog handlers and trainers', *Journal of Forensic Sciences* 49:2, 1–7.

Ross, N. 2010. *A Review of Archaeological Sieving and its Potential for Use in a Forensic Context*. Unpublished MA dissertation. Institute of Archaeology and Antiquity, University of Birmingham.

Rossmo, K. 2006. 'Geographic profiling in cold case investigations' in Walton, R. H. (ed.), *Cold Case Homicides: Practical Investigation Techniques*. Boca Raton: CRC Press, 537–60.

Rothschild, M. A. and Schneider, V. 1997. 'On the temporal onset of postmortem scavenging "motivation" of the animal', *Forensic Science International* 89, 57–64.

Roux, C., Huttunen, J., Rampling, K., and Robertson, J. 2001. 'Factors affecting the potential for fibre contamination in purpose-designed forensic search rooms', *Science & Justice* 41:3, 135–44.

Rowe, W. F. 1997. 'Biodegredation of hairs and fibres' in Haglund, W. D. and Sorg, M (eds.), 337–51.

RTPI (The Royal Town Planning Institute). 2000. *IT in Local Planning Authorities 2000*. London: The Royal Town Planning Institute.

Ruffell, A. 2005. 'Searching for the IRA "Disappeared": Ground-penetrating radar investigation of a churchyard burial site, Northern Ireland', *Journal of Forensic Sciences* 50:6, e1224.

Ruffell, A. 2010. 'Forensic pedology, forensic geology, forensic geosciences, geophysics and soil forensics', *Forensic Science International* 2010, 202, 9–12.

Ruffell, A. and McKinley, J. 2008. *Geoforensics*. Chichester: Wiley.

Ruffell, A., McCabe, A., Donnelly, C., and Sloan, B. 2009. 'Location and assessment of an historic (150-160 years old) mass grave using geographic and ground penetrating radar investigation, NW Ireland', *Journal of Forensic Science* 54:2, 382–94.

Rutty, G. N., Robinson, C. L., BouHaidar, R., *et al*. 2007. 'The role of mobile computed tomography in mass fatality incidents', *Journal of Forensic Sciences* 52:6, 1343–49.

Saunders, N. 2001. 'Excavating memories: Archaeology and the Great War 1914-2001', *Antiquity* 76, 101–8.

Scheuer, L. and Black, S. 2000. *Developmental Juvenile Osteology*. London: Elsevier.

Scheuer, L. and Black, S. 2006. 'Osteology' in Thompson, T. and Black, S. (eds.), *Forensic Human Identification*. London: Taylor & Francis, 199–219.

Schmitt, S. 2002. 'Mass graves and the collection of forensic evidence: Genocide, war crimes, and crimes against humanity' in Haglund, W. and Sorg, M. H. (eds.) 2002a, 277–92.

Schotsmans, E. M. J., Denton, J., Dekeirsschieter, J., *et al.* 2012. 'Effects of hydrated lime and quicklime on the decay of buried human remains using pig cadavers as human body analogues', *Forensic Science International* 217, 50–59.

Schrag, B., Uldin, T., Mangin, P. and Froidevaux, P. 2012. 'Dating human skeletal remains using a radiometric method: Biogenic versus diagenetic ^{90}Sr and ^{210}Pb in vertebrae', *Forensic Science International* 220, 271–78.

Schultz, J. J. 2008. 'Sequential monitoring of burials containing small pig cadavers using Ground Penetrating Radar', *Journal of Forensic Sciences*, 53:2, 279–87.

Schultz, J. J. 2012a. 'The application of ground-penetrating radar for forensic grave detection, in Dirkmaat, D. (ed.), 85–100.

Schultz, J. J. 2012b. 'Determining the forensic significance of skeletal remains' in Dirkmaat, D. (ed.), 66–84.

Schultz, J. J. and Martin, M. M. 2011. 'Controlled GPR grave research: Comparison of reflection profiles between 500 – 250 MHz', *Forensic Science International*, 209:1–3, 64–69.

Schute, I. and Wijnen, J. A. T. 2010. *Archeologisch Onderzoek in Eenchuldig Lanschap: Concentratiekamp Amersfoort*. RAAP-Rapport 2197. Weesp: RAAP.

Scollar, I., Tabbagh, A., Hesse, A. and Herzog, I. 1990. *Archaeological Geophysics and Remote Sensing*. Cambridge: Cambridge University Press.

Sellers, B. and Chamberlain, A. 1998. 'Cave detection using ground penetrating radar', *The Archaeologist* 31, 20–21.

Shaw, R. and Corns, A. 2011. 'High resolution LiDAR specifically for archaeology: are we fully exploiting this valuable resource? In Cowley, D.C. (ed.) 2011b, 77–86.

Siegel, J. A., Saukko, P. J. and Knupfer, G. C. (eds.) 2000. *Encyclopaedia of Forensic Sciences*, Vol 3. London: Academic Press.

Skinner. M. 1987. 'Planning the archaeological recovery of evidence from recent mass graves', *Forensic Science International* 34:4, 267–87.

Skinner, M. and Sterenberg, J. 2005. 'Turf wars: Authority and responsibility for the investigation of mass graves', *Forensic Science International* 151, 221–32.

Skinner, M. Alempijevic, D. and Djuric-Srejic, M. 2003. 'Guidelines for international forensic bio-archaeology monitors of mass grave exhumations', *Forensic Science International* 132, 81–92.

Skinner, M., York, H. P. and Connor, M. A. 2002. 'Postburial disturbance of graves in Bosnia-Herzegovina' in Haglund, W. and Sorg, M. H. (eds.) 2002a, 293–308.

Smith, K. (ed.). 2012. *Homicides, Firearm Offences and Intimate Violence 2011/12*. Home Office Statistical Bulletin. London: Home Office.

Sorg, M. H., Dearborn, J. H., Monahan, E. I., *et al.* 1997. 'Forensic taphonomy in marine contexts' in Haglund, W. D. And Sorg, M. H. (eds.), 567–604.

Spalding, K. L., Buchholz, B. A., Bergman, L-E., *et al.* 2005. 'Age written in teeth by nuclear tests', *Nature* 437, 333–34.

Staff, D. 2008. *The Lost Boy*. London: Bantam.

Steadman, D. 2005. *Hard Evidence: Case Studies in Forensic Anthropology*. New Jersey: Prentice Hall.

Steadman, D. W. and Worne, H. 2007. 'Canine scavenging of human remains in an indoor setting', *Forensic Science International* 173:1, 78–82.

Steele, C. 2008. 'Archaeology and the forensic investigation of recent mass graves: Ethical issues for a new practice of archaeology', *Archaeologies: Journal of the World Archaeological Congress* 4:3, 414–28.

Sterenberg, J. 2009. 'Dealing with the remains of conflict: An international response to crimes against humanity, forensic recovery, identification and repatriation in the former Yugoslavia', in Blau, S. and Ubelaker, D. (eds.), 416–25.

Steyn, M., Nienaber, W. C., and Iscan, M. 2000. 'Anthropology: Excavation and retrieval of forensic remains, in Siegel, J. A. *et al.* (eds.), 235–42).

Stover, E., Haglund, W. and Samuels, M. 2003. 'Considerations for forensic investigations, humanitarian needs and the demands of justice', *Journal of the American Medical Association* 290:5, 663–66.

Sturdy, C. 2008. *The Past is History? The Investigation of Mass Graves of the Holocaust Using Archaeological and Forensic Archaeological Techniques*. Unpublished MPhil(B) Thesis, University of Birmingham, UK.

Sturdy Colls, C. 2012a. 'Holocaust Archaeology: archaeological approaches to landscapes of Nazi genocide and persecution', *Journal of Conflict Archaeology* 7:2, 71–105.

Sturdy Colls, C. 2012b. *Holocaust Archaeology: Archaeological Approaches to Landscapes of Nazi Genocide and Persecution*. Unpublished PhD Thesis. University of Birmingham.

Sturdy Colls, C. 2012c. 'Gone but not forgotten: Archaeological approaches to the landscape of the former extermination camp at Treblinka, Poland', *Zagłada Zydow. Studia i Materiały and Holocaust Studies and Materials* 2013, 77–112.

Sturdy Colls, C. and Colls, K. (in press) 'Reconstructing a painful past: a non-invasive approach to reconstructing Lager Norderney in Alderney, the Channel Islands' in Ch'ng, E., Chapman, H., and Gaffney, V. (eds.), *Digital Heritage*. New York: Springer.

Sullivan, M. 2006, 'Evil Parent Killer at Large', [WWW] http://www.thesun.co.uk/article/0,,2-2006470644,,00.html (Accessed 20 December 2006).

Susa, E. 2007. 'Forensic anthropology in Hungary' in Brickley, M. and Ferlini, R. (eds.), 203–15.

Sweibocka, T. (ed.). 1995. *Auschwitz: A History in Photographs*. (2nd edition). Warsaw: The Polish Ministry of Information.

Swift, B., Lauder, I., Black, S. and Norris, J. 2001. 'An estimation of the post-mortem interval in human skeletal remains: A radionuclide and trace element approach', *Forensic Science International* 117:1–2, 73–87.

Szibor, R.., Schubert, C., Schöning, R., *et al.* 1998. 'Pollen analysis reveals the murder season', *Nature*, 395, 449–50.

Telling, A. E., Duxbury, R. M. C. and Duxbury, R (eds.). 1993. *Planning Law and Procedure*. London: Butterworths.

The Guardian. 2006. 'Guilty of murder - the man who police believe may have fed his wife to pigs'. http://www.guardian.co.uk/uk/2006/nov/14/ukcrime.uknews2 (14 November 2006).

Theune, C. 2010. 'Historical archaeology in national socialist concentration camps in Central Europe', *Historische Archäologie* 2, 1–13.

Thompson, T. J. 2004. 'Recent advances in the study of burned bone and their implications for forensic anthropology', *Forensic Science International* 146S, 203–05.

Thompson, T. J., Islam, M., Piduru, K. and Marcel, A. 2011. 'An investigation into the internal and external variables acting on crystallity index using Fourier Transform Infrared Spectroscopy on unaltered and burned bone', *Palaeogeography, Palaeoclimatology, Palaeoecology* 299, 168–74.

Tibbett, M. and Carter, D. O. (eds.). 2008. *Soil Analysis in Forensic Taphonomy: Chemical and Biological Effects of Buried Human Remains*. Boca Raton: CRC Press.

TPA (Town and Country Planning Act). 1909. [WWW] Available on: www.parliament.uk/about/living-heritage/transformingsociety/towncountry/towns/overview/townplanning/ (Accessed April 2013).

Trier, Ø. D., Larsen. S. Ø. and Solberg, A. 2009. 'Automatic detection of circular structures in high-resolution satellite images of agricultural land', *Archaeological Prospection* 16. 1–15.

Tsokos, M., Lessig, R., Grundmann, C., *et al.* 2006. 'Experiences in tsunami victim identification', *International Journal of Legal Medicine*, 120, 185–7.

Tuller. H. and Djuric, M. 2006. 'Keeping the pieces together: comparison of mass grave excavation methodology', *Forensic Science International* 156, 192–200.

Turton, S. 2003. *The Scavenging of Human remains in Forensic Contexts*. Unpublished MPhil thesis, Institute of Archaeology and Antiquity, University of Birmingham, UK.

Ubelaker, D. H. 1997. 'Taphonomic applications in forensic anthropology' in Haglund, W. D. and Sorg, M. H. (eds.), 77–90.

Ubelaker, D. H. 2001. 'Artificial radiocarbon as an indicator of recent origin of organic remains in forensic cases', *Journal of Forensic Sciences* 46:6, 1285–87.

Ubelaker, D. H. and Scammal, H. 1992. *Bones: A Forensic Detective's Casebook*. New York: Harper Collins.

Ubelaker, D. H., Buchholz, B. A., and Stewart, J. E. B. 2006. 'Analysis of artificial radiocarbon in different skeletal and dental tissue types to evaluate date of death', *Journal of Forensic Sciences* 51:3, 484–488.

UN (United Nations). 1948. *The Universal Declaration of Human Rights*, [WWW] http://www.un.org/ Overview/rights.html (Accessed 21 January 2008).

UN (United National General Assembly). 1974. Resolution 3220: Assistance and co-operation in accounting for persons who are missing or dead in armed conflicts. 6th November 1974.

UN (United Nations). 1991. United Nations Manual on the Effective Prevention and Investigation of Extra-Legal, Arbitrary and Summary Executions. U.N. Doc. E/ST/CSDHA/.12.

USGS. (United States Geological Survey). 2010. [WWW] www.usgs.gov.

Van Doorm, N. L., Wilson, A., Willerslev, E. and Gilbert, M. T. P. 2011. 'Bone marrow and bone as a source for postmortem DNA', *Journal of Forensic Sciences* 56:3, 720–25.

Vanezis. P. 1999. 'Investigation of clandestine graves resulting from human rights abuses', *Journal of Clinical Forensic Medicine* 6, 238–42.

Vass, A., Barshick, S. A., Sega, G., Caton, J., *et al.* 2002. 'Decomposition chemistry of human remains: a new methodology for determining postmortem interval', *Journal of Forensic Sciences* 47:3, 542–53.

Vass, A. A., Smith, R. R., Thompson, C. V., *et al.* 2004. 'Decompositional Odor Database – Phase 1', *Journal of Forensic Sciences* 49:4, 1–10.

Vitale, K., Reynolds, R., O'Shea, J., and Meadows, G. 2011. 'Exploring ancient landscapes under Lake Huron using cultural algorithms', *Procedia Computer Science* 6, 303–10.

Walsh, K. A. J. and Horrocks, M. 2008. Palynology: Its position in the field of forensic science, *Journal of Forensic Sciences* 53:5, 1053–60.

Walton, R. H. (ed.). 2006. *Cold Case Homicides: Practical Investigation Techniques.* Boca Raton: CRC Press.

Watters, M. 2003. *Results of Ground Probing Radar survey on several suspected mass gravesites in Bosnia.* Unpublished report, Sarajevo: International Commission on Missing Persons.

Watters, M. and Hunter, J. R. 2004. 'Geophysics and burials: Field experience and software development' in Pye, K. and Croft, D. J. (eds.), 21–31.

Wehr, A. and Lohr, U. 1999. 'Airborne laser scanning, An introduction and overview', *Journal of Photogrammetry and Remote Sensing* 54, 68–82.

Wessling, R. 2003. 'Various geological survey results' in *Site Assessment Summaries.* Unpublished CPA Documentation. Bournemouth: Inforce Foundation.

White, P. (ed.). 2010. *Crime Scene to Court – The Essentials of Forensic Science* (3rd edition). Cambridge: Royal Society of Chemistry.

White, T. D. and Folkens, P. A. 2005. *The Human Bone Manual.* London: Elsevier.

Wilkinson, C. 2004. *Forensic Facial Reconstruction.* Cambridge: Cambridge University Press.

Williams, E. D. and Crews, J. D. 2003. 'From dust to dust: Ethical and practical issues involved in the location, exhumation, and identification of bodies from mass graves', *Croatian Medical Journal* 44:3, 251–58.

Wilson, A. S. 2008. 'The decomposition of hair in the buried body environment' in Tibbett, M. and Carter, D. O. (eds.), 123–52.

Wilson, A., Janaway, R. C., Holland, A., *et al.* 2007. 'Modelling the buried human body environment in upland climes using three contrasting field sites', *Forensic Science International* 169, 6–18.

Wiltshire, P. E. J. 2006a. 'Consideration of some taphonomic variables of relevance to forensic palynological investigation in the United Kingdom', *Forensic Science International*, 163:3, 172–82.

Wiltshire, P. E. J. 2006b. 'Hair as a source of forensic evidence in murder investigations', *Forensic Science International* 163:3, 241–48.

Wiltshire, P. E. J. 2010. 'Forensic ecology', in White, P. (ed.), 54–85.

Wiltshire, P. E. J. and Black, S. 2006. 'The cribriform approach to the retrieval of palynological evidence from the turbinates of murder victims, *Forensic Science International* 163:3, 224–30.

Wright, R. 1995. 'Investigating war crimes – The archaeological evidence', *The Sydney Papers* 557:3, 39–44.

Wright, R., Hanson, I. and Sterenberg, J. 2005. 'The archaeology of mass graves' in Hunter, J.R. and Cox, M., 137–58.

Yehuda, R., Elkin, A., Binder-Brynes, K., Kahana, *et al.* 1997. 'Dissociation in aging Holocaust survivors', *American Journal of Psychiatry* 154:5, 720–21.

Young, J. E. (ed.). 1994. *The Art of Memory: Holocaust Memorials in History*. Munich and New York: Prestel-Verlag.

Zapata, J., Perez-Sirvent, C., Martinez-Sanchez, M. J. and Tovar, P. 2006. 'Diagenesis, not biogenesis: Two late Roman skeletal examples', *Science of the Total Environment* 369, 357–68.

Zawodny, J. K. 1962. *Death in the Forest: The Story of the Katyn Forest Massacre*. New York: Hippocrene Books.

Index

Forensic Approaches to Buried Remains, First Edition. John Hunter, Barrie Simpson and Caroline Sturdy Colls.
© 2013 John Wiley & Sons, Ltd. Published 2013 by John Wiley & Sons, Ltd.